Pain

What Do I Do Now?: Palliative Care

SERIES EDITOR-IN-CHIEF

Margaret L. Campbell, PhD, RN, FPCN
Professor
Wayne University College of Nursing
Detroit, Michigan

OTHER VOLUMES IN THE SERIES
Pediatric Palliative Care
Respiratory Symptoms

Pain

Edited by

Christopher M. Herndon, PharmD, BCACP
Professor, School of Pharmacy
Southern Illinois University
Edwardsville, IL, USA

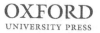
OXFORD
UNIVERSITY PRESS

OXFORD
UNIVERSITY PRESS

Oxford University Press is a department of the University of Oxford. It furthers
the University's objective of excellence in research, scholarship, and education
by publishing worldwide. Oxford is a registered trade mark of Oxford University
Press in the UK and certain other countries.

Published in the United States of America by Oxford University Press
198 Madison Avenue, New York, NY 10016, United States of America.

© Oxford University Press 2022

Library of Congress Cataloging-in-Publication Data
Names: Herndon, Christopher M., author.
Title: Pain / Christopher M. Herndon.
Other titles: What do I do now?
Description: New York, NY : Oxford University Press, [2022] |
Series: What do I do now? | Includes bibliographical references and index.
Identifiers: LCCN 2021045018 (print) | LCCN 2021045019 (ebook) |
ISBN 9780197542873 (paperback) | ISBN 9780197542897 (epub) |
ISBN 9780197542903 (online)
Subjects: MESH: Pain Management | Analgesics—therapeutic use |
Palliative Care | Case Reports
Classification: LCC RB127.5.C48 (print) | LCC RB127.5.C48 (ebook) |
NLM WL 704.6 | DDC 616/.0472082—dc23
LC record available at https://lccn.loc.gov/2021045018
LC ebook record available at https://lccn.loc.gov/2021045019

DOI: 10.1093/med/9780197542873.001.0001

9 8 7 6 5 4 3 2 1
Printed by Marquis, Canada

Contents

Contributors

Stephanie Abel, PharmD, BCPS
University of Kentucky HealthCare
Lexington, KY, USA

Nathan Boehr, DO
University of Kansas Medical
Center Division
Kansas City, KS, USA

Scot Born, MD, PharmD
Integrated Kidney Specialists
Nashville, TN, USA

Kate Brizzi, MD
Massachusetts General Hospital
Boston, MA, USA

Cara Brock, PharmD
College of Pharmacy
Roosevelt University
Chicago, IL, USA

Rachel Caplan, MD
Lewis Katz School of Medicine
Temple University
Philadelphia, PA, USA

Claudia Z. Chou, MD
Mayo Clinic
Rochester, MN, USA

Matthew D. Clark, PharmD
The University of Texas MD
Anderson Cancer Center
Houston, TX, USA

Noah Cooperstein, MD
Saint Louis University (Southwest
Illinois)
O'Fallon, IL, USA

Tim Cruz, PharmD, BCPS
HSHS St. Elizabeth's Hospital
O'Fallon, IL, USA

Alexis Dallara-Marsh, MD
Neurology Group of Bergen County
Ridgewood, NJ, USA

**Brandon Daniels, DC, CFMP,
FIACA, CCAc.**
Functional Health of St. Louis
St. Louis, MO, USA

Sandra DiScala, PharmD, BCPS
West Palm Beach VAMC
West Palm Beach, FL, USA

**Kourtney Engele, PharmD,
BCPS, BCCCP**
HSHS St. Elizabeth's Hospital
O'Fallon, IL, USA

Sarah Ermer, PharmD
University of Iowa College of
Pharmacy
Iowa City, IA, USA

Elyse A. Everett, MD, MOT
Washington University in St. Louis
School of Medicine
St. Louis, MO, USA

Jennifer Farrell, DO
Saint Louis University
St. Louis, MO, USA

Elise Fazio, DO
Intermountain Healthcare
Ogden, UT, USA

Jeffrey Fudin, PharmD, DAIPM,
FCCP, FASHP, FFSMB
Albany College of Pharmacy and
Health Sciences
Albany, NY, USA

Jessica Geiger, PharmD, MS,
BCPS, CPE
OhioHealth
Columbus, OH, USA

John Hausdorff, MD, FACP
Community Hospital of the
Monterey Peninsula
Monterey, CA, USA

Keith A. Hecht, PharmD, BCOP
Southern Illinois University
Edwardsville School of Pharmacy
Edwardsville, IL, USA

Christopher M. Herndon,
PharmD, BCACP
Southern Illinois University
Edwardsville
Edwardsville, IL, USA

Gary Houchard, PharmD
Ohio State University Wexner
Medical Center
James Cancer Hospital
Columbus, OH, USA

Michelle Krichbaum, PharmD
Nova Southeastern University
Fort Lauderdale, FL, USA

Jennifer Ku, PharmD, BCPS
MedStar Georgetown University
Hospital
Washington, DC, USA

Justin Kullgren, PharmD
Ohio State University Wexner
Medical Center
James Cancer Hospital
Columbus, OH, USA

Jane E. Loitman, MD,
MBA, FAAHPM
VA St. Louis Healthcare System
St. Louis, MO, USA

Erinn Louttit, MSN, FNP-BC
Wayne State University
Ann Arbor, MI, USA

Zachary Macchi, MD
University of Colorado Anschutz
Aurora, CO, USA

Erin McMenamin, PhD, CRNP
University of Pennsylvania School
of Nursing
Philadelphia, PA, USA

Mary Lynn McPherson, PharmD,
MA, MDE, BCPS
University of Maryland School of
Pharmacy
Baltimore, MD, USA

Ambereen K. Mehta, MD, MPH
UCLA Health
Los Angeles, CA, USA

Maura Miller, PhD,
GNP-BC, ACHPN
VA Medical Center
West Palm Beach, FL, USA

Neil Miransky, DO
Broward Health Medical Center
Fort Lauderdale, FL, USA

Dominic Moore, MD
McKay Dee Hospital Primary
Children's Hospital
Salt Lake City, UT, USA

Amanda Mullins, PharmD, BCPS
VA St. Louis Healthcare System
St. Louis, MO, USA

Patti Murray, DNP, HPCNP
Loyola University Medical Center
Maywood, IL, USA

Dharma Naidu, PharmD,
BCOP, APh
Community Hospital of the
Monterey Peninsula
Monterey, CA, USA

Lynn Nakad, MSN, RN
College of Nursing
University of Iowa
Iowa City, IA, USA

Theodore Pham Nguyen,
PharmD, BCPS
College of Pharmacy
University of Iowa
Iowa City, IA, USA

Daniel Paget, MD
Washington University of St. Louis
School of Medicine
St. Louis, MO, USA

Jayne Pawasauskas,
PharmD, BCPS
URI College of Pharmacy
Kingston, RI, USA

Amelia L. Persico, PharmD, MBA
Shields Health Solutions
Stoughton, MA, USA

Stefanie Pina-Escudero, MD
Global Brain Health Institute
University of California
San Francisco, CA, USA

Jennifer L. Rosselli, PharmD,
BCPS, BCACP, BC-ADM, CDCES
Southern Illinois University
Edwardsville School of Pharmacy
Edwardsville, IL, USA

Sandra Sacks, MD, MEd
UCLA Health
Los Angeles, CA, USA

Thomas M. Schelby, MD
Saint Louis University Southwest
Illinois Family Medicine Residency
St. Louis, MO, USA

Michael A. Smith,
PharmD, BCPS
University of Michigan College of
Pharmacy
Ann Arbor, MI, USA

Jessica L. Spruit, DNP, CPNP-AC
Wayne State University
Ann Arbor, MI, USA

Jonathan Thoma, MD
Saint Louis University (Southwest
Illinois)
O'Fallon, IL, USA

L. Toledo-Franco, MD, FACP
Saint Louis University Hospital
St. Louis, MO, USA

Ashley Unger, PharmD
HSHS St. Elizabeth's Hospital
O'Fallon, IL, USA

Tanya J. Uritsky, PharmD, CPE
Hospital of the University of
Pennsylvania
Philadelphia, PA, USA

Christine M. Vartan,
PharmD, BCPS
West Palm Beach VAMC
West Palm Beach, FL, USA

Julie Waldfogel, PharmD,
BCGP, CPE
Johns Hopkins Hospital
Baltimore, MD, USA

Erica L. Wegrzyn, BS, PharmD
Stratton VA Medical Center
Albany, NY, USA

Dokyoung S. You, PhD
Stanford Medicine
Palo Alto, CA, USA

1 Pain Assessment in Palliative Care

Tanya J. Uritsky

Case Study

A 54-year-old White woman presents to a follow-up clinic visit with her oncologist for treatment of stage IV metastatic breast cancer. She reports ongoing pain in her ribs and lower left thigh. Magnetic resonance imaging (MRI) revealed metastases in her lower three ribs on her right side as well as her lower left femur, for which she received radiation therapy that completed 1 month ago. She tolerated radiation well, with only slight nausea. Her pain never seemed to go away, however, and she feels her current analgesic regimen is not effective. A pain assessment reveals that she is in 7 out of 10 pain at worst and 5 out of 10 pain at best. She is not able to sleep well, and she has lost 10 pounds recently because her appetite is diminished. She reports the pain is dull and achy, localized to her rib cage. The pain is not completely relieved by oral oxycodone 5 mg tablets (she takes one or two tablets up to four times daily) or oral acetaminophen 500 mg tablets (she takes two tablets three times daily). The pain is most severe at night and seems better during the day when she is busy with work and helping to care for her new grandchild.

What Do I Do Now?

As a clinician approaching this patient case, the first question is "Why is this patient still reporting severe pain?" Is this appropriate or expected based on her treatment course? Is there potential disease progression? What else do you need to know to make that judgment?

A thorough pain assessment consists of gathering six essential pieces of information from the patient. If done correctly, a majority of what you need to know can be gathered just from this conversation. There will be additional information you may need to gather from the physical assessment, the patient's chart, or further diagnostic tests you will want to do when deciding on the appropriate treatment course, but the basic patient-reported information provides a significant amount of insight into the clinical presentation. For an explanation of the elements of a pain assessment, please refer to Box 1.1.

BOX 1.1 **Elements of a pain assessment: PQRSTU**

P: *Palliating or Precipitating*: What makes it better, and what makes it worse or brings it on?

Q: *Quality*: What does it feel like? Give it some words, preferably the patient's words, but providing some examples may be needed. Like burning, stinging, stabbing, shooting, etc.

R: *Radiating or Relief*: Does is start in one spot and radiate to another? If you forgot to ask about *Palliating*, it can also be covered here: "What have you tried to get relief, and what has worked or has not worked?"

S: *Site and Severity*: There may be more than one site, each requiring its own assessment. Severity is measured via pain rating scale based on the patient's age, cognitive status, and ability to communicate verbally.

T: *Timing/Temporal*: Is the pain worse at certain times: nighttime, morning?

U: "*U as in You*": How does the pain affect you? This includes functional and quality of life limitations as well as an assessment of the impact of the adverse effects of the medications on quality of life and the clinical situation.

If this patient reported severe burning pain, you would think about what could be causing her to have neuropathic pain. If she was reporting pain that is sharp after a recent fall, you would look for causes of somatic pain, and so forth. What is not included in the PQRSTU pain assessment is the "Y": Why does this patient have this pain? In a patient with current or recent malignancy, any new report of pain should be worked up to ensure there is not disease progression or recurrence. This would help establish the "why" from a physiologic perspective and possibly provide some answers to the patient's report of new or worsening pain. The pain should be treated with up-titration of the analgesic regimen while attempting to assess the underlying etiology.

Another element in the assessment of the "why" is the meaning of the pain. In patients with advanced disease, the experience of pain is often riddled with psychological and spiritual elements. A patient's purpose in life may have been challenged or eliminated entirely when the pain started or got too severe for them to continue working, for example. They may be grieving or suffering on a non-physical level that makes the physical experience that much more severe and intolerable. Assessing how the patient feels about the pain, what it means to them, and the impact it is having on their overall meaning and purpose is a critical element of the pain assessment.[1] This can be done by simply asking, "You are going through a lot, how is your spirit?" "Spirit" is not necessarily religious, even though people sometimes interpret it this way and may say they are not religious or that they do believe in God, or something to this effect. Getting at their spirit as an element of meaning and purpose in life can help redirect the conversation and help the clinician learn a tremendous amount about the patient's overall values and level of grief or suffering in light of a life-threatening diagnosis. This is sometimes referred to as "total pain."

Despite your best efforts, patients may still report pain scores in the high severity range. Pain scores are not always indicative of someone's experience of pain or their functional limitations. Patients living in chronic pain may be accustomed to living at a reported pain score of 6 out of 10. Remember that the bookends of the pain scale must be clearly defined: 0 is no pain and 10 should be defined as the worst pain imaginable, like getting hit by a bus or some other major event. Commonly, 10/10 pain is erroneously defined as the worst pain you have ever experienced, which certainly is not the same for every individual. Even despite defining these parameters, the patient's report may stay around a 6 or 7, but they appear comfortable and are able to meet their functional goals. What becomes apparent is the importance of defining those functional goals and assessing the patient's progress toward them on a regular basis. It may initially be something as simple as sitting on the side of the bed or walking to the bathroom. There are functional pain scales that can be incorporated into a standard assessment, such as the Defense and Veterans Pain Rating Scale or the Clinically Aligned Pain Assessment tool, or, in the absence of such a scale, simply qualifying a number by a correlating a function to a number for patients as you work through the numeric rating scale.[2,3]

Through establishing functional goals, clinicians can also help patients set realistic expectations. Expectation-setting takes into consideration the severity of the patient's condition and the patient's values and personal goals and pairs them with the possibilities and limitations of the medications and treatment options. If the patient still has advanced cancer and the tumor is still present, the pain medications are not likely to take all of the pain down to a level of zero. This is often a hard thing to say because a clinician's desire is often to fix a patient's reported problem. Saying this, however, is very important. Explaining to the patient that their pain will not likely go away and that we need to figure out a level at which they can continue to have an acceptable quality of life will help guide their treatment. Not uncommonly, patients may experience sedation from the pain medications, and, for some patients being a little sleepier (but in less pain) may be an acceptable tradeoff. For others, sleepiness may not be compatible with their lifestyle or goals, and so the limitations of safe and effective use of the medications will be a more significant limiting factor. It is also important for family members to be a part of these discussions because they may have different levels of acceptable pain or sedation, which can present conflict and tension between their loved ones and the care team.

Pain commonly impacts other parts of life, including sleep, mood, and appetite.[4] Depression and anxiety can also have similar effects, so assessing for these mood changes is part of a holistic assessment. A standardized assessment tool, like the Edmonton Symptom Assessment Symptom, can be utilized to assess for these symptoms.[4] Treating symptoms of mood disorders will generally improve pain outcomes. In this patient, it is important to assess why the patient is not sleeping well: Is it the pain, or is it anxiety about the pain and its effects on her life, or possibly worry that the disease is worsening? Is she worried about being able to work and being around to help care for her granddaughter? Addressing these concerns and referring for expert intervention and psychological support should be offered to help her learn coping strategies and process her fears and anxieties. Once the assessment is made, referrals can be made and medications can be trialed that would treat both pain and anxiety, such as a serotonin and norepinephrine reuptake inhibitor like duloxetine.

For a patient with bone pain, there is evidence supporting the use of nonsteroidal anti-inflammatory drugs (NSAIDs) as well as corticosteroids.[5] Patients may not report over-the-counter (OTC) agents when asked about what they have tried for the pain, so asking specifically about NSAIDs and providing OTC brand and generic name examples (like Motrin or ibuprofen; Aleve or naproxen) will help obtain this information from the patient. Herbals and cannabis should also be directly asked about since these are commonly not thought of as "medications." Corticosteroids provide significant relief from bone pain, and while patients may not be sure if they have taken any, asking about their pain level around receiving chemotherapy may provide some insight into their response to steroid therapy, which is commonly given prior to chemotherapy. If pain seems much improved for the 3–4 days after chemo, it is likely that the dexamethasone has been effective, and it may be best to consider a slower taper post-chemotherapy to prevent a rebound in pain. Patients receiving immunotherapy may not have this experience, and oncologists may not be willing to consider the use of corticosteroids in these patients.

In the case of our patient, we should check in with her about what she expected regarding the outcomes of radiation and the anticipated pain relief. She completed her treatment course a month ago and so pain relief should be expected at this point, at least to some degree. It would be prudent to check in with her radiation oncologist about the expected degree of relief he would hope for and when he feels that might be at its maximum potential. Also, a repeat scan to ensure there are no other new lesions or injuries to the bones would be indicated if we are to perform a thorough workup.

Exploring the meaning of the pain with the patient is also going to help to establish the level of grief and suffering associated with the pain. She may be fearful of losing her job or about the potential for disease progression and what that could mean for her prognosis. She may not be sleeping because of the pain, or because she is worried and anxious, or both. The pain itself could be leading to a decreased appetite, but we should also assess for depression as part of her clinical presentation. It is not possible to know about these elements unless we ask. We also want to know what else she has tried for the pain, and explore the role of NSAIDs and steroids as possible therapies for relief. Finally, what is her tolerable level of pain? How much can we expect her to functionally be able to do versus what she feels she would like to do? Establishing realistic expectations for her pain control will help get everyone on the same page and also allow for her to express her values and goals.

KEY POINTS TO REMEMBER

- Pain severity and patient-reported acceptable pain level may not always align. Patients may report high pain scores that are still considered tolerable and not limiting to function.
- The meaning of the pain is often a driver of anxiety. Understanding what the pain means to the patient can help target therapeutic interventions.
- Anxiety and pain often come hand and hand. Treating concomitant anxiety will help with pain management and coping with painful episodes.
- Setting expectations at the beginning of any therapy is important in setting and attaining achievable goals.
- Pain is a moving target. A new report of pain in any patient with an oncologic diagnosis should be reevaluated with imaging to assess for further progression of disease while providing adjustments to the pain regimen in the meantime to allow for full workup of the pain report.
- Do not forget to assess for utilization of, access to, or ability to engage with nonpharmacologic interventions and over-the-counter medications as part of the pain treatment regimen.

References

1. Gordon DB. Acute pain assessment tools: Let us move beyond simple pain ratings. *Curr Opin Anesthesiol.* 2015;28:565–569.
2. Blackburn LM, Burns K, DiGiannantoni E, Meade K, O'Leary C, Stiles R. Pain assessment: Use of the Defense and Veterans Pain Rating Scale in patients with cancer. *CJON.* 2018;22(6):643–648.
3. Topham D, Drew D. Quality improvement project: Replacing the numeric rating scale with a Clinically Aligned Pain Assessment (CAPA) Tool. *Pain Manage Nurs.* 2017;18 (6)363–371.
4. Burton AW, Chai T, Smith LS. Cancer pain assessment. *Curr Opin Support Palliat Care.* 2014;8:112–116.
5. NCCN Guidelines. Pain management. 2019. https://www.nccn.org/guidelines/guidelines-detail?category=3&id=1413

Further Reading

American Pain Society. *Principles of Analgesic Use.* 7th ed. Chicago; 2016.
Cluxton C. The challenge of cancer pain assessment. *Ulster Med J.* 2019;88(1):43–46.

2 Pain in the Noncommunicative Adult

Claudia Z. Chou

Case Study

An 88-year-old woman with a history of hypertension, diabetes, osteoarthritis, and Alzheimer's dementia is being admitted from home hospice for respite care at the nursing facility where you work. She has been restless, resisting care, and calling out for the last few hours. Vital signs: T 37.3, BP 144/80, HR 96, RR 12. She vocalizes "help me" repeatedly but is unable to give appropriate answers to questions. No focal neurologic abnormalities are noted. Her family is not in the room with her, and none of the nursing home staff has cared for her before.

What Do I Do Now?

The patient is unable to verbalize what is leading to distress, but her behaviors warrant further investigation, including for potential sources of pain. Evidence suggests that impaired communication leads to substantial unmet needs in individuals with dementia, and one such need may be pain control. *Persistent pain*, or *chronic pain*, is defined as pain that continues for a prolonged period of time, often 3–6 months or more, and may or may not be associated with a well-defined disease process. Persistent pain is common in the elderly population, affecting up to half of older adults, with similar estimates in those with dementia. Etiology of pain in the elderly is often multifactorial, with common causes being related to musculoskeletal, neuropathic, genitourinary, gastrointestinal, vascular, and respiratory etiologies. Despite recognition, pain is often undertreated in the elderly, especially in those with cognitive impairment. Chronic pain has been associated with depression and often affects activities including sleep, ambulation, sitting, bending over, completing household chores, and participating in activities such as religious services, recreational activities, and social events.

Assessment of pain should begin with patient report. Patients may refer to "pain" using other terms, including "burning," "discomfort," "aching," "soreness," "heaviness," or "tightness." Numerous scales for the assessment of pain exist for both communicative and noncommunicative populations although there is often a lack of validation and consistency across care settings and a lack of a gold standard scale for use in dementia. Although cognitive impairment presence, it should not be assumed that all patients with cognitive impairment are unable to endorse pain or participate in completion of pain scales. For those who cannot self-report, scales which utilize caregiver rating, observational, or interactive approaches are used to assess pain. However, these scales often cannot determine intensity of pain as they have not been tested for this. A recently developed scale, the Pain Assessment in Impaired Cognition (PAIC15) aligns with the American Geriatric Society guidelines for common pain behaviors in cognitively impaired older adults and uses items from existing scales to create a meta-tool that integrates the best items for pain assessment in this population. Other useful pain assessment tools for noncommunicative adults include the Pain Assessment in Advanced Dementia (PAIN-AD) and Checklist of Nonverbal Pain Indicators (CNPI). Consistency is key when using these tools: make sure the same tool is used in the same patient. A comparison of common assessment tools for this patient population may be found in Table 2.1.

If patients are unable to report pain, surrogates can help to identify pain and provide information on the patient's pain history. Patients should be observed at rest and with activity. Facial expressions of pain are commonly used in pain scales and can serve as an alternative for self-report of pain. Surrogates, including caregivers and family, often can identify the presence of pain, utilizing knowledge of the patient and nonverbal cues, including changes in expression in the face and eyes; however, gauging the intensity of pain is often less accurate. Clinical manifestations of persistent pain can vary among individuals and even over time in the same individual. In patients with dementia, expressions of pain can manifest as confusion, social withdrawal, aggression, or subtle behavioral changes.

Once a potential source of pain is identified, treatment is considered. Guidelines from the American Geriatric Society suggest starting with acetaminophen, given its relative safety profile. In select individuals, nonsteroidal anti-inflammatory drugs (NSAIDs) can also be considered. Patients with moderate to severe pain, which leads to functional impairment or diminished quality of life despite more conservative management, can be considered for a trial of opioids after established therapeutic goals have been determined. Adjuvant analgesics can be considered in those with certain types of refractory, persistent pain, including neuropathic pain.

TABLE 2.1 **Common pain assessment tools for use in the noncommunicative adult**

Tool	Number of items	Source/Validation
PAINAD	5	Warden V et al. *J Am Med Dir Assoc.* 2003;4(1):9–15.
CNPI	6	Ersek M et al. *Pain Med.* 2010;11:395–404.
PAIC 15	15	Kunz M et al. *Eur J Pain.* 2020;24(1):192–208.

Clinicians can consider using multiple medications that have complementary mechanisms of action, as opposed to a single medication that might lead to toxicity and side effects at higher doses when used as monotherapy. Following initiation of any pharmacotherapy, careful monitoring of response and side effects is recommended. In patients whose cognitive and functional status allow for participation, involvement of a multidisciplinary team for nonpharmacologic management including cognitive-behavioral therapy and physical therapy can be beneficial options.

On examination of the patient in our case, there was tenderness to palpation over the anterolateral aspect of her left shoulder and a used lidocaine patch was found among the bedsheets. Nursing home staff contacted family, who shared that her behaviors were unusual because she was usually cooperative with care needs. They also reported that she had chronic left shoulder pain attributed to an old rotator cuff injury. She had slumped during a transfer prior to nursing home admission and bumped the shoulder on the edge of the bed. The family had placed the lidocaine patch, which was not part of her normal medication regimen. Because the lidocaine patch appeared to have controlled pain adequately prior to admission, this was continued. During the course of her respite stay, she was noted to still appear restless with care, so as-needed acetaminophen was added prior to care to treat incidental pain.

KEY POINTS TO REMEMBER

- Pain is common in the elderly population with dementia and should be considered as a potential etiology for behavioral changes.
- Evaluation should begin with history, physical examination, evaluation of psychologic and cognitive function, and diagnostics, including laboratory and imaging data as appropriate.
- Pain assessment should include patient self-report, surrogate report, and observation of behaviors at rest and with activity.
- If pharmacologic therapy is initiated, it should target the identified source of pain and be followed by frequent and careful reassessment for benefits and side effects.

Further Reading

American Geriatrics Society Panel on Pharmacological Management of Persistent Pain in Older Persons. Pharmacological management of persistent pain in older persons. *J Am Geriatr Soc.* 2009;57(8):1331–1346.

Herr K, Bjoro K, Decker S. Tools for assessment of pain in nonverbal older adults with dementia: A state-of-the-science review. *J Pain Symptom Manage.* 2006;31(2):170–192.

Kunz M, et al. The Pain Assessment in Impaired Cognition scale (PAIC15): A multidisciplinary and international approach to develop and test a meta-tool for pain assessment in impaired cognition, especially dementia. *Eur J Pain.* 2020;24(1):192–208.

3 A Behavioral Approach to Pain Control

Dokyoung S. You

Case Study

JJ was diagnosed with breast cancer 2 years ago. Prior to the onset of cancer, she was a healthy working woman and busy mother of two school-aged children (8 and 10 years old). Upon completion of chemotherapy and radiation therapy, she attempted to return to work, but she quit her job shortly after because pain, fatigue, and anxiety symptoms made it difficult for her to work as a software engineer. She underwent a right mastectomy and completed a course of intravenous chemotherapy and radiation. Unfortunately, now her cancer has recurred and metastasized to the spine. JJ is reluctant to initiate a new chemotherapy regimen because she developed chemotherapy-induced neuropathic pain (CIPN) on her hands and feet. She describes the pain and associated symptoms as numbness and tingling sensations that are quite debilitating because they limit her daily activities and disrupt her sleep. She has tried multiple analgesics and co-analgesics with relatively poor efficacy. Her oncologist has referred JJ to an outpatient palliative care service.

What Do I Do Now?

UNDERSTANDING THE PATIENT'S BELIEF ABOUT PAIN AND TREATMENT GOALS

The most important first step is to understand JJ's belief about pain and her treatment goals. She expresses a desire to be pain-free. Is her treatment goal attainable? To date, the evidence-based treatment for neuropathic and cancer pain is individualized as well as multimodal treatments, of which goals are to optimize pain and symptom management, physical function, and quality of life and prevent related symptoms. Subsequently, a clinician should acknowledge and validate her effort and desire to find an effective treatment but also partner with the patient to establish a realistic and optimistic expectation about available treatments and likely outcomes. To help patients understand treatment strategies, a clinician can offer education on pain neuroscience, which has shown to be effective in reducing pain and improving physical function. Neuroscience education generally covers how pain works in the nervous system, how factors (e.g., biological, psychosocial, and lifestyle factors) affect the pain experience, and which treatment strategies obtain optimal outcomes. Such education can be offered by a clinician and through online resources. Once the patient understands the treatment strategy, a clinician can discuss specific treatment options.

COMPLEMENTARY AND ALTERNATIVE MEDICINE APPROACH

The patient has tried massage therapy, which offered some temporary pain relief. The patient visited her home country to get a traditional deep tissue massage, which she found even more helpful. The patient is interested in complementary and alternative medicine (CAM) approaches, which are more common treatment options in her home country. Additionally, she is asking if acupuncture is worth attempting. Some evidence supports that acupuncture is effective in reducing pain and improving quality of life. Acupuncture is a safe treatment without serious side effects and may help JJ manage pain with less opioids. Therefore, a clinician can encourage the patient to explore acupuncture as well as other CAM approaches like vitamins, herbals, massage, and aromatherapy.

PHYSICAL THERAPY

Due to pain, JJ has significantly reduced her physical activity. Although exercise is a top priority, she finds it hard to do because of increased pain and fatigue afterward. Over time, she has avoided increasingly more activities which cause her pain. At present, she has become fairly inactive and has lost significant strength. Her goal for exercise is to improve muscle tone so she can play with her children. A physical therapy consultation can help the patient develop individual exercise programs and engage in group-based movement programs such as yoga. Physical therapy programs have been found to be effective in improving not only physical function, pain, and fatigue, but also sleep quality, depression, and quality of life among patients with neuropathic pain and recurrent breast cancer.

BEHAVIORAL MEDICINE APPROACH

So far, JJ has used rest, activity avoidance, sleep, eating sweets, and spending time on the computer to search cancer treatments as her main pain coping strategies. These strategies can be characterized as passive coping. Examples of active pain coping strategies are using relaxation techniques, mindfulness, activity pacing, and finding a way of engaging in fun and meaningful activities. The patient completed two questionnaires assessing pain coping. The first one was the 13-item Pain Catastrophizing Scale (PCS). Pain catastrophizing is a tendency to ruminate on pain, think about worst-case scenarios about pain, and feel helpless about pain. Her PCS total score was a 42, with PCS scores of 30 or higher (the top 25% of chronic pain population) considered elevated levels of pain catastrophizing. Cumulative evidence indicates that higher levels of pain catastrophizing are associated with higher pain ratings and worse upper limb dysfunction in patients who have had a surgery for breast cancer. The 10-item Pain Self-Efficacy Questionnaire (PSEQ) was also administered to assess her level of perceived ability to control and cope with pain. JJ obtained a total score of 13, with scores of 15 or lower (the bottom 25% of the chronic pain population) indicating low levels of pain self-efficacy. Lower pain self-efficacy is associated with higher pain levels and greater pain interference.

Several behavioral medicine approaches have proved effective in improving pain catastrophizing and pain self-efficacy. Such evidence-based treatments are cognitive-behavioral therapy (CBT) and mindfulness-based stress reduction (MBSR). One important point to discuss is the time commitment of CBT and MBSR programs. Pain management behavioral medicine programs generally require attending a 2-hour session weekly over 8–12 weeks (total of about 16–24 treatment hours). To reduce treatment burden, alternative options like a single-session class covering pain neuroscience education and CBT skills, internet-based CBT, mindfulness, or self-paced online learning of pain self-management skills can be proposed to the patient. These alternative behavioral medicine approaches are effective in improving fatigue, emotional distress, and quality of life in patients with cancer. Finally, self-help books and personal device apps are available for patients to learn these important self-management skills.

LIFESTYLE MANAGEMENT

Lifestyle factors associated with pain are diet, substance use, sleep patterns, and exercise. JJ reports no appetite, does not eat much on a daily basis, and has lost approximately 28 pounds over the past 2 years. She reports emotional eating about 3–4 times per month and consuming large amounts of sweets and ice cream when she is highly distressed or lonely. She stays home often and usually does not have many social interactions when her children are in school and her husband is at work. Furthermore, she eats sweets to manage emotional distress and she feels shameful about her emotional eating. JJ may benefit from working with a psychologist/therapist to develop healthy adaptive coping strategies.

Last, JJ has recently started drinking alcohol once or twice a month and reports drinking one glass of wine when she is unable to relax and/or fall asleep. While she only drinks small amounts of alcohol, the patient also takes daily opioids, pregabalin, and a benzodiazepine. All may interact with alcohol and increase the risk of adverse consequences (e.g., respiratory or central nervous system suppression). Although she reports never drinking alcohol when she takes her anxiety or pain meds, she drinks alone after her husband and children are in bed and she thinks alcohol is helpful for her sleep. Subsequently, JJ may benefit from a brief sleep hygiene evaluation and education or CBT for insomnia.

SUPPORT GROUP

JJ reports that her husband of 12 years is the only support she has in the United States. The patient describes their relationship as good, but not intimate. She avoids sexual activity due to pain. She has a few close friends at work from her ethnic community; however, JJ has disconnected with many of them because she typically cannot tolerate social gatherings due to pain and frequent unsolicited advice regarding her condition. She feels that nobody understands her suffering, and, over time, has developed symptoms of depression. Social isolation and loneliness are known to be associated with higher levels of pain. Engaging in a support group should be discussed with JJ to reduce social isolation and get connected with people who share similar experiences. Several support groups are available for patients and their family. Also, a clinician may assess JJ's need for faith and spirituality and encourage her to talk to a spiritual leader, join a religious group, or read related books.

ONGOING MONITORING OF PROGRESS AND CHECKING BARRIERS

Generally, medical treatments, CAM approaches, and physical therapy are understandable options, but a psychosocial approach to pain may not make sense to patients, especially those with life-limiting illness. Therefore, after making recommendations and providing resources, the clinician needs to assess the patient's progress. Helping patients to identify and address barriers to engage in a biopsychosocial approach is paramount. More importantly, it will take some time for a patient to make decisions for treatments, try them out, and find the best treatment strategy. Therefore, *motivational interviewing* techniques should be employed to help patients stay motivated for making changes. For example, a clinician can validate the patient's effort to find the best pain care options, repeat pain neuroscience education, and provide positive affirmation about the patient's progress. Additionally, in our case, depression symptoms should be closely monitored as JJ reports moderate depression symptoms at this time. As mentioned earlier, depression symptoms predict worse progress over time in patients with breast cancer. Therefore, pharmacological treatment or psychotherapy options need to be discussed as needed in the future. When reporting or observing worsening depression symptoms, the patient may benefit from working with a psychiatrist to consolidate central nervous system and mood-altering medications and optimize medication management for depression and persistent neuropathic pain. While psychosocial approaches to JJ's pain may not result in complete alleviation of symptoms, offering these modalities and explaining the potential benefit could certainly improve JJ's quality of life.

KEY POINTS TO REMEMBER

- Patient's belief and treatment goals need to be evaluated first as these are critical to developing an individualized pain care plan.
- Both multidisciplinary and biopsychosocial treatments are evidence-based approaches for persistent neuropathic and cancer pain.
- A simple intervention like pain neuroscience education is effective in reducing pain and improving physical function.
- A biopsychosocial approach to pain care includes medical treatments, CAM treatments, physical therapy, behavioral medicine, lifestyle management, and social support.
- Addressing barriers to engage in biopsychosocial treatments and using motivational interviewing techniques are paramount to the development of a patient-centered, multimodal treatment plan.

Further Reading

Chan CW, Cheng H, Au SK, Leung KT, Li YC, Wong KH, Molassiotis A. Living with chemotherapy-induced peripheral neuropathy: Uncovering the symptom experience and self-management of neuropathic symptoms among cancer survivors. *Eur J Oncol Nurs.* 2018 Oct 1;36:135–141.

Liu WC, Zheng ZX, Tan KH, Meredith GJ. Multidimensional treatment of cancer pain. *Curr Oncol Rep.* 2017;19(2):10.

Lopez G, McQuade J, Cohen L, et al. Integrative oncology physician consultations at a comprehensive cancer center: Analysis of demographic, clinical and patient reported outcomes. *J Cancer.* 2017;8(3):395.

Novy DM, Aigner CJ. The biopsychosocial model in cancer pain. *Curr Opin Support Palliat Care.* 2014;8(2):117–123.

Youtube: Understanding pain in less than 5 minutes and what do about it. 2013. https://youtu.be/C_3phB93rvl

4 Cultural Competence in Pain and Palliative Care

Noah Cooperstein and
Chienyem Adaobi Nweke

Case Study

ML is a 65-year-old African American woman who presents through the emergency department with dyspnea, productive cough, fever, weakness, headache, and pain. She is currently receiving chemo for chronic lymphocytic leukemia (CLL). Additionally, she has chronic back pain, hypertension, atrial fibrillation, and chronic kidney disease requiring hemodialysis. Initial evaluation is significant for tachypnea, hypotension, and rhonchi in her left lower lung fields. Labs and a chest x-ray confirm a diagnosis of pneumonia. During the initial assessment, the patient's daughter identifies herself as holding the patient's power of attorney and states that she "wants everything done." The patient is transferred to the intensive care unit, where she receives antibiotics and vasopressors. The team arranges a meeting with the patient and her family to discuss goals of care and ultimately recommends palliative care. Here her daughter stops the discussion, stating "we're not ready to give up."

What Do I Do Now?

At first this may not seem like a case where culture plays a central role in patient care. However, the medical team has done little to learn about the patient's understanding of her illness and has failed to gain the trust of the patient or her family. As a result, the patient and her family are uncertain that the treatment options offered will help the patient or are even in her best interest.

A patient's background will likely influence their interaction with the medical system. Patients belonging to a minority group, or patients who are recent immigrants or refugees, may be skeptical of the US medical system for various reasons including historical inequities and injustices, cultural differences, and personal experiences of discrimination. Given that every patient combines a unique mix of cultural and personal experiences, there is no one-size-fits-all approach to addressing culture in medicine.

The principles of patient-centered care should guide the treatment of patients from any race or cultural background. Using a framework of culturally relevant concepts can further aid clinicians in building a relationship of mutual respect and trust with patients and their families.

CULTURE AND CULTURAL COMPETENCE

The concept of culturally competent medical care emerged during the US civil rights movement of the 1960s and 1970s, as a response to systemic disparities between racial, ethnic, and cultural groups in the delivery and outcomes of medical care. The definition of cultural competence has evolved significantly over time. Recent work has de-emphasized the overt and superficial trappings of cultural difference such as ethnicity, language, and dress, and instead focused on broader, more dynamic notions related to the social determinants of health. Cultural competence can be thought of as "the ability of (clinicians) to establish effective interpersonal and working relationships that supersede cultural differences by recognizing the importance of social and cultural influences on patients, considering how these factors interact, and devising interventions that take these issues into account." This understanding of culturally competent care avoids the impossible task of "disaggregating" the heterogenous mix of multicultural practices in the modern world and is thereby better suited to caring for a contemporary patient. Mirroring our evolving understanding of culture, there are two distinct approaches to cross-cultural care: categorical and patient-centered.

CATEGORICAL APPROACH

Early efforts of multicultural/categorical approaches focused on knowledge about cultures. The categorical approach involves learning about the attitudes, values, beliefs, and behaviors of certain cultural groups such as traditional medicine, cultural taboos, and non-Western conceptions of illness, healing, and health. While this methodology might be more easily conceptualized, it oversimplifies culture. This strategy ignores the heterogeneity and diversity within any cultural group or the reality that cultural groups often overlap with each other. Furthermore, defining and reinforcing cultural boundaries and norms runs the risk of bolstering racial and ethnic stereotypes by focusing intently on the differences of other cultures. Something as complex as a patient's cultural background cannot be reduced or solved by a formulaic approach or reduced to a check list of cultural considerations.

PATIENT-CENTERED APPROACH

In contrast to a categorical strategy, a patient-centered approach provides clinicians with a functional and effective model of cultural competence. Based on openness, empathy, curiosity, and respect, this method is representative of the universal principles of patient-centered care. This is a conceptualization of a patient's culture as a series of overlapping life experiences which blend cultural components into a unique and singular worldview. These experiences are informed by ethnicity, race, and language but also by family, religion, age, gender, education, and socioeconomic status. It also avoids the pitfalls associated with defining and then learning so-called "cultural norms." Instead, the clinician must ask the patient and their family for insight into their beliefs and wishes to define the plan of care. Rather than categorize the patient and provide care based on assumptions, the clinician must work with the patient to understand their unique story.

Culturally competent care must navigate, at minimum, three distinct cultures: that of the clinician, that of Western medicine, and that of the patient. Clinicians must be cognizant of how their own background, values, and beliefs influence their approach to patient care and medical decision-making. Western medicine, with an emphasis on evidence, autonomy, and truth-telling, provides another conceptual and cultural frame for medical decisions. Last, the patient's own unique experience and perspectives must guide shared decision-making so that the clinician and the patient can enter a productive dialogue grounded on personal insight and mutual understanding.

ML's African American heritage and her personal experiences in the medical system as an African American woman likely influence her medical decision-making. Her decision not to enter palliative care may stem from a belief that palliative care amounts to giving up or perhaps not receiving the same quality of care as a Caucasian counterpart. These beliefs would be justifiably grounded in the historical inequities faced by African Americans both in the medical system and society at large. Without exploring the patient's unique experience, the medical team will remain unable to partner with the patient in developing a plan of care.

THE IMPORTANCE OF CULTURALLY COMPETENT PAIN MANAGEMENT IN PALLIATIVE CARE

Pain, death, and dying bring issues of culture to the forefront in a way that routine medical care might not. Cultural beliefs, traditions, values, and personal experiences shape each patient's definition of a "good death." A patient's cultural background will strongly influence decisions at the end of life, such as who makes medical decisions, whether to pursue aggressive and invasive treatment, or whether to receive care at all.

There exist numerous systemic and structural barriers to accessing palliative care for culturally diverse patients. These include limited access to primary care, reliance on emergency departments for care, a lack of reflective diversity in the healthcare community itself, limited outreach to diverse communities by hospice organizations, and a lack of cultural competence training within hospice organizations. While hospice care is underutilized by the US population at large, patients belonging to racial or ethnic minorities, particularly African Americans, are underrepresented in hospice and palliative care. Minority and culturally diverse patients also face significant disparities in pain management. Culturally diverse patients are less likely to receive adequate pain management at any age, in any medical setting, compared to their Caucasian counterparts.

While correction of structural barriers to accessing care must take place at the organizational and societal levels, clinicians should ensure they deliver equitable and appropriate management by implementing the strategies of culturally competent care. Unlike other encounters where a clinician may have multiple opportunities to establish a relationship with a patient, at the end of life there are limited opportunities to get the encounter right.

A FRAMEWORK FOR CULTURALLY COMPETENT CARE

Patient-centered culturally competent care can be structured around four key components:

1. Core cultural issues
2. Social context
3. The explanatory model
4. Plan of care

Each of these components has its own subset of questions and elements (see Table 4.1). This approach seeks to make explicit the key elements that are already implicit in most encounters, with the aim of bringing the typical stumbling blocks of a cross-cultural encounter to the forefront so that they can be consciously, conscientiously, and mindfully engaged.

CORE CROSS-CULTURAL ISSUES

Five core issues of cross-cultural care exist:

1. Communication
2. Trust
3. Family
4. Tradition
5. Sexuality

TABLE 4.1 **Framework of patient-centered culturally competent care structured around four key components, each with its own subset of questions and elements**

Key component	Subset of elements
Assess the five core cross-cultural issues	Styles of communication
	Trust
	Decision-making and family dynamics
	Traditions, customs, alternative therapies, and spirituality
	Sexuality and gender issues
Determine social context	Social stress and support networks
	Change in environment
	Life control
	Language and literacy
Explore the meaning of illness using the explanatory model	What do you call this problem?
	What do you believe is the cause of this problem?
	How serious is this problem?
	How does this problem effect your body?
	What do you fear most about your condition?
	What do you fear most about treatment?
Collaborate on the plan of care	Establish patient aims
	Introduce a plan of care
	Acknowledge patient–clinician differences
	Collaborate on common goals
	Develop a mutually accepted plan
	Assess for understanding

Not every domain will necessarily be applicable to a specific cross-cultural encounter, but each can be quickly considered and then assessed in more detail if needed. Note that this is not a categorical approach. The point is not to assume or ascribe characteristics from one of the domains to any specific culture but rather to understand that clinician–patient differences in any of these domains have the potential to complicate a cross-cultural encounter. What follows is a brief introduction to each of these domains as well as examples for how each domain plays into a cross-cultural pain management encounter.

Communication

This domain includes both verbal and nonverbal communication. Key considerations are the patient's level of assertiveness, degree of stoicism (especially regarding pain), and preferred channel of communication.

Consider the following during an encounter:

- Norms and etiquette regarding nonverbal communication can be hard to predict. Take cues from the patient regarding eye contact and personal space.
- On a spectrum from deferent to aggressive, consider the extent to which a patient is assertive. Deferent patients might not voice objection to a plan, but do not assume that silence indicates agreement. Assess agreement using open-ended questions and encourage patients to voice their concerns.
- Cultural norms and personal beliefs around pain and expressing discomfort vary greatly. Stoic patients may be in grave pain but refuse to show it for various reasons. Avoid assessing pain strictly through a cultural lens in which pain is indicated by crying, writhing, or moans.
- Determine the patient's preferred channel of communication. Not all cultures place the same value on autonomy and truth-telling as does Western medicine. If the patient has family members present who are involved in the patients care, ask the patient how they would like to be informed of test results or other new information and if they would prefer a family member to be the point of contact.

Trust

Mistrust of the medical establishment is deeply rooted in some communities. Given the long history of abuse and neglect by the medical system, mistrust of the medical community is especially pronounced among members of the African American community. Mistrust of the medical system is by no means limited to the African American community, however. The extent to which a patient trusts their clinician (or the medical system at large) will likely influence their compliance with medical care or their willingness to seek care at all.

Consider the following during an encounter:

- If the patient expresses mistrust of the medical system, explore this openly and elicit their experience if they are willing to discuss it.
- Ask if the patient has had a bad experience with the medical system or faced discrimination. Listen openly and actively to their answer should they choose to share their experience.
- Empower the patient. Give the patient as much control over their care as possible. Involve them in decisions and give them options whenever possible.

The statement that "the doctors probably just want to give her pain meds so she'll stop breathing" expresses underlying mistrust of the team and the medical system. Hearing this is understandably hurtful to clinicians who hold nonmaleficence as a guiding principle. Being mindful of their own feelings, clinicians on the team have a responsibility to discuss these sentiments with the patient and her family. In fact, after gaining an understanding of the patient's perspective, this may represent an opportunity to build trust through mutual understanding.

Family Dynamics and Decision-Making

Not all patients will wish to make their own medical decisions, preferring instead to defer to a family member or trusted friend. In other instances, family members will wish to shield the patient from potentially distressing information or decisions. In many cases, there will be multiple family members present during the clinical encounter.

Consider the following during an encounter:

- Introduce yourself to any family members who are with the patient and identify their relationship to the patient. Establish if there is a central family authority figure who will be involved in medical decisions.
- Determine the patient's desired level of autonomy. Establish the extent to which the patient wants to defer their medical decision-making. Ensure there is an appropriate power of attorney in place.
- In cases where a patient wishes to defer all medical decisions and does not want to discuss prognosis or the plan of care, there

is an option to waive the right-to-know. This requires legal documentation. In many cases, social work or pastoral care can help facilitate this process.

· In rare instances, a family may attempt to block clinicians from having any direct communication with the patient, even during an initial encounter. In these instances, be tactful but firm. Explain that the patient has the option to defer to family, but that the initial patient interview, however brief, is an essential step in patient care. This approach does not apply in cases where there is concern for abuse or neglect.

ML has capacity and autonomy, but her preference is to defer medical decisions to her daughter. In addition to continued family meetings, clinicians from the medical team should periodically check in with the patient without family present to assure that she agrees with their wishes as well.

Traditions, Customs, and Spirituality

This domain often garners the most attention in discussions of cross-cultural care. Here, it is important to explore and accommodate a patient's practices and beliefs as fully as possible. This is an opportunity to explore cultural taboos or dietary restrictions which may impact treatment. Many therapies which have traditionally been associated with a specific culture, such as acupuncture or cupping, are now commonly encountered as complementary or alternative therapies and should be integrated into the plan of care if the patient desires.

Consider the following during an encounter:

· Ask if the patient is a member of a religious community. If so, find out if they would like a member of that community to see them during their care. Determine if the patient has any specific spiritual needs they would like addressed.

· Inquire about the role of religion or spirituality in the patient's life and ascertain if their beliefs may influence their care in any way. Ascertain if there are any specific treatments the patient wants to avoid due to cultural taboos, and explore these in detail.

- Ask if there are any traditional or folk remedies the patient has found helpful in the past and offer these if possible.

Sexuality and Gender Issues

This domain runs the gamut from interacting with patients from cultures with strictly enforced traditional gender roles to caring for patients from the LGBTQ community. No matter the clinician's personal beliefs about human sexuality or gender roles, every encounter should be approached with the aim of providing the best possible care to the patient in the most open and nonjudgmental manner possible.

Consider the following during an encounter:

- Patients who ascribe to strict gender roles may refuse care from a clinician of the opposite gender. Try to accommodate patients as fully as possible. In these instances, defer the physical exam or ask a colleague to perform the exam if possible. Clinicians should remind themselves this is a function of the patient's background and beliefs, not a criticism of the clinician's abilities.
- Avoid judgmental language, and caution support staff to do the same. This of course applies to all patients, but clinicians and staff who are uncomfortable around LGBTQ patients may use inappropriate humor to distract themselves from their own feelings of unease. The clinician will likely never recover a therapeutic relationship with a patient who overhears someone mocking their gender identity or sexual orientation.
- In cases where there is an honest mistake or misunderstanding made in good faith (e.g., misgendering a transgendered patient), thank the patient for correcting the oversight, establish the patient's desired pronoun, and move on.

SOCIAL DOMAINS

A patient's cultural background is not the only factor that influences their experience with the healthcare system. In addition to the core cultural issues just described, clinicians should assess the impact of social domains. Note that many of these clearly overlap with issues of culture.

Ask the patient about sources of stress or worry. Do not take it for granted that the primary concern of the patient is for their own well-being. Often, even at the end of life, a patient's primary concern may be for a loved one or even a pet. Find out who the patient relies on for support and comfort, be it a religious community, family, or friends.

Life Control

This domain is primarily related to the patient's socioeconomic status and overlaps with other social stressors. Discuss with the patient the extent to which they feel in control of their own medical care. Empower the patient to voice their wishes. Additionally, determine if the patient feels that they have experienced discrimination or unfair treatment by the healthcare system in the past and assure the patient that the current team will strive to avoid such mistakes.

Language and Literacy

If the patient is a non-native English speaker (assuming an English-speaking care setting), let them know they have the option to request an interpreter. Avoid trying to assess a patient's language proficiency. Even patients who are proficient in English may have a limited vocabulary of medical terminology or may simply wish to discuss their care in their native language. Avoid relying on family members for translation, and never use minors to translate. Additionally, ask patients if they have difficulty reading or following written instructions in any language, as this has obvious implications for how well the patient will be able to follow written instructions or read documents such as a power of attorney or living will.

EXPLANATORY MODELS

The explanatory model of sickness has been widely adopted in cross-cultural care. An explanatory model can be thought of as a mode of understanding a medical condition. Classically, the Western medical explanatory model is that of *disease*, whereas a patient or lay person's explanatory model is that of *illness*.

Every patient, no matter their cultural or ethnic background, will have an explanatory model for their illness. The following questions can be used to better understand the patient's explanatory model. Understanding the patient's explanatory model permits the clinician to provide care in a manner that the patient desires and understands while mitigating cross-cultural misunderstandings and conflicts.

Consider the following questions:

. What do you call this problem?
. What do you believe is the cause of this problem?
. How serious is this problem?
. How does this problem affect your body?
. What do you fear most about your condition?
. What do you fear most about treatment?

These questions should be tailored to the patient and the situation. The clinician need not ask every question of every patient. Often, simply asking "What do you think is going on?" or "What matters most to you in the experience of illness and treatment?" will elicit most of the information captured by these six questions.

Returning to ML's case, the initial failure of the family meeting stemmed from the medical team's lack of knowledge about the patient, including her understanding of her condition, her fears, and her goals. The preceding questions can be used to facilitate a discussion in which medical team learns about the patient rather than just telling her about treatments.

THE PLAN OF CARE

Understanding the patient's experience vis-à-vis the core cross-cultural issues, social context, and explanatory model enables clinicians to more effectively develop and discuss the plan of care. These domains should not be thought of as quantifiable values or any sort of cultural diagnosis—they are not lab values or imaging results. The aim is not to merely identify a cultural phenomenon or diagnose a cross-cultural issue. The goal is to start a conversation, not end it.

Consider the following steps when developing the plan of care:

. Establish patient aims
. Introduce a plan of care

- Acknowledge differences
- Find common goals
- Develop a plan
- Assess for understanding

CONCLUSION

This chapter posits a universal approach to culturally competent care that organizes and makes explicit the sorts of questions that most clinicians are already asking during a patient encounter. This strategy avoids reinforcing cultural stereotypes and the pitfalls of applying categorical knowledge to something as dynamic as culture. Good patient care always comes back to simple, honest, open communication with the patient and their family. Community outreach by palliative care clinicians to culturally and ethnically diverse populations in the local area using the methods described here might be a good first step to bolstering mutual understanding and building trust.

RETURN TO THE CASE

By changing the way the team approached the ML's care, they were able to understand her and her family's views on palliative care and opioid pain medications. During subsequent family meetings, they listened to the patient's experience and elicited her fears and goals. The medical team was then able to discuss how these goals aligned with the hospice philosophy. The patient, her family, and the medical team were able to collaborate on a plan of care. The patient was discharged home with hospice and an adequate pain management plan. Rather than viewing this as a form of resignation, both the patient and her family were confident that the plan of care was in line with the patient's wishes and fully in her best interest.

> **KEY POINTS TO REMEMBER**
>
> - End of life discussions have the potential to bring issues of mistrust, fear, and skepticism to the forefront when caring for patients who belong to a minority group or who are recent immigrants or refugees.

- Given that every patient combines a unique mix of cultural and personal experiences, we recommend a patient centered approach to cross cultural care based on openness, empathy, curiosity, and respect.
- Providing culturally competent pain management in palliative and end of life care is especially important since there is limited time and opportunity to establish trust, build mutual understanding, and collaborate on a plan of care.
- While hospice care is underutilized by the US population at large, patients belonging to racial or ethnic minorities, particularly African Americans, are underrepresented in hospice and palliative care.
- Community outreach by palliative care clinicians to culturally and ethnically diverse populations in the local area is a good first step to bolstering mutual understanding, building trust, and ultimately providing this valuable service in a more inclusive and representative manner.

Further Reading

Betancourt JR, Green AR, Carrillo JE, Ananeh-Firempong O. Defining cultural competence: A practical framework for addressing racial/ethnic disparities in health and health care. *Public Health Rep.* 2003;118(4):293–302.

Betancourt JR, Cervantes MC. Cross-cultural medical education in the United States: key principles and experiences. *Kaohsiung J Med Sci.* 2009;25(9):471–478.

Bullock K. The influence of culture on end-of-life decision making. *J Soc Work End Life Palliat Care.* 2011;7(1):83–98.

Butler M, McCreedy E, Schwer N, et al. *Improving cultural competence to reduce health disparities.* Rockville, MD: Agency for Healthcare Research and Quality; 2016.

Dillon PJ, Basu A. African Americans and hospice care: A culture-centered exploration of enrollment disparities. *Health Communication.* 2016;31(11):1385–1394.

Jongen C, McCalman J, Bainbridge R, Clifford A. *Cultural competence in health: A review of the evidence.* 1st ed. New York: Springer; 2017.

Martin EM, Barkley TW. Improving cultural competence in end-of-life pain management. *Home Healthc Now.* 2017;35(2):96–104.

Spector RE. *Cultural diversity in health and illness.* 9th ed. New York: Pearson; 2016.

5 Acupuncture for Analgesia

Noah Cooperstein and Jonathan Thoma

Case Study

A 25-year-old Hispanic man with metastatic testicular cancer is admitted for symptom management due to a large metastatic tumor burden of the liver. He has been admitted seven times recently for symptom control. He experiences regular severe nausea with emesis, despite appropriate therapy, making pain control with oral medications challenging. Furthermore, his current opioid pain regimen, including fentanyl patch, results in significant sedation and marginal pain relief. He reports 10 out of 10 pain diffusely across his abdomen with radiation into his lower back, pelvis, and right shoulder. The patient is discharged to home hospice. The patient understands his prognosis and is anxious about how his family will fare once he is gone. He desires to be more functional so that he can spend time with his family. He remains concerned about his pain medications' adverse effects and asks "what else" can be done to lessen his pain without further interfering with his ability to interact with his family.

What Do I Do Now?

BACKGROUND

This patient has reached the preterminal phase of his disease and has elected to enter hospice care for management of his pain. Previous attempts to manage his pain have resulted in intolerable side effects, leaving him to choose between pain control and the ability to spend meaningful time with his family. It is also evident that this patient has other sources of distress beyond pure physiologic pain. Specifically, he is anxious about his own future and that of his family.

In the paradigm of allopathic medicine, management of physical pain is a major focus of treatment at the end-of-life. As this case illustrates, there is more to pain than just a physical sensation of discomfort. The most common symptoms impacting quality of life at end of life are pain, dyspnea, fatigue, nausea, vomiting, constipation, and anxiety. Dr. Cicely Saunders, one of the originators of the modern hospice movement, coined the term "total pain" to capture the multiple dimensions of pain. Total pain includes physical pain and its related symptoms as well as pain or suffering that is psychological, social, or spiritual in nature. The total pain model holds that the most effective analgesia for patients at the end of life is achieved through a holistic approach that addresses each of these domains.

KEY CONCEPTS

Acupuncture integrates especially well into palliative care given its implicit overlap with the total pain model. Based on Confucian and Taoist philosophies that emphasize balance and harmony, acupuncture is, by definition, holistic in its approach to the patient. Moreover, while holistic and integrative in nature, acupuncture simultaneously retains the ability to target and treat specific symptoms such as pain, nausea, and anxiety. The following is intended only as an introduction to a few key concepts so that clinicians without acupuncture training can orient themselves to some of the fundamental principles of an acupuncture treatment. While these concepts are prescientific in their origins, they are naturalistic rather than magico-religious. They are grounded in first-hand human experience, specifically that of the patient, and do not rely on or require mystical or supernatural thinking.

Yin and Yang. Much of Western thought is predicated on the axioms of Aristotelian logic that hold that two opposites states cannot both exist (or be true) at once. In classical Chinese philosophy, however, opposites are understood as two parts of the same whole. Yin and Yang can be understood as two opposing aspects, characteristics, or properties of an entity or phenomenon as it exists in space and time. They exist on a single continuum, with each containing the seed of the other. Light, for example, belongs to Yang, while darkness belongs to Yin. "Left" is Yang while "right" is Yin. This is, in fact, is consistent with our experience of the world: as the day progresses, light eventually yields to darkness; there can be no right, without a left for reference. In Chinese medicine, all aspects of anatomy and physiology belong to either Yin or Yang based on their location, function, properties, or qualities.

Qi. Qi (pronounced "chee") connects and balances Yin and Yang. It's tempting for Western thinkers to conceptualize Qi as belonging to one of three categories: an energy or force, a fluid or substance, or a metaphorical or experiential concept. The duality of energy and matter, however, is a Western concept that does not apply to the classical understanding of Qi. The Chinese logogram (i.e., written character) for Qi is the combination of the characters for "rice" and "vapor." This captures the opposite yet complementary properties of Qi. It is both nourishment derived from food, fluid, or respiration and a circulating source of protection and vitalization(Helms 1995).[1] Qi is both ephemeral and constant, abstract and material. In the human body, Qi is believed to move through classically defined acupuncture channels which connect acupuncture points. Qi connects and balances Yin and Yang. It is neither material nor metaphorical.

The Five Elements. Pairs of organs (one Yin and one Yang) are organized based on their association with one of the five traditional elements: Fire, Earth, Metal, Water, or Wood. For example, kidney (Yin) is paired with bladder (Yang) and both belong to the same element (Water). This is perhaps the most straightforward and concrete example of these associations. The pairing of Master of the Heart (MH; Yin) with Triple Heater (TH; Yang) under the same element (Fire) better captures the complexity and nuance of this system and illustrates its insight into human physiology. MH protects the heart, governs blood, controls heat, and modulates mood and emotional state. TH directs Qi, regulates digestion and excretion, and controls the visceral organs. Both MH and TH remain somewhat abstract in the traditional texts: both have broad functional control over the body, yet neither has a specific organ or structure to which it is attached. Looking at this through a modern lens, this appears to be a representation of the autonomic nervous system, with MH as the sympathetic division and TH as the parasympathetic division. In fact, contemporary practitioners working under an allopathic diagnosis will often access ancient MH and TH points specifically to modulate and balance the autonomic nervous system. Traditional acupuncture treatments are meant to restore balance between Yin and Yang by moving Qi within the framework of the Five Elements. This approach is grounded in the patient's experience and sensation. This is a human-centered (what might now be called *patient-centered*) approach to healing.

CONTEMPORARY EVIDENCE FOR ACUPUNCTURE

Basic Science

At first glance, acupuncture can seem counterintuitive to a modern practitioner of allopathic medicine. There is no immediately self-evident explanation for why placing needles in a patient's ankle might alleviate neck pain or placing needles in the ears would reduce back pain. There is, however, meaningful basic science that supports a mechanistically plausible explanation for the effectiveness of acupuncture treatment.

Early investigations identified lower electrical resistance in the skin at acupuncture points compared to controls as well as lower resistance between acupuncture points along the same classically defined acupuncture channel. Subsequent studies using Technetium99 tracing found topographical migration along classically defined acupuncture channels when injected into acupuncture points but not when injected into non-acupuncture controls. The rate at which the tracer migrated did not correspond to blood flow or lymph circulation, suggesting an alternative pathway, perhaps peri-muscular.

Morphologic examination of the skin at acupuncture points often demonstrates subtle skin changes, frequently in the form of a small depression. Histologic examination of these same points in the skin frequently demonstrates the presence of unique lymphatics and neurovascular bundles, including the presence of autonomic nerve fibers. Taken all together, these findings suggest that acupuncture points are "real" in the sense that they are consistently morphologically and histopathologically different from randomly chosen skin points and that they appear to communicate in some manner along classically defined acupuncture channels.

More recent research has focused on the influence of acupuncture points on the central nervous system. There is evidence suggesting that analgesic effects from acupuncture are initiated by needle stimulation of high-threshold, small-diameter nerves in the muscle body. Stimulation of these nerves is transmitted through the periphery into the central nervous system (CNS) with the ultimate downstream effect of releasing endogenous opioids. The role of endogenous opioids in acupuncture is further supported by the finding that acupuncture-induced analgesic effects are reversible by naloxone in a dose-dependent manner. Various animal models have demonstrated acupuncture's influence on autonomic outflow from the CNS and modulation of the hypothalamic-pituitary-adrenal axis, including effects on blood pressure, gut motility, and immune response. Neuroimaging using functional magnetic resonance (fMRI) showed increased activation of numerous deep brain structures, most notably the somatosensory cortex and the limbic system, with the placement of needles at acupuncture points compared to sham points. On whole, this more recent work supports the hypothesis that, in addition to local and regional effects, acupuncture can influence and modulate the CNS, including the release of endogenous opioids, hormonal regulation, and autonomic tone.

Clinical Research

As with any treatment or intervention, bench-top science or mechanistic evidence is unconvincing if it cannot be translated into a clinically meaningful outcome. In practical terms, the question of *why* a treatment works is less important than that of *if* it works. The efficacy of acupuncture for pain management has been sufficiently—if often imperfectly—studied in numerous randomized controlled trials (RCT). There are sufficient data to allow for multiple systematic reviews and meta-analysis of the evidence to date. Acupuncture poses several unique challenges to rigorous scientific investigation, and while there is a large amount of data, the overall quality of evidence is moderate. While older reviews typically found insufficient evidence to make recommendations, the most recently completed meta-analyses indicate that acupuncture is a safe and effective treatment for chronic pain, cancer-related pain, and other common symptoms associated with end-of-life care.

Pilot Studies

Several pilot studies have explored the use of acupuncture for symptom management and improvement in quality of life for patients receiving palliative care. These have been single-arm, unblinded, prospective studies intended to provide preliminary data and guide further study. The results from these studies appear promising, with patient reports of improvements in pain, anxiety, nausea, appetite, and dyspnea, among others. However, more rigorous study is needed in this domain.

Systematic Reviews and Meta-Analyses

The evidence for the efficacy of acupuncture as it relates to pain management and palliative care has been evaluated in multiple recent systematic reviews and meta-analysis. A 2017 meta-analysis evaluated 10 studies that investigated the use of auricular (ear) acupuncture for the immediate relief of any type of pain. Study authors found that ear acupuncture is safe and likely effective for immediate pain relief, though results were limited by heterogeneity across studies .[2] A 2018 individual patient meta-analysis published in *The Journal of Pain* identified 20,827 patients from 39 trials who were randomized to receive acupuncture or control (sham acupuncture or no acupuncture) for chronically painful conditions, including nonspecific musculoskeletal pain, osteoarthritis, headache, and shoulder pain. The study found that acupuncture has a clinically relevant effect on chronically painful conditions that cannot be explained by placebo effect alone.[3]

A 2015 Cochrane Review evaluated five RCTs with a total of 285 patients for the efficacy of acupuncture for the treatment of cancer-related pain. This systematic review concluded the data were insufficient to judge the efficacy of acupuncture therapy but noted that none of the studies reported any harm to patients.[4] These findings were corroborated by two additional systematic reviews.[5,6] Both reviews highlight a high-risk for bias in the study designs, and each recommends additional future research. Notably, there was minimal overlap in the selected studies included between these reviews, further emphasizing the difficulty in building effective RCTs to evaluate acupuncture.

A 2019 systematic review and meta-analysis published in *The Journal of the American Medical Association* (JAMA) evaluated the use of acupuncture and acupressure in treating cancer pain.[7] A total of 17 randomized control trials with a total of 1,111 patients were reviewed and were appraised using the Cochrane Collaboration risk-of-bias tool. The main outcome was pain intensity by various validated pain scales. In seven studies, acupuncture was associated with reduced pain intensity compared to sham acupuncture. In six studies, combination with acupuncture and analgesic therapy was associated with reduced pain intensity. Overall, the systematic review found that acupuncture was associated with reduced pain in cancer patients. The evidence for these findings was graded as moderate due to significant heterogeneity among the studies, including variation in the acupuncture method used.

Overall Evidence

Though there is some plausible basic science to support acupuncture, historically, poor study design and the imprecise use of sham procedures have created an ambiguous body of clinical evidence. It is possible that as the quality of individual acupuncture studies continues to improve, so will the overall evidence for acupuncture. Based on the most current literature, and specifically two recent, well-designed meta-analyses published in major peer-reviewed journals,[3,8] it is reasonable to discuss acupuncture with patients receiving palliative care as a viable and safe adjunct therapy for pain and other symptom management and to refer interested patients to an acupuncture practitioner for treatment.

THE ACUPUNCTURE ENCOUNTER

History and Physical

Like any patient encounter, acupuncture treatment begins with the patient interview. In many respects, initial history-taking, especially when performed by a physician acupuncture practitioner, will mirror a standard allopathic interview. The practitioner will gather a history of present illness; a medical, social, and family history; and a review of systems. While similar in content, the underlying process is different. In an allopathic interview, the clinician is generally attempting to identify a pattern in the history and symptomatology that corresponds to a cognitive model (illness script) for a known condition. In the acupuncture interview, rather than attempt to arrive at a specific diagnosis, the acupuncture practitioner seeks to form a model of the type of disharmony or disruption the patient is experiencing.[1]

Following the initial interview, the acupuncture encounter will depart to questions that are not typical of a standard medical interview. The practitioner might ask about things like favorite season, color, or food. The physical exam mirrors this departure: following a routine physical exam, some practitioners may exam the patient's tongue or radial pulses. Ultimately, the function of the history and physical is not to necessarily to diagnose a specific disease or disorder, but to better understand the type of patient vis-à-vis understanding which of the five elements figures most prominently in their makeup.[1]

Counseling on Risks

As with any invasive procedure, acupuncture patients will be counseled on treatment-associated risks. The most common adverse events associated with acupuncture include pain, bleeding, or bruising, which are reported in about 3% of treatments. Orthostatic changes (lightheadedness, dizziness) are typically transient and occur in about 0.5% of cases. Infection is typically discussed as a possibility, though it is extremely rare. Overall, less than 10% of patients receiving regular acupuncture treatments experience a minor adverse event. Major adverse events are extremely rare. Pneumothorax is likely the most serious adverse event and may be underreported in the literature due to delay in presentation. Special considerations for patients at the end of life, especially those with cancer, include complications associated with immunosuppression, thrombocytopenia, or pancytopenia.

For the patient in our case study, after discharge to home, he traveled to the office of a local acupuncture practitioner. In additional to gathering a medical and social history, the initial interview with the acupuncturist focuses on understanding the ways in which the patient's diagnosis has impacted his life. Symptoms of nausea, fear, and pain emerge as common themes. After obtaining appropriate consent, the practitioner proceeded with a global treatment meant to balance the autonomic nervous system by placing needles in the patient's hands, wrists, ankles, and knees. The patient reported feeling less anxious following this treatment and agreed to return for weekly sessions.

Treatment

The specifics of treatment will vary depending on when and where the acupuncture practitioner received their training. Numerous acupuncture traditions have arisen over the millennia. These include distinct schools throughout East Asia including Chinese, Japanese, and Korean. Subsequent Western styles emerged during the twentieth century, including specific French, British, and American schools.[1] Additionally, unique subsystems or microsystems have developed that focus on treatment using needles applied to a specific body part or region. These include auricular (ear), scalp, and hand acupuncture.

The treatment itself may consist of the placement of a single needle, though usually multiple needles are employed. Needle placement may be at the location of pain or discomfort or remote from it. Many practitioners combine microsystems with other acupuncture treatments and may place additional needles in the ear, scalp, hand, or foot. In some cases, needles will be stimulated using heat (including burning the herb moxa when possible) or by low-voltage electricity. Typically, needles are placed and allowed to reside for 10–20 minutes before being removed. Needles placed in the scalp may remain in place for hours, however, and some specialized needles for the ear (ASPs) remain in place for days. Contemporary acupuncture only uses single-use, sterile, individually packaged needles which are properly disposed of at the end of the treatment.

The goals of a specific acupuncture treatment will vary depending on the practitioner's impression of the overall patient presentation. Treatment may focus on specific symptom management or may attempt to address more profound psychological or spiritual concerns. In addition to pain control, acupuncture treatments in palliative care frequently address dyspnea, pruritus, depression, anxiety, nausea, and issues with salivation. In some instances, treatment will focus on restoring a deeper level of balance or harmony. These treatments are designed to reverse depletion from stress or illness, balance the autonomic nervous system, or address deep-seated trauma. These metaphorically deeper treatments may address the psychological, social, or spiritual components of total pain.

RETURN TO CASE

Following their initial encounter, subsequent sessions included treatments for

- Sleep and pain using the ear and scalp microsystems
- Anxiety with needles placed in the scalp, hands, and feet
- Liver pain secondary to metastatic disease, with needles placed at points on channels for the liver and gallbladder
- Referred pain of the abdominal and pelvic organs using needles placed on channels for liver, stomach, kidney, spleen, and autonomic nervous system connected by low-voltage electrical stimulation
- Global energy depletion, with needles placed on kidney and gallbladder channels and connected by low-voltage electrical stimulation

Over the course of these treatments, the patient reported modest improvement in his nausea, anxiety, and pain, usually lasting 1–2 days following the treatment and without any of the sedation he experienced as a side effect of many of his medications. After several weeks of treatment, the patient progressed to the terminal phase of illness. His final visit to the acupuncture practitioner included a treatment meant to induce a deep catharsis of the trauma of dying in hopes of freeing him to connect with his family more deeply during his final hours.

References

1. Helms JM. *Acupuncture Energetics: A Clinical Approach for Physicians.* 1st ed. Berkeley, CA: Medical Acupuncture Publishers; 1995.
2. Murakami M, Fox L, Dijkers MP. Ear acupuncture for immediate pain relief—A systematic review and meta-analysis of randomized controlled trials. *Pain Med.* 2017;18(3):551–564. https://doi.org/10.1093/pm/pnw215
3. Vickers AJ, Vertosick EA, Lewith G, et al.; Acupuncture Trialists' Collaboration. Acupuncture for chronic pain: Update of an individual patient data meta-analysis. *J Pain: Off J Am Pain Soc.* 2018;19(5):455–474. https://doi.org/10.1016/j.jpain.2017.11.005
4. Paley CA, Johnson MI, Tashani OA, Bagnall A-M. Acupuncture for cancer pain in adults. *Cochrane Database Syst Rev.* 2015b;10:CD007753. https://doi.org/10.1002/14651858.CD007753.pub3
5. Wu X, Chung VCH, Hui EP, et al. Effectiveness of acupuncture and related therapies for palliative care of cancer: Overview of systematic reviews. *Sci Rep.* 2015;5:16776. https://doi.org/10.1038/srep16776
6. Lau CHY, Wu X, Chung VCH, et al. Acupuncture and related therapies for symptom management in palliative cancer care. *Medicine.* 2016;95(9). https://doi.org/10.1097/MD.0000000000002901

7. He Y, Guo X, May BH, et al. Clinical evidence for association of acupuncture and acupressure with improved cancer pain: A systematic review and meta-analysis. *JAMA Oncol.* 2020;6(2):271–278. https://doi.org/10.1001/jamaoncol.2019.5233

Further Reading

Cac GM. *The Foundations of Chinese Medicine: A Comprehensive Text.* 3rd ed. Edinburgh: Churchill Livingstone; 2015.

Kaptchuk TJ. Acupuncture: Theory, efficacy, and practice. *Ann Intern Med.* 2002;136(5):374–383. https://doi.org/10.7326/0003-4819-136-5-200203050-00010

Romeo MJ, Parton B, Russo RA, Hays LS, Conboy L. Acupuncture to treat the symptoms of patients in a palliative care setting. *Explore.* 2015;11(5):357–362. https://doi.org/10.1016/j.explore.2015.06.001

Zeng YS, Wang C, Ward KE, Hume AL. Complementary and alternative medicine in hospice and palliative care: A systematic review. *J Pain Symptom Manage.* 2018;56(5):781–794.e4. https://doi.org/10.1016/j.jpainsymman.2018.07.016

Zia FZ, Olaku O, Bao T, Berger A, et al. The National Cancer Institute's Conference on Acupuncture for Symptom Management in Oncology: State of the science, evidence, and research gaps. *JNCI Monographs.* 2017;2017(52):68–73. https://doi.org/10.1093/jncimonographs/lgx005

6 Chiropractic Treatment of Cancer Pain

Brandon Daniels

Case Study

A 75-year-old White man presents with a chief complaint of mid back pain and points in the proximity of the fifth thoracic vertebra. He also complains of anterior rib pain on the right side, located in the fifth intercostal space aligned with the mid-clavicular line. He has been to the hospital three times in the last 45 days due to pain, which is rated as a 10 of 10. He claims he is desperate for some form of relief and has tried everything. Six years prior he was diagnosed with lung cancer. He has a 50-pack year history. Eight months ago, he was informed that the cancer had metastasized to the liver. He is depressed and angry over poor familial relationships. He refuses any medications. His temperature is 98.6, blood pressure is 135/90, heart rate is 94, respiratory rate is 43, and $SPO_2\%$ is 88. No history of cholecystitis; Murphy's sign is negative. Thoracic spine x-ray demonstrates degenerative disc disease and osteoarthritis throughout. There is no evidence of metastasis to the spine.

What Do I Do Now?

WHEN IS CHIROPRACTIC OR A CONSERVATIVE HEALTHCARE REFERRAL APPROPRIATE?

If you are not trained in chiropractic, the following information may be beneficial when considering if a consult is warranted. When chiropractic is mentioned, most clinicians immediately think of the spine. However, chiropractic care is not limited to the spine. It also includes the cranium and the extremities. If there is any manifestation of pain in a patient receiving palliative care, a chiropractor may be consulted to assess these areas of pain for potential treatments.

Many chiropractors are also trained in additional fields such as acupuncture, functional medicine, applied kinesiology, and functional neurology. Finding a chiropractor who is properly trained in these specialties is recommended because they have deeper training in the underlying physiology, neurology, and meridian function that is often associated with the complex conditions seen in palliative care.

It is also very important to keep the wishes of the patient in mind. If a patient prefers to follow a more conservative treatment route, then a chiropractor trained in acupuncture, functional medicine, or functional neurology may be consulted.

CONTRAINDICATIONS

The World Health Organization (WHO) has a list of absolute and relative contraindications for chiropractic manipulation therapy (CMT). It is important to note that many contraindications may apply to individual spinal segments, but CMT on other areas of the spine may be permissible. I recommend that every practitioner be very familiar with these guidelines. Contraindications include but are not limited to unstable os odontoideum, spinal tumor, malignancy of the spine, meningeal tumor, aggressive types of benign tumors, and syringomyelia. Some sources suggest that not all of these are absolute contraindications. However, abiding by the WHO recommendations and your state licensing board is strongly recommended. High-velocity low-amplitude (HVLA) CMT may be contraindicated, but lower force adjusting techniques or soft tissue work may still be permissible and beneficial. Research has shown that many low-force adjusting techniques will still attain the desired result.

In our case study, you must be able to answer an important question: Are these complaints related to or resultant from the underlying disease process, or are they from an unrelated musculoskeletal condition? The first possible answer is no, they're not related. This is a simple musculoskeletal scenario. Therefore, standard treatments may be successful.

To answer this question, we can look at several different factors. These factors are not 100% diagnostic or exclusive in their findings. Rather, when assessing for several different findings, we are able to surmise a much larger amount of information that helps the practitioner to gather a clear understanding of the patient's condition. A manual muscle test (MMT) is a valuable skill in assessing many of these findings. This can be utilized with therapy localization (TL) as a reliable and reproducible measure to evaluate many conditions and findings. TL is the process of having a patient touch an area of the body (usually of dysfunction) that will change the results of MMT, which aids in reaching a diagnostic conclusion. The best method of TL is for the patient to use their fingertips. Common applications for TL are to subluxations (in the CMT sense of the word), Chapman's reflexes, meridian/acupuncture points, areas of pain, etc. A positive TL indicates the involvement/location of a problem but does not necessarily indicate what is wrong or why it is occurring.

All certified applied kinesiologists are properly trained in this manner.

CHRONIC MANIPULATIVE THERAPY/SPINAL MANIPULATIVE THERAPY

The first treatment option is CMT, also referred to as spinal manipulative therapy (SMT). While there can be differences between the two depending on specific training, here they will be used synonymously. CMT is the most common available treatment provided by Doctors of Chiropractic (DC), Doctors of Osteopathy (DO), or Doctors of Physical Therapy (DPT). In each case, careful examination should be performed to determine the proper area to adjust. These should include some combination of static palpation, dynamic palpation, tenderness evaluation, hypertonicity evaluation, and range of motion, and they may include other methods of evaluation such as TL, leg length analysis, vertebral challenge, etc. Prior to treatment, all available imaging such as x-ray, magnetic resonance imaging (MRI), and computed tomography (CT), should be reviewed and assessed for any contraindications to CMT. It is also recommended to fully review the patient's case history, physician and examination notes, and blood work (if properly trained). Imaging in the past 12 months will suffice in most cases. However, if there is no imaging performed within the past 12 months, or if there is onset of a new chief complaint potentially related to the disease process, then new imaging is required before proceeding with CMT treatment.

In this patient's case, there is hypomobility noted throughout the T4–T7 spinal segments. Static palpation revealed a possible T4 posterior on the left and a retrolisthesis at T5. Vertebral challenge indicated the same findings as well as an additional fixation of T6–T7 vertebrae. The erector spinae on the right were hypertonic and hyperfacilitated when tested for autogenic inhibition. There is tenderness and allodynia of the T5 spinous process.

These findings determine a need for CMT, and they also give the needed information on how and where to adjust. The practitioner could perform CMT at this point and establish a care plan under the impression that it is solely a musculoskeletal problem. Some relief may be experienced due to the neurological benefits of CMT alone. However, there are more factors that must be addressed in a palliative care scenario in order to properly answer our question.

It has long been observed that autonomic dysfunction is a process involved in most disease states. *Somatoautonomic dysfunction* is described as aberrant sympathetic or parasympathetic activity associated with the vertebral subluxation complex. Korr states that the most detrimental effect of the vertebral subluxation is an associated and disproportional hyperactivity of the sympathetic nervous system, termed *sympatheticotonia*.

This autonomic nervous system dysfunction will manifest in many ways. The first is explained via the relationship of the spinal nerves. Sympatheticotonia is influenced via the lateral horn of the spinal cord, with preganglionic nerves to the sympathetic ganglion and postganglionic nerves giving rise to visceral innervations. Therefore, we can often see a relationship between vertebral segments and visceral disease (Table 6.1). It is important to note that modern research also suggests that these relationships are not solely related to individual vertebral segments, but instead arise from multiple vertebral segments. As seen in Table 6.1, the T5 vertebral tenderness and pain is associated with the liver via these visceral innervations.

TABLE 6.1 **Spinal nerves and innervations**

Vertebrae	Innervation
C1	Brain, vagus nerve, inner and middle ear, sympathetic nervous system
C2	Eyes, auditory nerves, sinuses, mastoid bones, tongue
C3	Outer ear, teeth, cheeks, diaphragm
C4	Nose, lips, mouth, Eustachian tube, diaphragm
C5	Vocal cords, neck glands, pharynx, diaphragm
C6	Neck muscles, shoulders, tonsils
C7	Thyroid gland, bursae in the shoulders, elbows
T1	Forearms, hands, wrists, fingers, upper respiratory (esophagus, trachea)
T2	Heart, heart valves, coronary arteries
T3	Lungs, bronchial tubes, pleura, chest, breast
T4	Gallbladder, common bile duct
T5	Liver, solar plexus, general circulation
T6	Stomach
T7	Pancreas, duodenum, spleen, thymus, lymphatics
T8	Spleen, thymus, lymphatics
T9	Adrenal glands
T10	Kidneys, bladder
T11	Kidneys, ureters, bladder, small intestine
T12	Small intestine, lymph circulation, Ileocecal valve
L1	Ileocecal valve, large intestine, inguinal rings
L2	Appendix, cecum, abdomen, upper leg
L3	Sex organs (ovaries, uterus, testicles, prostate), uterus, bladder, knees
L4	Prostate gland, muscles of lower back, sciatic nerve, cecum
L5	Lower legs, ankles, feet
Sacrum	Hips, buttocks
Coccyx	Rectum

VISCERO-SOMATIC AND SOMATO-VISCERAL REFLEXES

Another of these relationships is via viscero-somatic and somato-visceral reflexes. All practitioners are familiar with somato-somatic reflexes, such as the patellar reflex that stimulates the L4 nerve root. However, many are not familiar with the viscero-somatic and somato-visceral reflexes that also exist throughout the body. The most well-known of these are *referred pain viscero-somatic reflexes*. *Chapman's reflexes*, another example of a viscero-somatic reflex, are correlated with specific organs and glands and were discovered by Frank Chapman in the 1930s. These reflexes are located on the anterior and posterior thorax and the abdomen, as well as the medial and lateral thighs. There are two ways to assess these reflexes. The first is with palpation. Active Chapman's reflexes will usually be tender upon palpation. The severity of the tenderness will often coincide with the severity or chronicity of the condition. When these reflexes are more acute, they will palpate as a puffy, slightly risen, inflamed area. When these reflexes are chronic, the palpatory finding resembles a small nodule such as a bead. Another way to assess the involvement of Chapman's reflexes is via TL and MMT. These reflexes can be treated by the practitioner applying a rotary massage to the reflex, usually for around 1–3 minutes.

In this scenario, the patient exhibits tenderness over the right fifth intercostal space between the anterior-axillary and mid-clavicular lines. This is a location of both referred pain for the liver and the Chapman's reflex for the liver. In our patient scenario, it is also the location of one of his chief complaints. An MMT reveals a positive double TL of this reflex to the area of T5 pain.

FUNCTIONAL MEDICINE

From a functional medicine perspective, much can be done for palliative care. This is accomplished by supporting the underlying physiology and lessening the total stress load on an organ or the body as a whole.

The overall focus is to work toward finding the sources of inflammation in the patient. This can be the disease process itself or even findings that are secondary or unrelated to the disease process. The integrative team of practitioners must address these secondary or unrelated findings as they will often be the source of much relief once improved. In our example, a chronic, subclinical infection will promote a large amount of pro-inflammatory cytokine and interleukin activity. These must be broken down and metabolized. If the liver is under too high of a burden, then it cannot properly metabolize these cytokines and they will be recirculated, adding to the total stress load and contributing to increasing inflammation.

We have discussed the role of sympatheticotonia in the body. This fight-or-flight state is believed to originate in the locus coeruleus. Norepinephrine stimulates the locus coeruleus, which triggers the hypothalamus, amygdala, vagus nerve, preganglionic neurons, sympathetic neurons, and so on. Norepinephrine is metabolized slowly, and thus excessive norepinephrine from a chronic sympathetic drive will stimulate the brain for long periods of time. Methylation, using S-adenosyl methionine (SAMe) and magnesium, is needed to convert noradrenaline to adrenalin and vanilmandelate (VMA). These are then metabolized at a much faster rate. Imagine that our patient has a genetic methylation issue and/or is magnesium deficient, both of which are very common. The patient cannot methylate efficiently, thus causing any stressor to add to the fight-or-flight response and increase noradrenaline, which the patient is unable to methylate and metabolize it out of the body.

Functional medicine can be used to address the nuclear factor-kappa beta (NFKB) cycle. NFKB is a very powerful cytokine and is immensely pro-inflammatory; it will contribute to further advance pain and possibly even the disease itself. Resveratrol and turmeric are two nutrients that have the ability to decrease this cycle due to their anti-inflammatory properties.

ACUPUNCTURE

Acupuncture may also play a valuable role in alleviating pain in the palliative care setting. *Mu points*, often called *alarm points*, are diagnostic and therapeutic acupuncture points according to Traditional Chinese Medicine. Acupuncture points will also TL when used with MMT. We can utilize these points individually, as well as with a double TL to the area of pain. We can also assess for pulse and/or perform tongue diagnosis as other sources of confirmation. In our patient scenario, there is a positive liver pulse point diagnosis as well as a positive double TL of the vertebral pain against the liver mu point.

APPLYING THE INFORMATION

Remember, the greatest value from all of these tests is not in the individual findings, but the collective group of findings. In our scenario we now know the following: there is hypomobility noted throughout the T4–T7 segments. Static palpation revealed that T4 was posterior on the left and there was a retrolisthesis at T5. Vertebral challenge indicated the same findings as well as a fixation of the T6–T7 vertebrae. The erector spinae on the right were hypertonic and hyperfacilitated. There is tenderness and allodynia of the T5 spinous process. We now know the T5 segment of the spine has contributions to the liver via the spinal nerves. There is a positive visceral referred pain pattern and a positive Chapman's reflex. There is a positive pulse point for liver. There is double TL of the area of pain against the visceral referred pain pattern, the Chapman's reflex, the acupuncture mu point, and the acupuncture pulse point for liver. We can definitely answer our question that yes, both of these areas of pain are directly related to the underlying disease process. For treatment purposes, we have several options.

Many practitioners in this case would elect to simply begin CMT. This is an option, but will have decreased effectiveness because minimal effort is being placed to alleviate the stress on the liver, which is the underlying source of the musculoskeletal pain. Rather, CMT should be used as one component of the palliative care treatment plan. The treatment plan should also include treatment of the Chapman's reflex, acupuncture to support the meridian, and functional medicine to address the underlying NF-KB cycle, rid subclinical infections, support hepatic biotransformation, support methylation if needed, and much more. By addressing all of these factors, the patient will get better results as the total stress placed on the system is greatly reduced.

In this scenario, the patient did not want to take any medications or undergo treatment. However, in most cases, patients do. Does this change the approach from our example? No. For the conservative healthcare practitioner, a systematic approach such as this will always lead to more thorough findings and thus more detailed treatment leading to a higher quality of life for the patient.

KEY POINTS TO REMEMBER

- Subjective history is very important. Imagine if this patient had worked in a chemical plant for 50 years. How could that affect his current condition? (Hint: glutathione levels, barrier systems, and liver function.)
- Communicate with other clinicians who are involved in the patient's care. Inform them of your findings and of your concerns.
- Do not give cancer patients L-glutamine as it may fuel their cancer. With any cancer patient (or personal history of cancer) confirm *all* desired supplementation and herbs with their oncologist.

Further Reading

Kanga I, Steiman I. Chiropractic management of a patient with breast cancer metastases to the brain and spine: A case report. *J Can Chiropractic Assoc.* 2015;59(3):269.

Leach RA, Pickar JG. Chapter 9 segmental dysfunction hypothesis: Joint and muscle pathology and facilitation. In *The chiropractic theories: A textbook of scientific research.* 4th ed. Lippincott Williams & Wilkins; 2004: 151.

Maciocia G. *The foundations of Chinese medicine.* 3rd ed. New York: Elsevier; 2013.

Schneider J, Gilford, S. The chiropractor's role in pain management for oncology patients. *J Manipulat Physiol Therap.* 2001;24(1):52–57.

Souza T. *Differential diagnosis and management for the chiropractor.* 5th ed. Burlington: Jones & Bartlett Learning, LLC; 2014.

Walther D. *Applied kinesiology synopsis.* 2nd ed. Burlington, MA: Jones and Barlett; 2016.

Walther DS. General examination and treatment procedures. In Walther DS (Ed.), *Applied kinesiology: Synopsis.* 2nd ed. Shawnee Mission, KS: Triad of Health Publishing; 2000: 37–39.

World Health Organization. Contraindications to spinal manipulative therapy. WHO guidelines on basic training and safety in chiropractic. 2005. https://www.who.int/medicines/areas/traditional/Chiro-Guidelines.pdf

World Health Organization. Guidelines on basic training and safety in chiropractic https://www.who.int/medicines/areas/traditional/Chiro-Guidelines.pdf

Scar Deactivation as an Alternative Treatment for Pain Control

Jennifer Farrell and Thomas M. Schelby

Case Study

CK is a 72-year-old former active-duty man with a complex surgical history. Since 1999, he has had four separate cervical and lumbar spinal fusions, one scar revision, implantation of a spinal cord nerve stimulator, and, most recently, a non-small cell lung cancer resection. These surgeries have left him with numerous scars including multiple midline spinal scars forming a continuous line from C2 to the end of the sacrum, two 10 cm paraspinal scars from T10 to end of sacrum, and one elliptical 15 cm scar on the right thoracic cavity. CK was well-known to our outpatient clinic for pain control, and he is already treated with gabapentin, tramadol, and oxycodone/acetaminophen. After his lung cancer resection and while the family considered palliative care, CK's pain worsened. Already ambulating with a wheeled walker and right foot brace due to chronic foot drop, CK was hoping to avoid additional pain medication, but inquired about other options that might lessen his pain.

What Do I Do Now?

Chronic, postsurgical pain (CPSP) is defined as pain that arises after a surgical procedure and that lasts at least 2 months and cannot be attributed to an alternative cause. Epidemiologic studies estimate that between 10% and 30% of patients undergoing surgery report persistent pain 1 year postoperatively, with up to 5% of patients describing pain as severe and disabling. Certain surgeries common among patients seeking palliative care are associated with even higher rates of CPSP. Between 13% and 69% of patients undergoing mastectomy or breast conservation surgery with axillary dissection report CPSP 1–5 years postoperatively, with increased prevalence and duration of pain in those who additionally underwent reconstruction, adjuvant radiation, or chemotherapy. As seen in CK's case, patients who undergo thoracic surgery also report high rates of CPSP, including 33% after thoracotomy and 25% after video-assisted thoracic surgery.

The etiology of CPSP does not have a clearly established or widely accepted pathophysiological cause, but there are multiple hypotheses. These possible sources include development of adhesions restricting fascial planes, cutaneous nerve entrapment, and disruption of the autonomic nervous system within the intracellular fluid matrix known as an *interference field*. Diagnostic workups of CPSP can be extensive and costly to exclude visceral etiologies. Once an alternative cause of postoperative pain has been excluded, there are no well-established guidelines dictating standard of care, but the treatment approach can include analgesics (i.e., acetaminophen or nonsteroidal anti-inflammatory drugs [NSAIDs]). In refractory cases suggestive of neuropathic pain or in situations where analgesics are contraindicated, tricyclic antidepressants, gabapentinoids, and serotonin–norepinephrine reuptake inhibitors (SNRIs) can be considered. If pharmacologic therapy fails to manage symptoms, consultation for pain management specialists and/or further surgical evaluation is often sought.

Scar deactivation is used as a standard of care by medical acupuncturists for treatment and resolution of scar-associated pain in patients with a history of CPSP. Scar infiltration with lidocaine has been used in numerous clinical settings, masquerading under different names. Referred to as *neural therapy* in Germany, the technique of injecting short-acting local anesthetic into the dermal subcutaneous junction of scar tissue has been widely applied, although there is limited readily available clinical trial evidence supporting its effectiveness. Theoretically, the anti-inflammatory effects of local anesthetics play a role in mitigating the autonomic nervous system disruption of the interference fields caused by scar tissue. Local anesthetics promote anti-inflammatory activity through a variety of mechanisms including reversibly inhibiting leukocyte adhesion via interference with the action of integrins and leukocyte adhesion molecule-1, limiting leukocyte migration, reversibly inhibiting phagocytosis, inhibiting phospholipase A2, inhibiting prostaglandins, inhibiting thromboxane release, inhibiting leukotriene release, inhibiting histamine release, reducing free radical formation, and inhibiting release of cytokines interleukin (IL)-1β, IL-8, and tumor necrosis factor (TNF)-α. Additionally, lidocaine injection is proposed to alleviate nerve entrapment within fascia through hydrodissection, a technique being effectively utilized in the management of carpal tunnel syndrome.

Scar deactivation is the technique of inserting acupuncture needles at a 30–45 degree angle into the superficial fascia to surround a scar. Scar infiltration is performed by calculating a 3 mg/kg dose of 0.5–1% lidocaine without epinephrine and injecting it into the dermis, followed by a subcutaneous injection using a 25-gauge, 1.5-inch needle and syringe appropriately sized given the calculated dose. It is postulated that needle insertion into connective tissue produces analgesia through a multifaceted process encompassing the disruption and remodeling of extracellular matrix in loose connective tissue, altering gene expression affecting neurotransmitter levels, and changing cellular signaling pathways in response to fibroblast and mast-cell involvement. In Traditional Chinese Medicine, injuries resulting in scar tissue formation are thought of as areas of blood and, subsequently, Qi stagnation. Disruptions in the flow of Qi at the point of scar tissue can result in abnormal skin sensations such as pain, itching, and numbness in addition to systemic effects. A case report has demonstrated effective pain relief with an acupuncture protocol utilizing the scar deactivation technique.[1]

Ultimately, CK was treated with five rounds of scar infiltration over 6 months, involving all surgical sites listed, with repeat procedures along the paraspinal and thoracic scar. Greatest and longest lasting relief of pain was achieved with two treatments each along the thoracic and left paraspinal scars. Now, more than 1 year later, the patient has expressed significant reduction of pain and increased ambulation. CK has moved on to other acupuncture modalities to assist in other elements of pain not related to surgical scars, but he relates a majority of relief to his scar infiltration treatments.

KEY POINTS TO REMEMBER

- CPSP is very common in the general population and even more so in patients receiving palliative care.
- Surgical management of breast and lung cancers are associated with a higher rate of CPSP.
- There is not a clearly established pathophysiologic mechanism for CPSP.
- Scar deactivation and infiltration are used commonly among medical acupuncturists for the treatment of CPSP, with positive anecdotal clinical responses.
- Scar deactivation and infiltration are simple techniques that can be easily performed during an office visit.

Reference
1. Feng S. The successful treatment of pain associated with scar tissue using acupuncture *J Acupunct Meridian Stud.* 2014;7(5):262–264.

Further Reading
Cassuto J, Sinclair R, Bonderovic M. Anti-inflammatory properties of local anesthetics and their present and potential clinical implications *Acta Anaesthesiol Scand.* 2006;50:265–282.

Egli S, Pfister M, Ludin SM, et al. Long-term results of therapeutic local anesthesia (neural therapy) in 280 referred refractory chronic pain patients *BMC Complement Altern Med.* 2015;15:200.

Malone D, Clark T, Wei N. Ultrasound-guided percutaneous injection, hydrodissection, and fenestration for carpal tunnel syndrome: Description of a new technique. *J Appl Res.* 2010;10(3):116–123.

Wasserman JB, Steele-Thornborrow JL, Yuen JS, et al. Chronic cesarean section scar pain treated with facial scar release techniques: A case series. *J Bodywork Movement Ther.* 2016;20:906–913.

Weinschenk S. Neural therapy: A review of the therapeutic use of local anesthetics. *Acupuncture Related Ther.* 2012;1(1):5–9.

8 Virtual Reality for Pain in Palliative Care

Lynn Nakad

Case Study

SM is a 54-year-old woman diagnosed with metastatic breast cancer combined with a malignant fungating wound who presents to the emergency department with complaints of severe bone pain. She is admitted with a palliative care consult placed. Goals of care were discussed and plans to discharge to a hospice care center are made. She experiences moderate to severe pain at the wound site. During her first dressing change session, she reported pain levels of 8 out of 10 despite sublingual fentanyl 200 μg. SM also complains of moderate to severe breakthrough pain throughout the day, which she describes as throbbing and stabbing. She was prescribed scheduled oral immediate release (IR) morphine 15 mg every 6 hours, oral IR morphine 15 mg every 2 hours as needed, oral acetaminophen 1,000 mg every 8 hours as needed, and a topically applied lidocaine 5% patch. Pharmacological interventions have provided inadequate pain relief, and she expresses anxiety over breakthrough pain and pain during wound care.

What Do I Do Now?

One of the main goals of SM's care plan is pain management. She reports high levels of procedural pain during wound dressing changes, as well as moderate to severe breakthrough bone pain throughout the day due to her metastasis. Despite pharmacological intervention, the patient's procedural and breakthrough pain seems to be inadequately controlled, which has caused additional stress and anxiety. Patients with cancer suffer from several intense physical and psychological symptoms, including pain and anxiety, which are accompanied by declines in physical and psychological health. More than 50% of patients with cancer and terminal illness experience pain, with many patients' pain being undertreated. Based on a meta-analysis of 122 studies, it was found that pain prevalence rates were 66% in advanced, metastatic, or terminal disease, with moderate to severe pain reported by 38% of all cancer patients despite availability of potent analgesics. Pain in malignant breast wounds was present in about 77% of patients and described as continuous, throbbing, and tender pain. The pathology of pain in these wounds includes nerve damage, tissue ischemia, inflammation, and infection. Wound-associated pain is frequently experienced during dressing change, often evoked by dressing removal and wound cleansing.

As a clinician, it is important to consider nonpharmacological interventions and address psychological distress, especially when adequate pain control is not achieved with pharmacologic intervention. For both acute and chronic pain, mind-body therapies, such as distraction and relaxation techniques, are associated with slight to moderate improvements in pain. However, current mind-body distraction therapies do not engage enough attentional resources to provide significant pain relief. Virtual reality (VR) is a new treatment modality that has the potential to more effectively redirect patients' attention and distract from pain due to its ability to engage central cognitive resources and elicit a positive effect.

VR is a computer-generated simulation of 3-D images that individuals can interact with in a physical way using special equipment. Modern VR technology consists of a head-mounted display (HMD) using a headset or goggles to project an image. This technology can be further divided into high-end (higher quality and processing power, such as headsets powered by a computer) and low-end immersive VR (limited quality and processing power, such as headsets powered by a mobile device). This technology provides an immersive experience through visual and aural exclusion of the real-world environment using an occlusive HMD and headphones and through multisensory (audio, visual, and sometimes tactile) input that typically includes user interaction with the virtual environment through the use of controllers. VR interventions targeting pain management have involved a variety of mechanisms, such as distraction, mindfulness, relaxation, behavioral therapy, and hypnosis.

VIRTUAL REALITY FOR PROCEDURAL PAIN

Most VR therapies have been shown to relieve pain through distraction. Similar to music therapy and guided imagery, VR diverts a patient's conscious attention away from painful stimuli to reduce perceived pain. Current literature suggests the use of VR distraction can reduce the severity of pain experienced during and after a variety of medical procedures and therapies, such as wound care, burn and postoperative dressing care, labor, physical therapy, and venipunctures. In these studies, VR was often used as an adjunct therapy to pharmacologic treatment. A systematic review of evidence supporting the use of VR among patients in acute inpatient medical settings found that it helped reduce pain, distress, and anxiety in adult and pediatric patients undergoing unpleasant medical procedures. A review of the clinical efficacy of VR for acute procedural pain found that there was a statistically and clinically relevant improvement in pain scores following VR interventions. Due to her frequent and painful wound care, SM would be a good candidate for the use of VR as an adjunct therapy to her current pharmacologic interventions. A tailored VR experience can be administered to SM during her wound care to help reduce her pain and anxiety.

VIRTUAL REALITY FOR BACKGROUND AND BREAKTHROUGH PAIN

In addition to her procedural pain during wound care, SM complained of moderate to severe breakthrough pain. Breakthrough pain is defined as exacerbations of pain (either spontaneously or related to a specific trigger) that occur on a background of stable pain otherwise adequately controlled by pharmacologic interventions. VR also has the potential to assist with

SM's breakthrough pain. Some studies have investigated the use of VR in background and breakthrough pain in hospitalized patients. Recent studies found that VR distraction therapy significantly reduced breakthrough pain in hospitalized patients compared to standard care and active distraction controls. The effect of VR was more pronounced for patients with more severe baseline pain. Most of these studies investigated a single use of VR distraction as an adjunct therapy to pharmacological interventions for breakthrough pain. One study advised patients to use VR three times a day for 10 minutes at a time and as needed for breakthrough pain over the subsequent 48 hours.[1] SM could benefit from using VR distraction therapy for breakthrough pain right after a pharmacologic intervention is provided. The VR distraction has the potential to improve her pain relief.

VIRTUAL REALITY FOR PSYCHOLOGICAL DISTRESS AND OTHER PAIN-RELATED SYMPTOMS

In addition to pain intensity, certain VR interventions might be more effective in managing other outcomes or factors of chronic pain, such as psychological distress, physical function, and quality of life. Several studies have examined the use of VR-enhanced cognitive-behavioral therapy (CBT) for symptom management in chronic pain patients. VR-enhanced CBT was found to decrease pain and depression, increase positive affect and emotions, and improve motivation and self-efficacy. Studies have also investigated the use of VR with *mirror visual feedback therapy*, a commonly used therapy for phantom limb pain (PLP). VR-enhanced mirror visual feedback therapy was found to be effective at relieving pain in PLP, chronic low back pain, and complex regional pain syndrome. Additionally, a combination of VR-enhanced relaxation and biofeedback therapy significantly reduced perceived pain and improved daily functioning and quality of life in a pediatric population. Although not extensively studied in palliative care, these VR-enhanced psychosocial therapies show great promise for these patients.

CONSIDERATIONS FOR DESIGN AND ADMINISTRATION

There is a lack of established guidelines or recommendations for VR intervention dosage and administration. However, based on existing literature, there are a few important considerations to make regarding designing, selecting, and administering VR interventions for pain management. These considerations include (1) VR technology and simulation software, (2) patient physical and emotional adverse effects, and (3) intervention dosage.

VR technology and software for simulations can have a significant impact on the level of presence a patient feels in the virtual environment during the VR session, which can impact VR analgesia and therapeutic effect. Research has shown that the greater the perceived presence in a virtual environment by a patient, the greater the effect of VR analgesia. There are four major underlying factors of presence—involvement, immersion, control, and sensory factors (Table 8.1)—which can help guide the selection of VR hardware and software for pain management. *Involvement* (psychological state resulting from focused attention on certain stimuli) and *immersion* (psychological state resulting from the interaction with an environment providing continuous stimuli) are said to be necessary conditions to experience presence. *Control factors* refer to the degree of control, responsiveness, and point of view in a virtual environment. *Sensory factors* relate to perceived realism of and self-inclusion in the virtual environment. To achieve greater therapeutic effect, VR therapeutic environments should generally be isolating from the clinical setting, have visual graphics and audio effects that respond to patient interaction, have active interaction with the virtual environment through positional tracking or controllers, and be fun and enjoyable. High-end immersive (higher quality and processing power) VR can provide a greater sense of presence, which leads to greater analgesia, compared to low-end immersive VR (limited quality and processing power). Certain factors can be more subjective, so patient preferences should be considered, and providing choice in VR software is ideal. Additionally, it is also important to select hardware that can be properly sanitized for multiple patient use (i.e., hospital-grade germicidal wipes and headset covers).

Before introducing a VR intervention, it is important to evaluate a patient's tolerability of VR. Patients should be screened for contraindications and potential precautions (Table 8.2) prior to initiating a trial test for tolerability of VR. In a short trial, clinicians should measure physical and emotional adverse effects of VR as well as discomfort from VR equipment, such as an ill-fitting headset; facial, nasal, or neck pain; or an inability to explore the virtual environment fully due to limited mobility. Some users

TABLE 8.1 Major underlying factors of presence in virtual reality (VR)

Factor	Subdomain	Definition
Involvement	Significance	A user's perception of significance or meaning attached to any aspect of the virtual environment (i.e., the VR simulation involves playing golf, and the user greatly enjoys playing golf)
	Affect	A user's mood/affect during or after the VR simulation (i.e., the user might feel happy after experiencing a pleasant VR simulation)
	Comfort	A user's comfort in terms of equipment comfort and experienced side effect
Immersion	Isolation	A user's perception of isolation from their real-world environment
	Interface awareness	A user's perception of natural modes of interaction and control
Control	Degree of control	The level of control a user has over the virtual environment
	Immediacy of control	A user's perception of the virtual world's responsiveness (i.e., delays between an action and the result in the virtual environment might affect the effectiveness of the intervention)
	Active search	The extent to which a user can modify their point of view, explore the environment, or reposition their head
Sensory	Realism	A user's perceived realism of the virtual environment
	Self-inclusion	A user's perception of themselves in the virtual environment

have reported feeling negative symptoms like motion sickness after using VR, which is referred to as "cybersickness." Cybersickness results from a discrepancy in physical and visual motion perceived by the vestibular and oculomotor system. It involves one or more of following symptoms: eyestrain,

TABLE 8.2 Contraindications and precautions for virtual reality (VR) therapy

Contraindications and precautions	Description
History of motion sickness	Motion sickness is a potential predictor for the occurrence of cybersickness within virtual environments. Patients should be screened for a history of motion sickness.
Visual deficits	Patients with visual deficits may not receive adequate therapeutic benefit from VR therapy due to reduced presence and immersion.
History of seizures	VR is contraindicated in patients with history of photo-induced or photo-sensitive seizures due to strobe-like flashing, certain 3-D graphic renderings, and high contrast details.
Psychiatric disorders and/or cognitive impairment	Contraindicated in patients prone to delirium and patients unable to cooperate with VR use. Precautions should be taken for patients with mild cognitive impairment.
Claustrophobia	Sensory isolating effects of head-mounted display (HMDs) can cause anxiety in some patients.
Head trauma or mobility impairment	Patients with head (i.e., facial and neck) trauma and mobility impairment should avoid using VR as it can exacerbate these conditions.
Contact precautions	While certain VR hardware can withstand hospital-grade germicidal wipes and accommodate HMD covers, the use of VR is not recommended in patients under certain resistant infection precautions.

nausea, fatigue, headache, blurred vision, and postural instability. These symptoms have been shown to negatively affect user experience and reduce intended therapeutic effects. In addition to these physical adverse effects, patients can also have emotional adverse effects, such as fear and anxiety.

While some VR interventions intend to reduce stress and anxiety, they can sometimes exacerbate these symptoms in some patients.

The recommended dosage of VR will depend on a variety of considerations, such as pain etiology, tolerability of VR, and intended therapeutic effect. Therefore, tailored patient protocols regarding frequency and duration of VR are indicated. Based on existing literature, it is recommended to limit VR exposure to 30 minutes per session, with breaks of at least 10 minutes and with the optimal session duration being 15–20 minutes. For procedural pain, it is recommended to provide VR distraction therapy for the length of the procedure if possible. For VR-enhanced behavioral and mindfulness therapies, several VR sessions will likely be indicated for effectiveness.

KEY POINTS TO REMEMBER

- VR is an effective distraction intervention for a variety of painful medical procedures as well as background and breakthrough pain in trauma and cancer patients.
- VR therapies for pain are often used as an adjunct therapy to pharmacologic intervention.
- VR technology can also be used to enhance behavioral and mindfulness therapies, such as CBT, biofeedback, and mindfulness meditation to improve both pain and pain-related outcomes, such as anxiety, physical function, and quality of life.
- Careful consideration should be made to the VR technology and simulation software used in therapies to improve therapeutic effect and reduce incidence of adverse effects.
- Tailor protocols and dosage for VR therapies to individual patients, accounting for physical and emotional adverse effects.

Reference
1. Spiegel B, Fuller G, Lopez M, Dupuy T, Noah B, Howard A, . . . Dailey F. Virtual reality for management of pain in hospitalized patients: A randomized comparative effectiveness trial. *PloS One*, 2019;14(8). doi:10.1371/journal.pone.0219115

Further Reading

Birckhead B, Khalil C, Liu X, et al. Recommendations for methodology of virtual reality clinical trials in health care by an international working group: Iterative study. *JMIR Mental Health.* 2019; 6(1):e11973.

Chan E, Foster S, Sambell R, Leong P. Clinical efficacy of virtual reality for acute procedural pain management: A systematic review and meta-analysis. *PloS One.* 2018;13(7):e0200987. doi:10.1371/journal.pone.0200987.

Frey D, Sharar SR. Virtual reality therapy for acute/procedural pain. In Rhonda J. Moore (Ed.), *Handbook of pain and palliative care.* Cham: Springer; 2018: 581–600.

Gromala D, Tong X, Shaw C, Jin W. Immersive virtual reality as a non-pharmacological analgesic for pain management: Pain distraction and pain self-modulation. In Hershey PA (Ed.), *Virtual and augmented reality: Concepts, methodologies, tools, and applications.* IGI Global; 2018; 1176–1199.

Mallari B, Spaeth EK, Goh H, Boyd BS. Virtual reality as an analgesic for acute and chronic pain in adults: A systematic review and meta-analysis. *J Pain Res.* 2019;12:2053.

McSherry T, Atterbury M, Gartner S, Helmold E, Searles DM, Schulman C (2018). Randomized, crossover study of immersive virtual reality to decrease opioid use during painful wound care procedures in adults. *J Burn Care Res.* 2018;39(2):278–285.

Wittkopf PG, Lloyd DM, Coe O, Yacoobali S, Billington J (2019). The effect of interactive virtual reality on pain perception: A systematic review of clinical studies. *Disabil Rehabil.* 2019:1–12.

9 Selecting an NSAID

Julie Waldfogel

Case Study

NN is a 68-year-old man with a history of knee osteoarthritis, congestive heart failure (American College of Cardiology/American Heart Association [ACC/AHA] Stage B), and newly diagnosed metastatic non-small cell lung cancer (NSCLC). He was recently started on treatment with carboplatin, pemetrexed, and pembrolizumab and is tolerating treatment well. NN is seen in your palliative medicine clinic as part of recommended standard of care. His white blood cell and platelet counts have decreased to 6,000/mm^3 and 90,000/mm^3 respectively about a week after receiving chemotherapy but are now back to his normal baseline. NN's main complaint today is bilateral knee pain, described as a dull ache and severity of 6/10 on the numeric rating scale. He reports this pain as ongoing for years. In discussion, he has tried acetaminophen 1,000 mg every 6 hours, ibuprofen 200 mg every 8 hours, and a combination menthol 10% and methyl salicylate 15% cream in the past with no effect. His oncologist would like your advice on if nonsteroidal anti-inflammatory drugs (NSAIDs) are appropriate in his case and, if so, choosing which NSAID to start.

What Do I Do Now?

onsteroidal anti-inflammatory drugs (NSAIDs) are an important part of multimodal analgesia. Choosing which NSAID to prescribe is determined by three major components: efficacy, adverse effects, and adherence.

EFFICACY

First, confirm that the pain is expected to respond to NSAIDs. NSAIDs are most useful for nociceptive pain, particularly from an inflammatory source. Where possible, reference the guidelines to evaluate strength of evidence and use their recommendations to guide medication use. For NN's case, systemic and topical NSAIDs are strongly recommended for the treatment of knee osteoarthritis by the American College of Rheumatology/Arthritis Foundation guidelines. Of note, the guideline does not recommend any particular systemic NSAID over another, and, in general, NSAIDs are considered equally efficacious. If a patient considers an NSAID ineffective, confirm the dosing, frequency, and duration of use. One time use of a small dose of an NSAID should not be considered a sufficient trial. And consider that a single failed trial does not mean the patient does not respond to all NSAIDs—rotation to a different agent may be necessary.

ADVERSE EFFECTS

NSAIDs are known for a variety of significant adverse effects, primarily mediated by their mechanism of action. NSAIDs provide analgesia and decrease inflammation by inhibiting the production of prostaglandins. They do so as competitive, reversible inhibitors of prostaglandin G and H synthase (also known as cyclo-oxygenase [COX]-1 and -2), preventing the conversion of arachidonic acid to a variety of prostanoids including PGE_2, prostacyclin (PGI_2), and thromboxane A2 (TxA_2).

NSAIDs are classified as either nonselective or COX-2 selective (Table 9.1), and this distinction helps inform their side-effect profile.

Gastrointestinal/Bleeding Risk

NSAIDs can cause a variety of gastrointestinal adverse effects including dyspepsia, heartburn, and abdominal discomfort. More seriously, NSAIDs

TABLE 9.1 **Examples of nonselective and cyclo-oxygenase (COX)-2 selective nonsteroidal anti-inflammatory drugs (NSAIDs)**

Nonselective NSAIDs	COX-2 selective NSAIDs
Ketorolac	Celecoxib
Ibuprofen	Meloxicam
Naproxen	Etodolac
Indomethacin	Diclofenac

can cause gastric and duodenal ulcers and ultimately lead to serious complications such as bleeding or perforation, occurring in 1–2% of regular NSAID users each year.

Mechanistically, COX-1 is the dominant source of prostanoids in gastric epithelial cells and platelets, which inhibit stomach acid secretion and promote the secretion of mucus. Inhibition of COX-1 leads to a deficiency of these protective prostaglandins, allowing for acid-related damage.

The risk of gastrointestinal complications can be impacted by more than NSAID administration. Older age, a history of peptic ulcer, dyspepsia, or concurrent *Helicobacter pylori* infection all increase risk. Likewise, larger doses and longer duration of use of NSAIDs increase risk as does concomitant administration of medications which increase bleeding risk, such as anticoagulants and corticosteroids. Although rare, NSAIDs have also been implicated in an immune-mediated, drug-induced thrombocytopenia, potentially increasing bleeding risk via multiple mechanisms. In oncology patients, consider the role of chemotherapy in mediating this risk. For NN, carboplatin and pemetrexed are both myelosuppressive and can cause thrombocytopenia, increasing the risk of bleeding as well.

To reduce the risk of gastrointestinal events, start with acid suppression. Data support that proton pump inhibitors (PPIs) are more effective than H_2-receptor antagonists (H_2Ras). Consider twice-daily dosing of PPIs in patients with high risk. Treat *H. pylori* infection when identified. COX-2 selective NSAIDs have a reduced risk of gastrointestinal complications compared to nonselective NSAIDs. The combination of COX-2 selective NSAID and a PPI has been associated with the greatest risk reduction.

Cardiovascular Risk

NSAIDs have been associated with a variety of significant cardiovascular events. Both nonselective and COX-2 selective agents have been associated with higher rates of hospitalization for diseases such as congestive heart failure (CHF) and hypertension, and COX-2 selective agents have been associated with higher risk for thrombotic events. As with gastrointestinal adverse effects, risk increases with dose and with duration of NSAID use.

Mechanistically, COX-2 produces prostacyclin, a vasodilatory prostaglandin that inhibits platelet aggregation. For COX-2 selective agents, this lack of prostacyclin combined with uninhibited COX-1 production of thromboxane A2 leads to the theoretical development of a prothrombotic state.

The American Heart Association (AHA) released an updated scientific statement detailing a stepped care approach to the use of NSAIDs in patients with known cardiovascular disease or those who are at risk for ischemic heart disease. In this statement, they recommend not using NSAIDs where possible. If NSAIDs are indicated, they recommend nonselective NSAIDs first. Use COX-2 selective agents only if nonselective NSAIDs are ineffective. Regardless, use their lowest dose possible and consider adding aspirin 81 mg daily for patients at an increased risk for thrombotic events, although note this will likely negate any benefit to gastrointestinal/bleeding risk conferred by using a COX-2 selective agent.

The AHA guideline recommends naproxen as a preferred agent given that data from clinical trials and meta-analyses suggest that naproxen has no increased cardiovascular risk compared to placebo. Of note, the PRECISION trial published after the AHA guideline found no difference in cardiovascular risk in patients randomized to celecoxib, naproxen, or ibuprofen for arthritis.

Drug Interactions

Make sure to conduct a thorough medication reconciliation to determine the risk for clinically significant drug interactions associated with NSAID use. Some medications, when given concurrently with NSAIDs, can increase the risk for adverse effects, particularly bleeding. These include anticoagulants (such as warfarin), aspirin, corticosteroids, and potentially serotonin-active antidepressants. Ibuprofen has been shown to inhibit the cardioprotective effect of aspirin through competitive binding to the COX-1 receptor; this has not yet been shown with other NSAIDs. If patients are taking ibuprofen and aspirin daily, ensure the ibuprofen is taken at least 8 hours before or at least 30 minutes after the aspirin dose.

In NN's case, also consider that ibuprofen has a known interaction with his current chemotherapy regimen as it inhibits the renal secretion of pemetrexed, thus increasing overall systemic exposure and risk for adverse effects. This is particularly relevant in patients with a creatinine clearance between 45 mL/min and 79 mL/min. Due to this interaction, it is recommended to avoid ibuprofen 2 days before, the day of, and 2 days following administration of pemetrexed.

FACTORS THAT INFLUENCE ADHERENCE

Remember the importance of factors that influence all drug selection, including dosing frequency, cost, route, and pill burden. Depending on the drug chosen, NSAIDs can be dosed anywhere from once daily to four times daily. NSAIDs with less frequent dosing include meloxicam, celecoxib, and naproxen and may be preferred in patients with chronic pain to reduce pill burden. Consider route of administration: in those who cannot use the oral route or prefer to avoid additional pills, diclofenac is available in several topical formulations including solution, creams, and patches, and several are available in either a parenteral or intranasal formulation. Topical NSAIDs have the added benefit of reduced systemic absorption, which may reduce the risk for adverse effects.

And consider the additional pill burden of agents recommended to treat adverse effects. Data suggest that 80% adherence to a PPI is required to achieve the planned benefit, with risk of gastrointestinal events increasing by 16% for every 10% drop in adherence.

In NN's case, NSAIDs are strongly recommended for his knee osteoarthritis per guidelines. However, he has several comorbidities and potential drug interactions that make a selection challenging. For NN, consider topical NSAIDs as a next step to minimize systemic exposure.

- Given the adverse effect profile of NSAIDs, first ensure that an NSAID is appropriate. NSAIDs are most useful for nociceptive pain, particularly from an inflammatory source. Where possible, reference the guidelines to evaluate strength of evidence and use their recommendations to guide medication use.

- COX-2 selective NSAIDs are preferred in patients with an increased gastrointestinal/bleeding risk. Consider use of a PPI to help reduce risk.

- Nonselective NSAIDs are preferred in patients with an increased cardiovascular risk. Naproxen may be preferred. Avoid ibuprofen, if possible, in patients on aspirin.

- Consider drug interactions that increase bleeding risk or increase the risk for adverse effects of the other agent due to NSAIDs' effect on protein binding and renal secretion. Ibuprofen can have an increased risk in patients on pemetrexed due to reduced renal secretion and clearance.

- Consider pill burden, dosing frequency, route, and cost when selecting an NSAID. Longer acting NSAIDs may be preferred in patients with chronic pain to reduce pill burden. Topical NSAIDs are available in patients hoping to reduce pill burden or decrease systemic exposure.

Further Reading

Antman EM, Bennett JS, Daugherty A, Furberg C, Roberts H, Taubert KA. Use of nonsteroidal anti-inflammatory drugs: An update for clinicians: A scientific statement from the American Heart Association. *Circulation.* 2007;115:1634–1642.

Brunton L, Hilal-Dandan R, Knollmann B, eds. *Goodman & Gilman's the Pharmacological Basis of Therapeutics.* 13th edition. New York: McGraw-Hill Education; 2018.

Kolasinski SL, Neogi T, Hochberg MC, et al. 2019 American College of Rheumatology/ Arthritis Foundation guideline for the management of osteoarthritis of the hand, hip and knee. *Arthritis Care Res (Hoboken).* 2020;72(2):149–162.

Nissen SE, Yeomans ND, Solomon DH, et al. Cardiovascular safety of celecoxib, naproxen or ibuprofen for arthritis. *N Engl J Med.* 2016;375(26):2519–2529.

Scheiman JM. NSAID-induced gastrointestinal injury: A focused update for clinicians. *J Clin Gastroenterol.* 2016;50:5–10.

Van den Bemt, PM, Meyboom RH, Egberts AC. Drug-induced immune thrombocytopenia. *Drug Saf.* 2004;27(15):1243–1252.

10 Selecting the Antidepressant as an Adjuvant Analgesic

Tim Cruz and Chris Herndon

Case Study

BB is a 70-year-old woman with a 3-month history of nonpapillary adenocarcinoma. While in the hospital, a surgeon attempted a laparoscopic cholecystectomy, at which time a tumor was identified and biopsied. Abdominal computed tomography (CT) scan revealed metastasis to the liver. In addition to her cancer diagnosis, BB also has a long-standing history of diabetes with painful peripheral neuropathy as well as chronic low back pain. Her current pain regimen includes oral gabapentin 600 mg every 8 hours, oral extended-release morphine sulfate 20 mg every 12 hours, and oral immediate-release morphine sulfate 5 mg every 4 hours as needed. She reports the pain as burning in her feet and aching in her back with a range of 6–8/10 most days; this is unchanged from before her diagnosis. On review of systems, she endorses some constipation and confesses that she has been feeling down lately and sleeping a lot more than normal. She has decided on hospice referral versus curative treatment.

What Do I Do Now?

Depression is a common co-occurring condition that can be devastating for patients and their loved ones, causing a large detriment to the patient's quality of life. In BB's case, she does not currently have any suicidal ideation, but she is having family problems due to her depression. Additionally, chronic pain and depression are commonly seen as co-occurring conditions. This raises a couple of important questions for the clinician treating depression in the setting of palliative care and chronic pain.

- What medications can be recommended for treating depression *and* pain in a palliative patient?
- What patient-specific factors might confound safe and effective treatment of pain and co-occurring depression in a palliative care patient?

WHAT IS THE RELATIONSHIP BETWEEN PAIN AND DEPRESSION?

The short answer to this question is this: there is no clear answer. What is known, however, is that up to 85% of patients with chronic pain also present with depression. This is likely further amplified in cases of life-limiting illness. In addition to their role in depression, the neurotransmitters serotonin (5HT), dopamine (DA), and norepinephrine (NE) have been implicated in the pathogenesis of pain. Pain, in most patients, can be associated with an inflammatory response that can lead to depression and alter neurotransmitter metabolism, neuroendocrine function, and neuroplasticity.[1] Depression has been found to be a risk factor for developing chronic pain, and the inverse is true as well: chronic pain is a risk factor for depression.[2]

Pain and depression are both considered to be related to suffering. Brain imaging studies have shown that an emotional stimulus to invoke a negative reaction has been found to activate the same parts of the brain that are activated with a physical stimulus. Because of this, the pathways are thought to be similar. Additional imaging studies have found enhanced activation of sensory neurons when patients are in a depressed versus nondepressed state, thus showing a possible link between worsening pain with depression.

BB, the case patient, has a history of chronic pain and now seems to have developed depression surrounding her new diagnosis. This could present a problem and might cause worsening pain in the future. It is important to continually assess BB's mood and pain symptoms going forward to ensure we are treating both depression and pain.

DIAGNOSING DEPRESSION IN PALLIATIVE CARE

Diagnosis of depression in the palliative care setting can be exceedingly difficult. Most of the struggle can be attributed to the overlap of traditional depression symptoms and common end-of-life symptoms. Symptoms such as anorexia, concentration issues, and lack of energy are prevalent for both depression and end of life.[3]

The Science Committee of the Association of Palliative Medicine assessed multiple depression screening tools and found that, in the palliative care patient, asking the question "Are you feeling down, depressed, or hopeless most of the time over the past 2 weeks?" is the most effective assessment tool. Additionally, they validated other tools including the Edinburgh Postnatal Depression Scale (EPDS) and the Hospital Anxiety and Depression Scale (HADS) for palliative care patients. While the Patient Health Questionnaire (PHQ-9) is one of the most common tools in depression screening, it has not been fully validated in the palliative care population.

Looking back at BB, any of the given tools to assess her depression for diagnosis would be appropriate. She has already admitted to us that she has been feeling depressed recently. She also reports sleep disturbances, but it is not clear if this is due to depression or related to her cancer diagnosis.

SELECTING AN AGENT FOR PAIN IN PATIENTS WITH DEPRESSION

Depression treatment in palliative care is not unlike that of non–palliative care patients. Treating with antidepressants and referral for psychotherapy can have a major benefit in a patient's well-being. Additionally, the most common first-line medications for depression in a non-palliative setting are, usually, the same for palliative patients. These agents include selective serotonin reuptake inhibitors (SSRI), serotonin-norepinephrine reuptake inhibitors (SNRI), bupropion, and mirtazapine. While all these medications will have a benefit in depression, only some of the listed medications will also have meaningful change in a patient's pain severity as adjuvant analgesics.

SNRIs should be first-line in patients with depression and pain syndromes. Venlafaxine, duloxetine, milnacipran, levomilnacipran, and desvenlafaxine are the medications in this class. Several SNRIs have significant data for use in patients with chronic pain syndromes, and, as such, should be considered over SSRIs when a patient is experiencing chronic or neuropathic pain. Side effects of SNRI medications include gastrointestinal upset, sexual dysfunction, weight gain, increased bleed risk, blood pressure increases (due to norepinephrine), hyponatremia risk, and rarely, increased suicidality.

Low-dose tricyclic antidepressants (TCAs) can be used to augment antidepressant effects in patients and have good data to show benefit in treating chronic pain syndromes and migraine prevention. These medications are not without risks. TCAs are implicated in cardiotoxicity and QTc prolongation. A baseline electrocardiogram is recommended prior to initiating these medications in older patients, although this practice rarely occurs. This class of medications has a much higher overdose risk compared to other antidepressants. They also exhibit many anticholinergic effects, sedation, orthostatic hypotension, and dizziness. The doses used for pain and antidepressant augmentation are much lower than traditional dosing, leading to fewer adverse effects. For example, the standard dose of amitriptyline for pain usually ranges from 25 to 50 mg, whereas the dosing for depression ranges from 100 to 300 mg (note: exceptions to these doses exist). For use in the palliative care setting, these medications should only be used at lower doses. At these doses, there can be an enhanced antidepressant effect when used in combination with an SNRI or SSRI and will likely help with the patient's pain.

Bupropion is another commonly prescribed first-line agent for depression, but it has a different mechanism of action than the SSRIs and SNRIs. Bupropion prevents the reuptake of dopamine and norepinephrine but does *not* inhibit serotonin reuptake. Because of the norepinephrine effect of bupropion, it would make sense that it has utility in pain management. Very few studies have been published about the utility of bupropion for pain, unfortunately. One small study did find that bupropion improved pain scores in those with diabetic painful peripheral neuropathy. Bupropion is a very activating antidepressant, making it a good choice for patients who are dealing with drowsiness or sedation. Adverse effects include insomnia, headaches, seizures, and weight loss. Bupropion is contraindicated in patients with a history of eating disorders and seizure history.

SSRIs and SNRIs are commonly used in cancer patients as they have a good safety profile and efficacy data for depression. There are some data on the use of SSRIs in the treatment of diabetic peripheral neuropathy, but they are small studies that have conflicting outcomes. More studies are needed to definitively show a benefit of SSRIs in chronic pain syndromes. Side effects of SSRI are like that of SNRIs but with less risk for blood pressure increases. Another difference is that citalopram and escitalopram use should be limited in cardiac patients, especially at higher doses, as QTc prolongation is an additional side effect. Additionally, many of the SSRIs have CYP 2D6 interactions, and drug interactions should always be assessed.

Trazodone, an antidepressant known for its sedating properties, has been thought to have some pain benefit. Unfortunately, studies have not shown this in most patients. A 2020 study of low-dose trazodone compared to placebo found no significant difference in pain reduction. At this time, trazodone should be avoided if pain control is needed.

Referring to the case, BB has a lot going on besides depression. She is having significant issues, including having little energy, diabetic peripheral neuropathy, and chronic low back pain. While the use of an SSRI in this patient would not be inherently wrong for depression, there are better options given her co-occurring conditions. Similarly, while TCAs have benefit in pain management, she already reporting sedation; as such, it is recommended to avoid use at this time. An SNRI would be the best first-line option for this patient. The class has a very favorable side-effect profile, minimal sedation, and well-documented benefit for chronic pain.

KEY POINTS TO REMEMBER

- *All* antidepressants carry a warning for increased suicidal ideation, and patients should be monitored for the first few weeks of a new medication or dose increase for thoughts of suicide.

- When deciding on an agent, generally, an SNRI should be added first, given an adequate trail of 4–6 weeks, and then increased if needed.
- TCAs may be effective for chronic pain but should be used at low doses in palliative care patients.
- SSRIs and mirtazapine are first-line for depression but have minimal benefit in chronic pain. These agents should be reserved for those whose depression is not controlled with SNRIs or if they are used in conjunction with a TCA

References
1. Sheng J, Liu S, Wang Y, Cui R, Zhang X. The link between depression and chronic pain: Neural mechanisms in the brain. *Neural Plast.* 2017;2017:9724371. doi:10.1155/2017/9724371. Epub 2017 June 19. PMID: 28706741; PMCID: PMC5494581.
2. Doan L, Manders T, Wang J. Neuroplasticity underlying the comorbidity of pain and depression. *Neural Plast.* 2015;2015:504691. doi:10.1155/2015/504691. Epub 2015 February 25. PMID: 25810926; PMCID: PMC4355564.
3. Marks S, Heinrich T. Assessing and treating depression in palliative care patients. *Curr Psychiatry.* 2013 August;12(8):35–40.

Further Reading
Howard P, Shuster J, Twycross R, Mihalyo M, Wilcock A. Psychostimulants. *J Pain Symptom Manage.* 2010 November;40(5):789–795. doi:10.1016/j.jpainsymman.2010.09.004. PMID: 21075274.
Lee YC, Chen PP. A review of SSRIs and SNRIs in neuropathic pain. *Expert Opin Pharmacother.* 2010 December;11(17):2813–2825. doi:10.1517/14656566.2010.507192. Epub 2010 July 19. PMID: 20642317.
Lipone P, Ehler E, Nastaj M, et al. Efficacy and safety of low doses of trazodone in patients affected by painful diabetic neuropathy and treated with gabapentin: A randomized controlled pilot study. *CNS Drugs.* 2020 November;34(11):1177–1189. doi:10.1007/s40263-020-00760-2. PMID: 32936427; PMCID: PMC7658082.
Rayner L, Price A, Hotopf M, Higginson IJ. The development of evidence-based European guidelines on the management of depression in palliative cancer care. *Eur J Cancer.* 2011 Mar;47(5):702–712. doi:10.1016/j.ejca.2010.11.027. Epub 2011 January 4. PMID: 21211961.

11 Selecting the Anticonvulsant as an Adjuvant Analgesic

Zachary Macchi and Nathan Boehr

Case Study

A 62-year-old man with left frontoparietal glioblastoma receiving home hospice care experiences seizures at home. He previously failed multiple modes of treatment including chemotherapy, surgery, and radiation, and he continues to experience treatment-refractory headaches and neuropathic pain. Recently discharged after a prolonged hospital stay for worsening right hemiplegia and headaches, rated 10 out of 10 using a pain rating system, home hospice was elected following extensive goals-of-care discussions. He was stable on discharge but with ongoing headaches and pain. In the past week, while at home, he developed new-onset seizures with increasing frequency. Seizures are particularly bothersome to his caregivers. During these episodes he is acutely obtunded, flaccidly hemiparetic on the right, and proceeds to lose consciousness with tonic-clonic movements of all extremities, larger amplitude on the left. He regains consciousness interictally but now has had four seizures in a 24-hour period.

What Do I Do Now?

This case presents a number of issues regularly encountered in palliative care and is noteworthy for a number of reasons. First, the patient is experiencing multiple, complex symptoms that warrant a comprehensive palliative care approach, including neuropathic pain, migraines, and now breakthrough seizures. Second, the context in which the patient has experienced breakthrough seizures (home hospice) shapes clinical decision-making. Previous goals-of-care discussions are likely to influence the potential next steps for management, such as acute and long-term pain and seizure control. Finally, there is a transference of suffering to the patient's family, which can directly affect patient quality of life and end-of-life care.

There are multiple etiologies for new-onset seizures, including primary or metastatic brain neoplasms, stroke, preexisting epilepsy, or metabolic derangement. Patients with the highest seizure risk at end of life are those with a prior history of seizures, and the risk can be as high 76% in patients with late-onset epilepsy compared to 11% in patients with no prior seizure history. The patient in our case developed seizures as result of disease progression from glioblastoma. New-onset seizures can be present at any point in the course of glioblastoma but in later stages can suggest increasing mass effect, cerebral edema, infection, or intracranial hemorrhage. Management of seizures at end of life can be difficult. Poor control can have a detrimental impact on the patient's quality of life and cause significant distress for caregivers and families. Anticipatory education should be provided during advance care planning and goals-of-care communications, particularly for individuals who are felt to be at high risk of developing epilepsy. Many patients enrolled in home hospice do not have intravenous access, therefore other routes of administration, such as intranasal, rectal, and intramuscular dosing, may need to be available in case the oral route is lost.

Cognitive impairment can occur as a result of disease progression, causing patients to have increased difficulty with medical decision-making and potentially lose the ability to take oral medications. Patients with life-limiting illness should therefore have an advance directive and medical durable power of attorney (MDPOA) in place. Clinicians should recommend that patients regularly discuss their wishes with surrogate decision-makers to ensure they are acting on the patient's behalf should their MDPOA become active.

The decision to stop disease-directed therapy and shift goals of care to a comfort-focused approach should be shared by the patient (or their surrogate) and the clinician. Several factors are used to make this decision, including quality of life, treatment expectations, and functional status. Patients and clinicians should be aware that, in most cases, enrollment in hospice services cannot occur while disease-directed therapy is continued. Patients should be encouraged to consider what constitutes an acceptable quality of life for them. It is recommended that these conversations occur early in the disease course and are documented in an advance directive to avoid barriers to medical decision-making during a crisis.

In the next steps for management of our patient, special considerations should be made about selecting an anticonvulsant that can address multiple issues, including augmenting pain management and migraine prevention, while avoiding side effects or medication interactions.

ACUTE SEIZURE MANAGEMENT

For acute seizure management in our case, goals-of-care discussions should be reviewed with the patient or, if he is unable to participate due to postictal state or cognitive impairment, reliance on advance directive documentation and medical proxy decision-makers should be pursued. The first likely point of contact for our patient and his caregivers and/or family would be the on-call hospice nurse, who in turn could contact the physician or nurse practitioner for additional orders.

The palliative care clinician has a number of options for acute management of seizures in the ambulatory and home hospice setting. There are several anticonvulsants with routes of administration which do not require intravenous access. One option, sometimes included in home hospice "comfort kits," is midazolam, a short-acting benzodiazepine administrated intranasally. Dosing of intranasal midazolam is 5 mg for patients weighing less than 50 kg and 10 mg for patients weighing greater than 50 kg. The injectable form is used and divided into two doses using a mucosal atomization device, administering one spray in each nostril. Ease and comfort of administering this medication intranasally makes it an excellent choice for patients receiving specialized palliative care or hospice services. Alternatively, diazepam could be used and is available as a gel given rectally or an autoinjector for intramuscular administration. Drawbacks of these two routes include discomfort and the need to educate family or caregivers on administration. A final option if the patient is having breakthrough seizures but is interictally alert would be the addition of clonazepam, a long-acting benzodiazepine, which can be used as a bridge for initiation of another antiepileptic medication. Dosing of clonazepam in this situation would be 0.5–1 mg administered by mouth twice daily for a total of 3–5 days. These choices for acute seizure control may augment pain management because benzodiazepines have anecdotally been used as adjuncts in a variety of pain conditions. However, benzodiazepines are not a long-term solution for chronic seizure control or pain expected over weeks to months due to the potential for tolerance and loss of efficacy. Table 11.1 summarizes potential medications for acute seizure management in the home hospice setting.

TABLE 11.1. **Medications for acute seizure management in home hospice care**

Agent (Route)	Dosing [3]	Additional notes
Midazolam (IN, IM)	**Intranasal:** *If patient is >50 kg*: 5 mg IN once *< 50 kg*: 10 mg IN once. Dose divided into one spray in each nostril. **Intramuscular:** 5 mg IM once	Injectable form used with a mucosal atomizer for intranasal administration.
Diazepam (PR, IM)	**Rectal:** 0.2 mg/kg PR given once **Intramuscular:** 10 mg IM every 10–15 minutes PRN, *max* 30 mg/total dose	Can repeat one dose in 4–12 hours with no more than two treatments in 24 hours. Applicator devices deliver doses in 2.5 mg increments.
Clonazepam (PO)	0.5–1 mg PO BID for a total of 3 days	Can be used as a bridge to achieving therapeutic drug levels when starting a new antiepileptic and/or during periods of time when the seizure threshold is lowered (e.g., infection).

All benzodiazepines such as the medications listed above, can cause sedation and respiratory depression.
IN, intranasally; IM, intramuscular; PR, rectally; PRN, as needed; PO, by mouth; BID, twice daily.

SEIZURE MANAGEMENT AND ANALGESIA

Our case is a common scenario among patients with primary brain tumors because chronic pain from headaches and neuropathy are typical. There are several medications that offer a twofold benefit for seizure control while augmenting pain management, and both have been studied for efficacy as both an antiepileptic and analgesic. Antiepileptic monotherapy is preferred as 47% of patients will respond to a single agent with only an additional 13% achieving seizure freedom after a second agent is added. The benefits continue to decline when adding a third and fourth agent. Table 11.2 summarizes several antiepileptics that can be used adjunctively for pain management, including dosing and side effect profiles.

First-line for seizure control with additional indications for the treatment of mixed neuropathic pain (peripheral and central causes) are the gabapentinoids, gabapentin and pregabalin. Each is effective for treating pain, and dosing for seizure control is similar to that in pain management. Gabapentin is typically dosed at 100 mg by mouth administered three times daily and increasing the dose by 300 mg/day every 3 days to a maximum dose of 3,600 mg/day. For pregabalin, dosing should start at 75 mg by mouth twice daily, increasing the dose by 150 mg/day every 2 weeks to a maximum of 600 mg/day. There is a dose-dependent benefit to analgesia for pregabalin where doses near 600 mg/day can yield up to a 50% reduction in pain. Dose increases are based on reported pain relief or adverse effects. Adjustments for both are needed in the setting of renal dysfunction, and discontinuing either should be done slowly to avoid provoking breakthrough seizures. Common side effects for both gabapentin and pregabalin include somnolence, dizziness, peripheral edema, and, uncommonly, respiratory depression, especially when administered with other centrally acting medications like opioids. Slow titration over days can avoid these side effects. Caution should be taken when co-administering with opioids as one population-based study found an increased risk of mortality with concurrent use of opiates and pregabalin. Regarding seizure management, each of these agents has demonstrable benefits for treating focal epilepsy. In our case, either choice would be appropriate as a first-line medication for managing focal seizures given their low side-effect profile and potential for neuropathic pain relief.

TABLE 11.2 **Antiepileptic drugs (AEDs) adjunctively used in analgesia**

Agent	Dosing [3, 7]	Side effects	Additional notes
Gabapentin	**AED**: Start 100 mg POTID Increase 300 mg/day every 3–5 days **Max dose:** 3,600 mg/day	Drowsiness, dizziness, edema, respiratory depression when used with opioids	First-line for neuropathic pain Renally dosed
Pregabalin	**AED**: Start 75 mg PO BID Increase 150 mg/day every 2 weeks **Max dose:** 600 mg/day	Drowsiness, dizziness, edema, respiratory depression when used with opioids	First-line for neuropathic pain Renally dosed
Carbamazepine	**For pain**: Start 100–200 mg/day every 3–5 days to effect **AED**: Start 200 mg PO BID Increase 200 mg/day every 7 days **Max dose:** 1,600 mg/day	Leukocytosis, thrombocytopenia, hyponatremia dizziness, ataxia, somnolence, nausea, vomiting, blurred vision, aplastic anemia, Stevens-Johnson syndrome, DRESS	Metabolic inducer (CYP450 3A4) Renally dosed _Target total serum levels:_ **AED**: 4–12 μg/mL
Oxcarbazepine	**AED**: Start 300 mg PO BID Increase 300 mg/day every 3 days to effect **Max dose:** 2,400 mg/day	Leukocytosis, thrombocytopenia, hyponatremia, dizziness, ataxia, somnolence, nausea, vomiting, blurred vision, aplastic anemia, Stevens-Johnson syndrome, DRESS	Metabolic inducer (CYP450 3A4) Lower incidence of side effects than carbamazepine. Renally dosed _Target total serum levels:_ **AED**: 10–35 μg/mL

Lacosamide	**AED:** Start 50 mg twice daily Increase 100 mg/day every 7 days **Max dose:** 400 mg/day	Dizziness, nausea, headaches, diplopia	Can be administered intravenously Renally dosed
Valproic acid	**AED:** Start 15 mg/kg/day divided BID Increase 250–500 mg/day every 7 days to a maintenance dose of 40–60 mg/kg/day **Migraine:** Start 250 mg PO BID Increase to 500 mg/day after 7 days **Max dose:** 60 mg/kg/day	Liver dysfunction, dizziness, tremor, somnolence, nausea, hyperammonemia, tremors, depression, cognitive impairment (long-term)	Metabolic inhibitor (CYP450 3A4) Can be administered intravenously _Target total serum levels:_ **Migraine PPx:** <50 µg/mL **AED:** 50–100 µg/mL

PO, by mouth; TID, three times daily; BID, twice daily; DRESS, drug reaction with eosinophilia and systemic symptoms; CYP, cytochrome P450; CrCl, creatinine clearance.

Other antiepileptics have been studied for use in pain management. Carbamazepine and its analogue oxcarbazepine are approved for the treatment of focal epilepsy with off-label uses for neuropathic pain, especially trigeminal neuralgia. Either of these medications could be used in our case to treat the patient's neuropathy as well as seizures. The benefits do not stop there as both agents have weak effects on migraine prevention and may reduce our patient's migraine frequency. These agents have a number of limitations, including serial laboratory monitoring, effects on drug metabolism, and side effects including risk for neurotoxicity and serious skin reactions (e.g., Stevens-Johnson syndrome). Additionally, doses for seizure control are typically higher than those used for pain control. Lacosamide is another potential option for seizure management and analgesia. Although evidence is weak for its use in pain management, lacosamide has shown benefits for peripheral neuropathic pain at doses near the recommended maximum total daily dose (400 mg/day)[3]. Similar to other antiepileptics, slow titration to discontinuation is recommended as seizures can be provoked by abrupt discontinuation. Valproic acid is another commonly used antiepileptic that has evidence for treating peripheral neuropathic pain and preventing migraine, as well as managing behavioral disturbances such as mania, depression, or psychosis. For seizures, valproic acid dosing starts at 15 mg/kg/day divided twice daily and increased 250–500 mg/day every 7 days to a maintenance dose of 40–60 mg/kg/day. Target serum levels for migraine prevention tend to be lower (total level <50 μg/mL) than those desired for seizure management (total level 50–100 μg/mL) or mania (total level 85–125 μg/mL). Despite these benefits, valproic acid has several limitations to use in the palliative care context including the need for drug level monitoring, inhibition of drug metabolism, liver dysfunction, tremors, and neurotoxicity from the drug itself or disturbed metabolism (e.g., hyperammonemia). Patient's with Parkinson's disease or parkinsonian conditions can experience worsening motor symptoms while taking valproic acid. Also, patients using cannabidiol (CBD) or marijuana-containing products for pain management may be more prone to liver dysfunction when using valproic acid.

For patients on multiple antiepileptics, several considerations should be made when adding one for secondary pain control. As mentioned, valproic acid can inhibit hepatic metabolism (specifically through inhibition of cytochrome P450 activity) and raise levels of other antiepileptics (e.g., lamotrigine, phenytoin), anticoagulants (e.g., warfarin), and diabetic medications (e.g., glipizide). In fact, lamotrigine clearance reduced by 50% when used with valproic acid. Other antiepileptic medications that can influence the metabolism of other drugs include phenobarbital and phenytoin, both of which are inducers of cytochrome P450. The use of these metabolic interactions should be taken into consideration when choosing an anticonvulsant. Of the non-analgesic antiepileptic drugs, levetiracetam is least likely to interact with those listed in Table 11.2 and is a reasonable choice for seizure polytherapy but has little effect on pain control. A careful review of other concurrent medications, like immunosuppressants and chemotherapeutics, and medical comorbidities should ultimately inform the choice of anticonvulsant.

SPECIAL CONSIDERATIONS

When choosing the antiepileptic, other factors that might influence clinical decision-making include consideration of the underlying etiology and comorbidities. For patients with primary or metastatic brain tumors, a host of other issues, including neuropsychiatric disturbances and cognitive impairment, can complicate care at any point in the disease.

Medications that affect cognition, such as benzodiazepines, gabapentin, pregabalin, and valproic acid, can affect mood and cognition and potentially exacerbate preexisting problems. Patients with psychiatric comorbidities such as depression or generalized anxiety disorder might see worsening mood symptoms after starting these medications, while patients with bipolar disorder might see a benefit from the mood stabilization properties of valproic acid. Elderly patients or those with comorbid dementia or metabolic encephalopathies (e.g., hepatic encephalopathy) may be hypersensitive to anticonvulsants that affect cognition and are more likely to develop medication-induced delirium.

As previously stated, many of these medications influence the metabolism of other substances. For patients with hepatic or renal dysfunction, dosing and side effects should also be weighed when selecting an antiepileptic. Individuals with primary headache conditions like migraine or trigeminal neuralgia may also see a compounded benefit from using anticonvulsants like carbamazepine and oxcarbazepine for seizure and headache prevention.

CONCLUSION

In the end, the next steps in management for our case include initial acute seizure control with a benzodiazepine followed by initiation of pregabalin. Additionally, the best choice of medication should also be one which the clinician feels most comfortable prescribing. The patient's decision to pursue home hospice suggests that his wishes and desires are to remain at home receiving care focused on comfort and quality of life. Seizure control and pain management at the end of life serve to benefit quality of life while minimizing invasive interventions and undue harm. Palliative care specialists should ensure that patients receiving home hospice have access to anticonvulsants for acute seizure management, and these should be easy to administer for caregivers and healthcare providers alike.

Control of seizures has a direct effect on quality of life, and discussions about the risks and benefits of each should inform the choice of long-term antiepileptic that aligns with the patient's goals of care. Certainly, pain management is a major palliative need for the individual in our case, and likely the anticonvulsant with the greatest potential for benefit is the one which simultaneously treats multiple problems ("killing two birds with one stone"), thus avoiding polypharmacy, and personalized to the patient's condition and comorbidities.

KEY POINTS TO REMEMBER

- Seizures are common end-of-life problems for patients with primary and metastatic brain tumors.
- Benzodiazepines are first-line in acute seizure treatment and come in forms for use in the ambulatory setting that can be administered by informal caregivers or healthcare providers (e.g., intranasal midazolam, rectal diazepam).
- Several anticonvulsants, including gabapentin, pregabalin, oxcarbazepine, and carbamazepine, can be used as adjunctive neuropathic analgesics and should be considered as options for addressing both pain control and seizure management simultaneously.

- Gabapentin and pregabalin are first-line choices for management of mixed neuropathic pain. Slow titration to effect/pain relief is recommended to avoid common side effects like somnolence and dizziness.
- Some anticonvulsants used in analgesia can influence drug metabolism through enzyme induction (carbamazepine and oxcarbazepine) and inhibition (valproic acid). This includes reducing or increasing levels of immunosuppressants, chemotherapeutics, and other anticonvulsants.
- Special considerations should be made if choosing anticonvulsants which affect cognition, especially in comorbid dementia, metabolic derangements, and concomitant use of other centrally acting medications (e.g., opioids and benzodiazepines).

Further Reading

Anti-Epileptic Drugs for Pain. Fast Fact #271. Palliative Care Fast Facts and Concepts. Palliative Care Network of Wisconsin. https://www.mypcnow.org/fast-fact/anti-epileptic-drugs-for-pain/

Chang BS. Cannabidiol and serum antiepileptic drug levels: The ABCs of CBD with AEDs. *Epilepsy Curr.* 2018;18(1):33–34. doi:10.5698/1535-7597.18.1.33

Clouston PD, DeAngelis LM, Posner JB. The spectrum of neurological disease in patients with systemic cancer. *Ann Neurol.* 1992;31(3):268–273. doi:10.1002/ana.410310307

Epocrates, Version 20. Epocrates, Inc. home page. www.epocrates.com.

Gomes T, Greaves S, van den Brink W, et al. Pregabalin and the risk for opioid-related death: A nested case-control study. *Ann Intern Med.* 2018;169(10):732–734. doi:10.7326/M18-1136

Grönheit W, Popkirov S, Wehner T, Schlegel U, Wellmer J. Practical management of epileptic seizures and status epilepticus in adult palliative care patients. *Front Neurol.* 2018;9(595):1–8. doi:10.3389/fneur.2018.00595

Kinze S, Clauss M, Reuter U, et al. Valproic acid is effective in migraine prophylaxis at low serum levels: A prospective open-label study. *Headache.* 2001;41(8):774–778. doi:10.1046/j.1526-4610.2001.01142.x

Kwan P, Brodie MJ. Epilepsy after the first drug fails: Substitution or add-on? *Seizure.* 2000;9(7):464–468. doi:10.1053/seiz.2000.0442

Nemire R. Valproate. Epilepsy Foundation. https://www.epilepsy.com/sites/core/files/atoms/files/epilepsy_valproate_0.pdf

12 Ketamine as an Analgesic Adjuvant in Palliative Care

Sandra Sacks and Ambereen K. Mehta

Case Study

FS is a 27-year-old female patient with a history of Ewing's sarcoma of the left scapula who had it surgically resected 1 year ago. She now presents with recurrence, with metastases to her lung, spine, bilateral hips, ribs, and left femur and is admitted for uncontrolled pain. It was previously controlled with an outpatient pain pump with hydromorphone 2 mg every 15 minutes and increased to 6 mg every 15 minutes without relief. She was also on a multimodal oral regimen consisting of methadone 20 mg three times daily, gabapentin 600 mg three times daily, duloxetine 30 mg daily, meloxicam 7.5 mg daily, and scheduled acetaminophen 650 mg every 6 hours. In the hospital, the palliative care and pain consult services attempted to increase her opioids, but were limited by side effects of sedation and confusion.

What Do I Do Now?

As a clinician approaching this case, it is important to first complete a thorough pain assessment because understanding what kind of pain FS has will help identify what kind of medication she may respond to. Neuropathic pain is best managed by neuropathic analgesics, musculoskeletal pain responds to anti-inflammatories, and visceral and somatic pain often responds to opioids. Many patients experience mixed pain, thus, as a result, a combination of medications is often a more successful, safe, and effective pain management plan. FS had neuropathic, nociceptive somatic, and nociceptive visceral pain, but the palliative care team was reaching limits with the more commonly used medications.

An immediate concern was her change in mental status while continuing to have severe pain. One possibility for this is opioid-induced neurotoxicity (OIN). OIN is a multifactorial syndrome that causes a spectrum of symptoms from mild confusion or drowsiness to hallucinations, delirium, and seizures. It can occur with any opioid but is more likely to occur when using opioids with active metabolites, such as meperidine, codeine, morphine, and hydromorphone.[1] In this situation, the palliative care clinician is faced with a difficult situation with multiple possible options. One option is to do an opioid rotation, stop the offending agent, and start a medication with less active metabolites, such as intravenous fentanyl. In this case, the patient did not have successful pain control previously with alternative opioids, thus making rotation less attractive.

Another option is to utilize an analgesic adjuvant, such as ketamine, which can help restore normal pain processing in patients with complex pain syndromes and decrease a patient's opioid requirement. For severe, complex pain as often seen in palliative care, we rely on a combination of these methods.

KETAMINE

Ketamine is a dissociative anesthetic that noncompetitively blocks the N-methyl-D-aspartate (NMDA) receptor, a ligand-gated calcium channel activated by glutamate. Activation of this channel contributes to the "windup" phenomenon, which leads to central sensitization. As it can potentially inhibit this process, ketamine has been used to treat numerous chronic pain states, including cancer pain.

In addition, activation of the NMDA channel plays a major role in cognition, chronic pain, opioid tolerance, and mood regulation. At higher doses, ketamine also activates a variety of opioid receptors as well as a multitude of other non-NMDA pathways that play integral roles in pain and mood regulation. These include antagonistic effects on nicotinic and muscarinic cholinergic receptors, activation of D_2 dopamine receptors, and enhancement of descending modulatory pathways.[2,3]

PHYSIOLOGIC AND PSYCHOMIMETIC EFFECTS

Ketamine can be administered via intravenous, intramuscular, oral, intranasal, sublingual, topical, or rectal routes. When taken orally, a greater amount is converted to norketamine after first-pass metabolism through the liver. Norketamine is less effective because it has a lower affinity to the NMDA receptor.[3] Intravenous administration is by far the most common and well-studied.

On the cardiovascular system, ketamine can increase arterial blood pressure, heart rate, and cardiac output, particularly after a rapid bolus injection. These indirect cardiovascular effects are due to central stimulation of the sympathetic nervous system and inhibition of the reuptake of norepinephrine after release at nerve terminals. These changes are accompanied by increases in the pulmonary artery pressure and myocardial work. While these sympathomimetic effects may benefit patients with hypotension and borderline vital signs, it is important to remember that large bolus injections of ketamine should be administered cautiously in patients with coronary artery disease, uncontrolled hypertension, congestive heart failure, or arterial aneurysms. Ketamine also acts as a direct myocardial depressant through inhibiting calcium transients and may be unmasked by sympathetic blockade or exhaustion of catecholamine stores, such as end-stage shock.

Ketamine has multiple beneficial effects on the respiratory system, which is one of the reasons why it is so frequently utilized in the perioperative settings by anesthesiologists. It has minimal effects on depressing the central respiratory drive while maintaining upper airway muscle, pharyngeal, and laryngeal reflexes. It also acts as a potent bronchodilator, which can be helpful in patients with obstructive airway diseases. While its use may cause sialorrhea, this effect can often be mitigated through administering concurrent antisialagogues, such as glycopyrrolate or atropine.

The psychomimetic effects of ketamine are well-known. It is these psychomimetic effects that have resulted in its misuse as a recreational drug because it is related to phencyclidine (PCP) as a derivative. These effects are seen with the use of perioperative ketamine at subanesthetic doses and include hallucinations, visual disturbances, unpleasant dreams, and dysphoria. These psychomimetic effects are usually mitigated by using low-dose benzodiazepines. Memory impairment as well as difficulty with judgment may be seen.[3]

Ketamine is also associated with urinary toxicity, especially in patients who use the medication for months to years, but this can occur after days of use as well. Patients can experience frequency, urgency, urge incontinence, dysuria, and hematuria. Less specific symptoms of lower abdominal pain may be more subtle but equally important. These symptoms may suggest interstitial cystitis, papillary necrosis, and hydronephrosis. Serious, irreversible damage may result, including renal failure. When patients taking ketamine report urinary symptoms, if there are no signs of bacterial infection, ketamine should be held and a referral to urology may be necessary.[3]

Practitioners should regularly check liver function (LF) while patients are taking ketamine for a longer period of time to monitor for hepatobiliary toxicity. If there are elevations in LFs, abdominal pain, or biliary duct dilation, holding ketamine usually results in resolution.[3]

CONSENSUS GUIDELINES

Different institutions have different protocols for initiating ketamine infusions. There is no established protocol, but, in 2018, the American Society of Anesthesiology, American Society of Regional Anesthesia, and the American Academy of Pain Medicine prepared consensus guidelines for the use of ketamine in acute pain management and chronic pain management.[4]

When used in chronic pain, many physicians will often administer higher doses in an effort to "reverse central sensitization," preferring to utilize pharmacologic agents to counteract potential adverse effects rather than tapering down the infusion. In contrast, in acute pain management, often in perioperative settings, ketamine dosages are more often titrated to effect, balancing analgesic properties with adverse effects, often requiring a reduction in dosages to mitigate unwanted effects.

The consensus guidelines recommend a bolus dose up to 0.35 mg/kg and infusion doses of 0.5 to 2 mg/kg/hr. Relative contraindications include patients with poorly controlled cardiovascular disease, pregnancy, active psychosis, severe hepatic disease, elevated intracranial pressure, elevated intraocular pressure, and active substance abuse.[4]

In healthy individuals, the guidelines do not recommend any preinfusion testing. However, in patients with suspected or high risk of cardiovascular disease, a baseline electrocardiogram should be used to rule out ischemic heart disease. In patients with baseline liver dysfunction or at risk of liver toxicity, such as patients with chronic hepatitis or alcohol use, preinfusion and postinfusion LF tests should be considered on a case-by-case basis.

The supervising clinician and administering clinician should be certified in Advanced Cardiac Life Support (ACLS), be familiar with ketamine, anticipate possible adverse effects, and be able to quickly administer treatment options. For doses greater than 1 mg/kg/hr, it is recommended that the infusion take place in a monitored setting containing resuscitative equipment and immediate access to rescue medications and personnel who can treat emergencies. A positive response should include objective measures of benefit in addition to satisfaction, such as a greater than 30% decrease in pain score. For responders, oral ketamine, dextromethorphan, or intranasal ketamine can be tried in lieu of serial infusions.

ANTIDEPRESSANT EFFECTS

The antidepressant effects of ketamine have generated high interest in recent years in the psychiatric community. Given the high rate of chronic pain coexisting with depression and other psychiatric morbidities, there has been much interest in this area. However, despite the surge in use for mood disorders, there is a relative paucity of clinical data compared to its use as an analgesic and anesthetic agent.

Ketamine's inhibition of the NMDA receptor is thought to be the reason for its effects as an antidepressant. The mood-enhancing effects appear to emerge in approximately 4 hours, after most of the drug has been cleared from circulation, and persist for up to 2 weeks, long after the acute analgesic effects have dissipated.

While the optimal dose of intravenous ketamine has not been established for treatment-resistant depression, small randomized trials that compared different doses have shown efficacy at 0.5 mg/kg administered over 40 minutes. Other routes of ketamine administration, oral and intranasal, have positive results but are more varied in regards to time to onset of relief.[5]

CANCER PAIN

Cancer-associated pain, either from disease progression or sequelae of treatment, may sometimes be difficult to treat. While opioid medications make up the cornerstone therapy, these medications may not always provide adequate pain control in certain patients, as in our case with FS. These medications may also cause tolerance, hyperalgesia, and other adverse effects, including but not limited to sedation, myoclonus, confusion, and respiratory depression. In cases of intractable cancer pain, when there may be a narrow therapeutic window between pain relief and opioid side effects, ketamine infusions may be considered and are an excellent adjuvant.

Refractory cancer pain that is neuropathic in nature and opioid-tolerant presents two situations that can be very difficult to treat. In these instances, a low-dose ketamine infusion as an analgesic adjuvant can be considered to improve pain control.

When a patient is already taking opioids and ketamine is added to their regimen, practitioners may need to reduce the opioid by 25–50% because opioid receptor activation also affects the NMDA receptor activation. Specifically, if a patient becomes drowsy, develops dyspnea, or begins hallucinating, the dose of opioids should be decreased. A benzodiazepine should also be started.

CONCLUSION

A ketamine infusion was started for FS. She was started on 0.1 mg/hr with slow increases every 24 hours up to 2 mg/hr, at which she had enough pain control to provide relief. While she remained on the same amount of systemic opioid, her pain was stable and she was alert enough to be able to be discharged home with hospice, per her wishes. Recommendations were provided to the hospice program to consider compounded ketamine troches if refractory pain recurred.

KEY POINTS TO REMEMBER

- Ketamine works on the NMDA receptors and can be used as an adjunct for cancer-related pain.
- Ketamine is an excellent neuropathic agent and has been shown to reduce opioid tolerance and hyperalgesia.
- Ketamine is most well-studied and most effective in IV form.
- Short-term side effects to be aware of include tachycardia, hypertension, increased intracranial pressure, hallucinations, and delirium.
- Psychomimetic effects of hallucinations, visual disturbances, unpleasant dreams, and dysphoria can often be mitigated using low-dose benzodiazepines.
- Long-term side effects to be aware of include urinary and hepatobiliary toxicities that often are reversible with stopping ketamine.
- Relative contraindications for ketamine administration include patients with poorly controlled cardiovascular disease, pregnancy, active psychosis, severe hepatic disease, elevated intracranial pressure, elevated intraocular pressure, and active substance abuse.

References

1. Gallagher, R. Opioid-induced Neurotoxicity. *Can Fam Physician.* 2007;53(3):426–427.
2. Visser E., Schug SA. The role of ketamine in pain management. *Biomed Pharmacother.* 2006;60(7):341–348.
3. Quibell R, Fallon M, Mihalyo M, Twycross R, Wilcock A. Ketamine. *J Pain Symptom Manage.* 2015;50(2):268–278.
4. Cohen SP, Bhatia A, et al. Consensus guidelines on the use of intravenous ketamine infusions for chronic pain from the American Society of Regional Anesthesia and Pain Medicine, the American Academy of Pain Medicine,

and the American Society of Anesthesiologists. *Region Anesth Pain Med.* 2018;43(5):521–546.
5. Goldman N, Frankenthaler M, Klepacz L. The efficacy of ketamine in the palliative care setting: A comprehensive review of the literature. *J Palliat Med.* 2019;22(9):1154–1161.

Further Reading

Schwenk ES, Viscusi ER, et al. Consensus guidelines on the use of intravenous ketamine infusions for acute pain management from the American Society of Regional Anesthesia and Pain Medicine, the American Academy of Pain Medicine, and the American Society of Anesthesiologists. *Region Anesth Pain Med.* 2018;43(5):456–466.

13 Lidocaine as an Analgesic in Palliative Care

Jessica Geiger and Dharma Naidu

Case Study

RM is a 54-year-old woman being admitted with increasing pain down her right arm. The pain originates in the neck area and travels down her right hand, into her fingers. The pain is described as tingling and burning. She is unable to lift her hand, and currently has her arm in a sling to provide some comfort by decreasing any movement. Over the past week, her pain has remained at 9 out of 10 on the numeric pain scale. RM weighs 68 kg. RM has estrogen receptor positive, HER2- negative metastatic breast cancer and is currently on third-line treatment. She is diagnosed with brachial plexopathy, which explains the right arm pain. RM received a nerve block and is currently taking the following medications: methadone 10 mg oral three times daily, pregabalin 200 mg oral twice daily, duloxetine 60 mg oral daily, and hydromorphone 4 mg oral every 3 hours as needed for pain (using approximately 6 doses/day). Despite the current therapies and breakthrough utilization, RM's pain remains uncontrolled.

What Do I Do Now?

idocaine was developed as a local anesthetic in 1943, and the earliest report of pain relief was published in 1961. Lidocaine blocks sodium channels, which makes the medication a useful anesthetic and anti-arrhythmic. Its proposed mechanism includes the systemic effect of lidocaine in damaged and dysfunctional nerves, inhibiting depolarization of the neuronal membranes. Systemic lidocaine may also reduce and/or prevent the proliferation of active sodium channels and thus prevent their firing. Intravenous lidocaine can also reduce sensitivity and activity of spinal cord neurons and decrease N-methyl-D-aspartate (NMDA) receptor-mediated post-synaptic depolarization. Lidocaine infusion has been utilized in perioperative pain, sickle cell disease, neuropathic pain, and refractory cancer pain. Local anesthetic use in neuropathic pain was reported in a Cochrane Database review in 2005. Thirty-two controlled clinical trials met the selection criteria, which included 16 trials with lidocaine and 1 trial with lidocaine plus mexiletine sequentially. In this analysis, lidocaine and mexiletine were superior to placebo, and limited data showed no difference in efficacy or adverse effects versus carbamazepine, amantadine, gabapentin, or morphine. In these trials, systemic lidocaine was safe, with no deaths or life-threatening toxicities. In a systematic review and meta-analysis of lidocaine use in cancer pain, the authors identified one positive ($n = 50$) and three negative ($n = 10$ each) crossover trials evaluating lidocaine versus placebo, and one trial ($n = 16$) compared lidocaine with dexmedetomidine. Meta-analysis of pooled data in 60 patients demonstrated a significant benefit of lidocaine infusion of 4–5 mg/kg over 30–80 minutes compared with placebo for more than 50% reduction in cancer pain. A recent study has also shown that lidocaine infusion has similar effects as morphine for treating pain.

DOSING

In reviewing the trials for lidocaine's use in neuropathic pain, the doses ranged from 1 to 5 mg/kg infused over 30 minutes to 6 hours.[1] In studies evaluating perioperative and postoperative pain, doses range from a 1–2 mg/kg bolus followed by an infusion of 1–2 mg/kg/hr given for up to 48 hours postoperatively.[2] Reeves and colleagues published a retrospective chart review to evaluate the effect of use of continuous lidocaine infusion for pain management in an inpatient setting. Twenty-one patients were included in this analysis. Eighteen patients were female and 3 were male, average age was 53 years, and majority had an oncologic diagnosis. Of these, 43% had a component of neuropathic pain. The infusion doses ranged from 0.25 to 1.8 mg/kg/hr, with a median infusion of about 64 hours.[3] In this study, none of the patients received a bolus dose.

Given this evidence, most institutions have adopted dosing that includes a bolus dose of 1 to 3 mg/kg administered over 10–20 minutes followed by an infusion of 1–2 mg/kg/hr for pain management. Patients can be transitioned from lidocaine to mexiletine if an oral agent is desired as mexiletine has a similar mechanism of action. Recommended starting dose of mexiletine is 150 mg every 8 hours with a target dose of 200 mg every 8 hours as long as the patient tolerates it.[4]

OUTCOME

Lidocaine infusion can result in decreased pain as well as decreased opioid requirement. One study reported 8 of the 21 patients (38%) experienced a pain response that was described as a 20% reduction in pain score during the infusion compared with prior to the infusion. This pain response was immediate post infusion and was maintained for 24 hours after discontinuation of the infusion. In terms of decrease in opioid use, this study was able to show a significant dose decrease (874 mg MEDD, based on average daily usage during the infusion).[3]

Thomas et al.[5] reported on experiences at an inpatient hospice setting. Of the 61 patients evaluated (two-thirds were women, average age, 69), 50 (82%) had major relief from their pain; a major response was defined as a move from severe pain to moderate or mild pain or a move from moderate to mild pain.[5] Five (8%) patients had a partial response while 6 patients (10%) showed no benefit. Additionally, researchers were able to demonstrate that patients with neuropathic pain or opioid-refractory pain benefitted most from the addition of lidocaine infusion. Of the subset with neuropathic pain, 82% had a major response. Opioid-refractory patients were defined as those still having pain despite of a MEDD of greater than 200 mg. In the opioid-refractory patients, 91% reported a major response.

Peixoto et al.[6] reported that lidocaine infused at 5 mg/hr over 1 hour, with the option to increase subsequent doses up to 10 mg/kg, had provided a major response to pain in 49% of patients evaluated. A major response was defined as a change in pain score of 3 or greater. A majority of the patients were experiencing neuropathic pain.

SAFETY

Lidocaine infusion results in toxicity including perioral numbness, sedation, light-headedness, tinnitus, and headache. Interesting to note that in the Peixoto study,[6] where patients received 5 mg/kg doses over 1 hour, only 1 patient (1.9%) needed the infusion discontinued because of a tightening feeling in the throat. The most common observed side effects temporally related to lidocaine infusion were drowsiness (30.7%), perioral numbness (13.4%), nausea (5.7%), and minor fluctuations of blood pressure (3.8%). Lidocaine infusion is well tolerated, and, in most circumstances of adverse effects, the infusion can be stopped or dose decreased to manage the toxicity. Whereas lidocaine levels can predict toxicity, in the clinical setting, the lidocaine levels do not guide treatment and thus lidocaine levels are usually not monitored.

While it is usual to have electrocardiographic (EKG) monitoring in patients with cardiac issues on lidocaine infusion, there is always the question of use of EKG monitoring for patients receiving palliative care. Most institutions have policies that dictate if lidocaine infusion needs to be with concurrent EKG monitoring; however, given current literature, in patients with clear hospice or palliative goals and not having high risk of cardiac issues, lidocaine infusions are administered without EKG monitoring.

CONCLUSION

Due to the neuropathic nature of RM's pain, she may benefit from treatment with lidocaine. As RM weighs 68 kg, an appropriate bolus dose would be 68–200 mg, followed by an infusion of 68–136 mg/kg/hr. For simplicity, RM can be given a 100 mg bolus, followed by a 100 mg/hr infusion. RM should be monitored for potential side effects, and EKG monitoring could be considered.

KEY POINTS TO REMEMBER

- Consider lidocaine in cancer pain, neuropathic pain, opioid-resistant pain, postoperative pain, and sickle cell crisis.
- Initiate bolus dose at 1–3 mg/kg over 20 minutes and then start infusion at 1–2 mg/kg/hr. Dose duration can range depending on goals.
- For patients on concurrent opioids, reduce long acting opioids by 30–50% at initiation of lidocaine given its opioid-sparing effects.
- Outpatient infusions can be given at 5 mg/kg over 1 hour, given every 3 weeks for patients considered as responders post initial infusion.
- Lidocaine levels do not guide dosing for pain.
- Close monitoring can address most adverse effects.
- EKG monitoring may not be necessary given clear goals of care in select palliative and hospice patients; however, it can be considered in patients with comorbid cardiac issues.

References

1. Challapalli V, Tremont-Lukats IW, McNicol ED, Lau J, Carr DB. Systemic administration of local anesthetic agents to relieve neuropathic pain. *Cochrane Database Syst Rev.* 2005;4:CD003345
2. Kandil E, Melikman E, Adinoff B. Lidocaine infusion: A promising therapeutic approach to chronic pain. *J Anesth Clin Res.* 2017 January;8(1):1–14. doi:10.4172/2155-6148.1000697
3. Reeves DJ, Foster AE. Continuous intravenous lidocaine infusion for the management of pain uncontrolled by opioid medications. *J Pain Palliat Care Pharmacotherapy.* 2017 Sep-Dec 31(3–4):198–203.
4. Atayee R, Naidu D, Geiger-Hayes J, et. al. A multi-centered case series highlighting the clinical use and dosing of lidocaine and mexiletine for refractory cancer pain. *J Pain Palliat Care Pharmacother.* 2020;34(2):90–98.
5. Thomas J, Kronenberg R, Craig M, et al. Intravenous lidocaine relieves severe pain: results of an inpatient hospice chart review. *J Palliative Med.* 2004;7(5):660–667.
6. Peixoto RD. Hawley P. Intravenous lidocaine for cancer pain without electrocardiographic monitoring: a retrospective review. *J Palliat Med.* 2015;18(4):373–377.

Further Reading

Bartlett EE, Hutserani O. Xylocaine for the relief of postoperative pain. *Anesth Analg* 1961;40:296–304.

Clattenburg EJ, Nguyen A, Yoo T, et al. Intravenous lidocaine provides similar analgesia to intravenous morphine for undifferentiated severe pain in the emergency department: A pilot, unblended randomized controlled trial. *Pain Med.* 2019;20:834–839.

Eipe N, Gupta S, Penning J. Intravenous lidocaine for acute pain: An evidence based clinical update. *BJA Education.* 2016 September;(16)9:292–298.

Kranke P, Jokinen J, Pace NL, et al. Continuous intravenous perioperative lidocaine infusion for postoperative pain and recovery. *Cochrane Database Syst Rev* 2015:CD009642

Lee JT, Sanderson CR, Xuan W, et al. Lidocaine for cancer pain in adults: A systematic review and meta analysis. *J Palliat Med.* 2019 Mar;22(3):326–334.

14 Non-Opioid Analgesic Side Effects

Matthew D. Clark

Case Study

WC is a 34-year-old transgender man with cecal cancer and L2/L3 spinal lesions who presents for an appointment with supportive care services. He is currently complaining of pain in his lower back with radiation to his right knee and rates his pain at 6 on a 10-point numeric rating scale. He is very hesitant to try opioids due to a family history of opioid use disorder. Duloxetine 30 mg twice daily was initiated along with a transcutaneous electrical nerve stimulation (TENS) unit to be placed on the painful areas. Two weeks later, the patient presents to the clinic with complaints of profuse diaphoresis and uncontrolled diarrhea unrelieved by loperamide. Onset of symptoms was 1 week ago, with no relieving or exacerbating factors. The patient reports that the painful neuropathy symptoms have improved. However, his current symptoms have greatly decreased his quality of life.

What Do I Do Now?

Many non-opioid analgesic drug classes may be useful in managing various pain syndromes. Non-opioid analgesics include acetaminophen, nonsteroidal anti-inflammatory drugs (NSAIDs), antidepressants, anticonvulsants, muscle relaxants, and corticosteroids. These agents may be useful for managing pain associated with headaches, osteoarthritis, neuropathy, and bone pain. In some cases, patients may be controlled solely with these analgesics. Typically, they are easily titrated, can be rotated to other non-opioids, or used concomitantly with other analgesics in the event that a patient's pain is not adequately controlled.

Compared to opioids, non-opioids have a lower risk for abuse and addiction. However, non-opioids can be associated with unfavorable adverse events. Generally, these agents are well tolerated. However, some adverse events may lead to the discontinuation of the analgesic or even hospitalization. In the case of the patient WC it is clear that he is experiencing an adverse reaction from the duloxetine that was initiated 3 weeks prior to this office visit. WC also has a past medical history of major depressive disorder along with anxiety for which he was also taking sertraline. The addition of duloxetine, also a serotonergic agent, may have predisposed WC to symptoms of serotonin syndrome. Conducting a thorough examination of a patient, including past medical history, current home medications, and social history is imperative when deciding on a certain therapy to initiate. This chapter looks at the common non-opioid medications prescribed for pain along with their adverse effects, warnings, and contraindications.

ACETAMINOPHEN

Acetaminophen is a widely used analgesic and antipyretic. It comes in various formulations and is useful for treating symptoms of mild to moderate pain and fever. Acetaminophen's over-the-counter status has led to its common everyday use for many patients. Although tolerated by most patients, acetaminophen can result in adverse reactions. In adults, this medication may cause nausea, vomiting, headache, and insomnia. Additionally, acetaminophen has shown to cause agitation, atelectasis, and pruritus in pediatric patients. Acetaminophen has a recommended dose limit of 4 g per 24-hour period, although some guidelines suggest a limit of 3 g per day based on risk of liver transaminase elevations, even in healthy adults.

As acetaminophen shares a glucuronidation metabolic pathway with many opioids, combination may increase this risk. Caution should be exercised when administering acetaminophen to patients with hepatic impairment, alcoholism, chronic malnutrition, severe hypovolemia, and renal impairment. The use of acetaminophen in patients with severe hepatic impairment or severe active liver disease is contraindicated.

ANTICONVULSANTS

Anticonvulsants are useful adjuvant analgesics that may be quite effective as monotherapy for pain of neurogenic origin or for their synergistic or opioid-sparing effect. Commonly used anticonvulsants include gabapentin and pregabalin. These agents work by blocking subtypes of calcium channels, ultimately reducing the release of glutamate. Gabapentin and pregabalin have similar side-effect profiles. They may cause dizziness, somnolence, ataxia, difficulty concentrating, peripheral edema, and weight gain. Respiratory depression may occur when gabapentinoids are used concomitantly with other strong central nervous system (CNS) depressants, especially opioids. While extremely rare, these agents should be discontinued if angioedema occurs.

Another group of anticonvulsants work by blocking sodium channels, resulting in the prevention of initiation and propagation of action potentials. These includes carbamazepine, lamotrigine, oxcarbazepine, topiramate, and zonisamide. Lamotrigine may cause dizziness, headache, diplopia, ataxia, nausea, blurred vision, somnolence, and rash. Most notable is the low but real risk of Steven-Johnson syndrome. Common side effects of topiramate include somnolence, abnormal vision, ataxia, dizziness, paresthesias, nephrolithiasis, metabolic acidosis, and weight loss. Carbamazepine and oxcarbazepine may cause aplastic anemia, diplopia, dizziness, ataxia, hyponatremia, and rash. All of the anticonvulsants have been associated with neurocognitive dulling, although this adverse effect appears to be most common with topiramate at higher doses. Class-wide warnings for increased risk of suicidal ideation exists for these agents.

Clinicians should be cognizant of withdrawal symptoms when anticonvulsants are abruptly discontinued. These symptoms can range from short-term malaise up to and including seizures.

ANTIDEPRESSANTS

Pain commonly co-occurs with depression and anxiety, making antidepressants a potentially attractive option as adjuvant analgesics. The serotonin-norepinephrine class of drugs are especially useful given that their dose ranges for pain are similar to those used to treat depression and anxiety. Duloxetine may cause nausea, constipation, and hyperhidrosis. Liver transaminases should be monitored periodically as there have been reports of hepatic dysfunction associated with duloxetine. Venlafaxine may cause CNS reactions such as somnolence, dry mouth, dizziness, and insomnia. Also, venlafaxine may cause adverse gastrointestinal effects like nausea, constipation, and anorexia. Tricyclic antidepressants (TCAs) like amitriptyline and nortriptyline can have anticholinergic effects such as constipation, dry mouth, orthostatic hypotension, and urinary retention. Prolongation of the QTc interval has been well-documented with TCAs and should be considered, especially in older patients.

An important consideration when initiating antidepressants is the possibility of developing *serotonin syndrome*. This potentially life-threatening condition may occur when the dose of a serotonergic agent is increased or when multiple serotonergic agents are administered simultaneously. Mild cases of serotonin syndrome include hypertension, tachycardia, diaphoresis, shivering, tremor, myoclonus, and hyperreflexia. In more severe instances, patients will have the aforementioned symptoms in addition to hyperthermia, hyperactive bowel sounds, dramatic fluctuations in pulse and blood pressure, delirium, and muscle rigidity. Complications of serotonin syndrome can lead to seizures, rhabdomyolysis, metabolic acidosis, renal failure, acute respiratory distress syndrome, coma, and death. Management involves discontinuing serotonergic agents, supportive care, sedation with benzodiazepines, and observation.

CORTICOSTEROIDS

Corticosteroids are often used in the settings of both malignant and nonmalignant pain syndromes. Additionally, they are indicated for inflammatory and autoimmune conditions. Mechanistically, they inhibit the synthesis of prostaglandins and leukotrienes. Adverse events of corticosteroids are

TABLE 14.1 **Acute and chronic adverse effects of corticosteroids**

Acute adverse effects	Chronic adverse effects
Acne	Acne
Hyperglycemia	Amenorrhea
Hypertension	Cataracts
Hypokalemia	Cushing syndrome
Immunosuppression	Dermal thinning
Impaired wound healing	Diabetes
Indigestion	Gastrointestinal bleeding
Increased appetite	Glaucoma
Infection	Growth retardation
Myopathy	Hirsutism
Weight gain	Osteoporosis/fractures

determined based on dose and duration of therapy. Acute and chronic adverse effects are listed in Table 14.1.

KETAMINE

A general anesthetic commonly used for short procedures, ketamine provides analgesia by antagonizing N-methyl-D-aspartate (NMDA) receptors. Patients may experience fluctuations in blood pressure and heart rate upon administration of ketamine. Likewise, if an elevation of blood pressure poses a serious hazard for a patient, ketamine should be avoided. Ketamine may also manifest psychological effects. This includes pleasant dream-like states, vivid imagery, hallucinations, and delirium. Severity of symptoms may vary, and symptom resolution normally occurs within a few hours after administration.

MUSCLE RELAXANTS

There are mechanistically different classes of muscle relaxants. Likewise, each muscle relaxant has a slightly different side-effect profile. Antispasticity muscle relaxants include baclofen and tizanidine. Baclofen may cause dizziness, confusion, and sedation. Patients who abruptly discontinue baclofen may experience withdrawal symptoms.

Tizanidine, a centrally acting alpha-2 agonist, may cause hypotension, dry mouth, and weakness. Additionally, rebound hypertension may occur if tizanidine is abruptly discontinued. Tizanidine is associated with a risk of hepatic injury, and periodic monitoring of liver transaminases is recommended. Strong CYP1A2 enzyme inhibitors should be avoided when taking tizanidine.

Other skeletal muscle relaxants include carisoprodol, metaxalone, orphenadrine, chlorzoxazone, cyclobenzaprine, and methocarbamol. These primarily act by depressing the CNS. Carisoprodol may have a higher risk of abuse owing to its metabolism to meprobamate, a barbiturate. In addition to its CNS effects, metaxalone can cause dose-limiting gastrointestinal upset. Metaxalone should be avoided in patients with significant liver impairment.

Cyclobenzaprine is a muscle relaxant that works centrally in the brainstem and reduces tonic somatic motor activity. Structurally similar to the TCAs, common adverse effects include drowsiness, dry mouth, and dizziness. Patients in the acute recovery phase of myocardial infarction and patients with arrhythmias, heart block, or congestive heart failure should avoid cyclobenzaprine.

NONSTEROIDAL ANTI-INFLAMMATORY DRUGS

Another class of analgesics commonly used is the nonsteroidal anti-inflammatory drugs or NSAIDs. There are several agents in this class of analgesics with various routes of administration. NSAIDs are useful for inflammatory pain and headaches. They exert their mechanism of action by inhibiting cyclo-oxygenase (COX-1 and COX-2), and their adverse effects depend on their selectivity for which COX enzyme they inhibit. COX selectivity of each NSAID is displayed in Table 14.2.

NSAIDs that selectively inhibit COX-1 are more likely to cause gastrointestinal bleeding and ulcerations. This is due to the inhibition of the gastric protectant, prostaglandin E2, resulting from the inhibition of COX-1. Patients who are at an increased risk for adverse gastrointestinal events include patients with a history of peptic ulcer disease,

TABLE 14.2 **Cyclo-oxygenase selectivity of each nonsteroidal anti-inflammatory drug (NSAID)**

COX-1 selective	Nonselective	COX-2 Selective
Ketorolac	Ibuprofen	Sulindac
Flurbiprofen	Fenoprofen	Diclofenac
Ketoprofen	Diflunisal	Celecoxib
Indomethacin		Meloxicam
Aspirin		Etodolac
Naproxen		
Tolmetin		
Piroxicam		

age 60 years or older, male, and concurrently taking a corticosteroid or anticoagulation.

On the other hand, NSAIDs that are more selective for COX-2 increase a patient's risk for cardiovascular events, such as stroke or myocardial infarctions. This results from vasoconstriction and platelet aggregation caused by these agents. Patients with a history of cardiovascular disease are at risk for developing NSAID-induced cardiac toxicity. NSAIDs should be discontinued if heart failure or hypertension develops or worsens after administration. All NSAIDs increase the risk for renal impairment, most notably in those with preexisting renal compromise.

TOPICAL AGENTS

Sometimes analgesia can be achieved without the use of systemic analgesics. Topical agents like capsaicin, lidocaine, and diclofenac can be helpful for managing both local and radiating musculoskeletal and arthritic pain. These agents are normally very well tolerated, and adverse effects are typically local. This includes local skin irritation, erythema, and pruritus. Additionally, capsaicin may cause pain at the application site. These adverse effects should resolve after removal and discontinuation of the topical agent. Lidocaine patches should only be applied for 12 consecutive hours in a 24-hour period as systemic absorption leading to systemic adverse effects is possible.

SUMMARY

Non-opioid analgesics are an effective option for treating various pain syndromes when opioids may not be warranted. Although non-opioid analgesics are typically well tolerated, healthcare professionals should be aware of potential adverse reactions associated with these agents. Potential life-threatening side effects like those experienced by the patient in this case can be avoided with proper understanding of the side-effect profiles, contraindications, warnings, and drug interactions of each analgesic. Ultimately, acknowledging the safety considerations of non-opioid analgesics can optimize a patient's quality of life.

> **KEY POINTS TO REMEMBER**
>
> - Acetaminophen should be limited to a dose of 4 g per 24 hours. Exceeding this limit may lead to hepatic injury.
> - Patients on serotonergic antidepressants for pain management should be monitored for signs and symptoms of serotonin syndrome.
> - Side effects from corticosteroids are based on the dose and duration of therapy. These agents should be tapered prior to discontinuation following high dose or prolonged periods.
> - Ketamine may lead to an increased blood pressure and should be avoided in patients with risk of cardiac injury with high blood pressure.
> - The side effects of NSAIDs depend on the cyclo-oxygenase selectivity of the agent. NSAIDs with COX-1 selectivity have potential for gastrointestinal-related adverse effects while those with COX-2 selectivity have potential for cardiovascular events.

Further Reading

Bottenmiller S. Opioid-induced hyperalgesia: An emerging treatment challenge. *US Pharm.* 2012;37(5):HS-2-HS-7.

Drini M. Peptic ulcer disease and non-steroidal anti-inflammatory drugs. *Australian Prescriber.* 2017;40:91–93.

Perry LA, Mosler C, Atkins A, et al. Cardiovascular risk associated with NSAIDs and COX-2 inhibitors. *US Pharm.* 2014;39(3):35–38.

Volpi-Abadie J, Kaye AM, Kaye AD, et al. Serotonin syndrome. *Ochsner J.* 2013;13:533–540.

Yasir M, Goyal A, Bansal P, et al. Corticosteroid adverse effects. Updated April 13, 2020. StatPearls. Treasure Island, FL: StatPearls Publishing; 2020 Jan. https://www.ncbi.nlm.nih.gov/books/NBK531462/

15 Cannabis for Pain Management in Palliative Care

Christopher M. Herndon and Tim Cruz

Case Study

MT is a 64-year-old man with T4N1M1 metastatic cholangiocarcinoma diagnosed 18 months ago. He is currently receiving immunotherapy (pembrolizumab) and has experienced a 32-pound weight loss over the past 6 months. He receives paracentesis as needed and takes spironolactone 50 mg daily. He has refused hospice referral. His pain control is currently managed by his primary care team and consists of oral controlled-release morphine 100 mg every 8 hours and immediate release oral hydromorphone 8 mg every 4 hours as needed for breakthrough pain. MT was on chronic opioid therapy prior to his cancer diagnosis for the treatment of chronic low back pain with radiculopathy. In addition, MT takes oral pregabalin 200 mg every 8 hours, oral carbamazepine 200 mg every 12 hours, and endorses daily use of cannabis for pain, anxiety, and appetite. He reports his pain as deep, aching, and stabbing and states that severity ranges from 6/10 to 10/10 depending on activity and time since last paracentesis.

What Do I Do Now?

his scenario is unfortunately more common than one might anticipate. In a growing number of US states, medical and recreational use of cannabis is legal and becoming more socially acceptable. In MT's case, both medical and recreational cannabis are cost-prohibitive for him to obtain and possess legally. He purchases his cannabis as flower from an acquaintance for smoking and does note on several occasions that quality or quantity of his supply is an issue. This raises several important questions for the clinician treating pain in the setting of serious illness:

- Is recommending cannabis for the treatment of pain evidence-based?
- What is the concentration of the active cannabinoids in the product?
- What drug-drug interactions might confound safe and effective treatment of pain?
- What regulatory and financial barriers exist to the safe and effective use of cannabis for pain?

ENDOCANNABINOID SYSTEM

The endocannabinoid system has broad functions within the central and peripheral nervous systems. The two primary, biologically active endocannaboids in the body are anandamide and 2-arachidonylglycerol (2-AG). Both are produced postsynaptically and released into the synapse, where they bind to one of two currently known cannabinoid receptors. Cannabinoid receptor-1 (CB_1) is primarily located within the central nervous system (CNS), whereas cannabinoid receptor-2 (CB_2) is more widely expressed within the immune and gastrointestinal systems. When cannabinoids are obtained from a plant they are considered phytocannabinoids, and there are numerous unique, biologically active cannabinoids described.

Tetrahydrocannabinol (THC), specifically delta-9-tetrahydrocannabinol, is the psychoactive cannabinoid most commonly sought and serves as a partial agonist at the CB_1 receptor. THC additionally binds the CB_2 receptor, but to a comparatively lesser extent. Cannabidiol (CBD) is also widely found in variable concentrations within different strains of cannabis and produces an inverse-agonist (and potentially an antagonist) effect at the CB_1 receptor and antagonist effect at CB_1.[1] Many strains and hybrids of cannabis result in variable concentrations of these two distinctly different cannabinoids, thus complicating research and, more importantly, selection or recommendation from a clinician. Given the unknown source of MT's cannabis, little can be offered in terms of recommending dosing or titration.

GENERAL SUPPORTING EVIDENCE

In addition to the difficulty in recommending specific cannabinoids for patients obtaining their cannabis from unregulated sources, high-quality controlled studies demonstrating efficacy specifically for cancer pain are largely lacking. Questions remain for the optimal cannabinoid (THC, CBD, or varying combinations of both) and the optimal delivery route (oral, sublingual, smoked, or vaporized) in the treatment of pain in general and cancer pain specifically.[2] For instance, dronabinol has largely been disappointing anecdotally as a stand-alone analgesic in cancer pain; however, a two-part study did show improvement in pain intensity compared to placebo in patients with refractory pain.[3] Older studies also showed both a reduction in pain as well as a correlation with higher doses of THC and reduced pain intensity. Oromucosal spray, commercially available as a 50:50 mix of THC and CBD, has been more widely studied for the treatment of cancer pain. Results for the 50:50 THC/CBD oromucosal spray have been equivocal, with two of the studies showing no significant difference in pain relief compared to placebo and one study showing improvement with low and moderate doses, but not high doses. The European Pain Federation does recommend that the oromucosal spray may be considered in cancer pain refractory to opioids. While smoked/vaporized cannabis has been studied more extensively for cancer-related nausea and cachexia, studies specifically evaluated cancer pain are largely absent.

CANNABINOID CONCENTRATIONS

Traditional cannabis obtained through unregulated channels has changed dramatically over the past two decades. Previous *Cannabis sativa* possessed THC concentrations ranging from 3% to 9%. Today, hybridization of cannabis has resulted in THC concentrations as high as 25%. Considering the variable pharmacologic properties of this cannabinoid as dosage changes, this may confound clinicians' ability to recommend in a widespread manner. Additionally, the over-the-counter CBD preparations that can be found almost anywhere have been proved to have inconsistent concentrations when tested against stated ingredients. It is important to remember that as the dose of THC or CBD increases, the risk of harms may also increase. When available, medical and recreational cannabis obtained through regulated dispensaries are clearly preferred for patient care. These typically have clearly defined THC and CBD concentrations which may allow for more accurate dose titration.

DRUG-DRUG INTERACTIONS

Drug interactions are commonplace when providing palliative care. Drug interactions specifically involving cannabinoids involve those that impact the exposure to the cannabinoid itself or when the cannabinoid either inhibits or induces the metabolism of another substrate drug being used.[4,5] Both THC and CBD are metabolized via cytochrome P450 (CYP) 3A4, and THC is also metabolized via CYP 2C9. Medications either inhibiting or inducing these enzymes have been shown to significantly impact THC and CBD serum drug levels. Individually, THC and CBD have varying effects on other drugs commonly used in palliative care. For instance, THC may inhibit CYP 2C9 and 3A4 whereas CBD may inhibit CYP 2C19 and 3A4. Traditionally, CBD is considered a more potent inhibitor of CYP 3A4. While not specifically tied to THC itself, smoking of cannabis has shown induction of CYP 1A1 and 1A2. Glucuronidation-based drug interactions also exist that are clinically relevant. CBD inhibits UDP-glucuronosyltransferase (UGT) 1A9 and 2B7. Representative interactions and their corresponding clinical outcomes are provided in Table 15.1. Returning to MT, recall that he is on morphine and hydromorphone and has also been stable on carbamazepine. Numerous drug interactions may exist with his cannabis use.

REGULATORY AND FINANCIAL BARRIERS

Medical or recreational cannabis use by patients receiving palliative care has been a contentious point of discussion to say the least. Prescribers are

TABLE 15.1 Representative drug-drug interactions with cannabinoids in palliative care

Enzyme	Modifiers	Targets
CYP 3A4 inhibition	Clarithromycin, erythromycin, diltiazem, itraconazole, ketoconazole, ritonavir, verapamil, CBD	THC: Increased effect CBD: Increased effect Alprazolam: Increased effect Carbamazepine: Increased effect Diltiazem: Increased effect Verapamil: Increased effect Fentanyl: Increased effect Buprenorphine: Increased effect Cyclosporine: Increased effect Simvastatin: Increased effect
CYP 3A4 induction	Carbamazepine, phenytoin, rifampin, efavirenz, phenobarbital, primidone	THC: Reduced effect CBD: Reduced effect
CYP 2C9 inhibition	Amiodarone, fluconazole, co-trimoxazole, fluoxetine	THC: Increased effect
CYP 2C9 induction	Rifampin	THC: Decreased effect
CYP 2C19 inhibition	CBD	Aripiprazole: Increased effect Clopidogrel: Decreased effect Citalopram: Increased effect Diazepam: Increased effect
CYP 1A2 induction	Smoked THC	Tizanidine: Reduced effect Duloxetine: Reduced effect Alosetron: Reduced effect Clozapine: Reduced effect
UGT 1A9 inhibition	CBD	Acetaminophen: Increased effect Propofol: Increased effect Canagliflozin: Increased effect Etodolac: Increased effect Indomethacin: Increased effect Irinotecan: Increased effect
UGT 2B7 inhibition	CBD	Buprenorphine: Increased effect Diclofenac: Increased effect Valproic acid: Increased effect Morphine: Variable (decreased conversion to morphine-3-glucuronide and morphine-6-glucuronide)

often hesitant to greenlight patient cannabis use when also providing controlled substances such as benzodiazepines and/or opioids. In fact, when performing routine or random drug toxicology screening in patients, many prescribers will consider a positive THC as a treatment agreement violation or red flag for abuse. Continued scheduling of cannabis as a schedule 1 controlled substance by the US Drug Enforcement Agency (DEA) also causes many prescribers angst given the potential for problems with ongoing DEA provider registration. Clear policies on how to approach medical or recreational cannabis use by patients receiving palliative care should guide prescribers and ensure a consistent message. Financial barriers are likely even more burdensome for patients seeking symptom palliation. Cannabis is not covered by third-party payers and very unlikely to be covered as part of the hospice per diem for patients at the end of life. In fact, many hospice administrators voice concern that publicly recommending to patients or covering medical cannabis may somehow jeopardize their Medicare reimbursement.

In some states, having a medical cannabis card may decrease costs to the patient (primarily from reduced tax liability) compared to recreational cannabis. While potency and content is unpredictable, rarely is cannabis obtained from unregulated sources as expensive as that obtained from dispensaries.

Returning to MT, we encouraged him to obtain his cannabis from a licensed recreational dispensary to ensure known cannabinoid concentrations. We are unable to sign the qualifying condition attestation papers for medical cannabis as our administrators are concerned that our Federally Qualified Healthcare Center status may be jeopardized if the providers engage in this practice. We additionally continued to practice prudent opioid risk mitigation practices.

KEY POINTS TO REMEMBER

- Evidence to support the efficacy of cannabis for the treatment of cancer pain is still equivocal; however, cannabis may be beneficial for other non-pain symptoms.

- When possible, cannabis should be obtained from regulated sources to ensure predictable concentrations of expected cannabinoid.
- Cannabis has numerous clinically relevant drug-drug interactions that should be considered prior to recommending cannabis or when changing drug therapy for patients already on cannabis.

References

1. Narouze S. Antinociception mechanisms of action of cannabinoid-based medicine: An overview for anesthesiologists and pain physicians. *Reg Anesth Pain Med.* 2020 November 25:rapm-2020-102114.
2. Inglet S, Winter B, Yost SE. Clinical data for the use of cannabis-based treatments: A comprehensive review of the literature. *Ann Pharmacother.* 2020;54(11):1109–1143.
3. Narang S, Gibson D, Wasan AD, Ross EL, Michna E, Nedeljkovic SS, Jamison RN. Efficacy of dronabinol as an adjuvant treatment for chronic pain patients on opioid therapy. *J Pain.* 2008;9(3):254–264.
4. Alsherbiny MA, Li, CG. Medicinal cannabis: Potential drug interactions. *Medicines.* 2019;6(1):3. doi:10.3390/medicines6010003
5. Antoniou T, Bodkin J, Ho JM. Drug interactions with cannabinoids. *CMAJ.* 2020;192(9):E206. doi:https://doi.org/10.1503/cmaj.191097

16 Supplement Use in Pain Treatment

Jennifer L. Rosselli

Case Study

WS is a 56-year-old Black woman who presents to the palliative care clinic with type 2 diabetes for 20 years, hypertension, distal symmetric polyneuropathy, and end-stage chronic kidney disease requiring hemodialysis. The patient reports jolts of pain that move from the toes to the knees of both legs off and on several times per day, most noticeable at night. The patient declines prescription medication for neuropathy; she would rather take a vitamin or something natural for the pain. Findings from the foot exam are significant for lacking pressure sensation with monofilament testing bilaterally. Pinprick sensation is not perceived on the hallux bilaterally. Tuning fork vibratory sensation and pedal pulses are intact. The A1C today is 8.9%. The primary care physician requests your recommendation for a "natural" product for this patient's neuropathic symptoms, information on how the patient can purchase a supplement that is safe and reliable, and where to access reputable information about vitamins and herbals.

What Do I Do Now?

Conventional pharmaceuticals used in the treatment of pain may have limited therapeutic utility when patients experience insufficient efficacy and unwanted adverse effects, or risks are present that preclude the use of allopathic medication. Because of these limitations to the use of conventional therapies along with the opioid overdose epidemic, complementary and alternative medicine (CAM) may be appealing or preferred for pain treatment. Vitamins and herbal therapies, sold as dietary supplements, are the most widely utilized type of CAM modalities. Supplements may provide benefit as part of an integrative approach to pain treatment but are not without risks. Health professionals involved in the care of patients who consume dietary supplements should have general knowledge and utilize reputable resources related to the efficacy and safety of products used in pain treatment.

REGULATION OF DIETARY SUPPLEMENTS

Vitamins, minerals, amino acids, and herbs are classified as dietary supplements in the United States. Regulated by the Food and Drug Administration (FDA) as food products, they are not required to undergo rigorous testing for efficacy or safety as is required of products classified as drugs, and they are allowed to be marketed for public use without approval by the FDA.

Independent third-party organizations, such as the United States Pharmacopeia (USP), have developed good manufacturing practices auditing programs and have conducted product verification testing to ensure the quality of dietary supplements. The USP awards the USP Verified Mark to be displayed on the label of dietary supplements that have met its identity, strength, purity, and quality criteria.

A dietary supplement can only be removed from the market if the FDA determines it to be of significant or unreasonable harm. The Dietary Supplement and Nonprescription Drug Consumer Protection Act requires that manufacturers of dietary supplements and nonprescription medications report serious adverse events that result in death, are life-threatening, cause birth defects, or require medical treatment such as hospitalization or surgery. Due to the knowledge gaps in safety created by the limited regulatory oversight and monitoring of dietary supplements, it is important that consumers and health professionals report suspected adverse events to the FDA through the MedWatch Program.

CLINICAL RESOURCES

Providing current information about the potential benefits and risks associated with treatment options is an important step to engage patients in when selecting optimal pain therapies. The degree to which dietary supplements are regulated is very different compared to the regulatory oversight of conventional medications. Consumers of supplements should be cautioned that products will vary in the accuracy of labeling and claims of health benefits made by manufacturers. Clinicians and patients should obtain research-based information from reputable resources, such as those outlined in Table 16.1.

SUPPLEMENTS USED FOR COMMON PAIN CONDITIONS

5-Hydroxytryptophan

5-hydroxytryptophan (5-HTP) is derived from the seeds of the *Griffonia simplicifolia* plant and is a precursor to serotonin, a neurotransmitter believed to play a significant role in fibromyalgia symptoms. 5-HTP 300–400 mg/day has been evaluated as a treatment in fibromyalgia and observed to improve the number of tender points, pain, sleep quality, morning stiffness, anxiety, and fatigue compared to placebo, and it has shown similar efficacy when compared to tricyclic antidepressants and monoamine oxidase inhibitors (Table 16.2). In 1989, there were cases of eosinophilia-myalgia syndrome associated with contaminated 5-HTP supplements imported from Japan. This led to an FDA-directed product recall and limited the importation of 5-HTP. Nausea is a common adverse effect, is typically transient, and can be mitigated by dividing 5-HTP doses into three daily doses and initiating at low doses followed by a slow titration. Patients with bipolar disorder should use 5-HTP cautiously due to the potential for inducing mania. 5-HTP can interact with other serotonergic medications increasing the risk of serotonin syndrome.

TABLE 16.1 Dietary supplement resources

Resource	Contents
Free-access resources for consumers and health professionals	
HerbList™	Mobile application developed by NCCIH Brief clinical summaries of herbal supplements Links to other resources
Herbs at a Glance	Web-based version of HerbList™ app available on the NCCIH website Brief clinical summaries of herbal supplements
Memorial Sloan Kettering Cancer Center's About Herbs	Concise product overviews
NIH MedlinePlus Herbs and Supplements	Concise product overviews
Resources for health professionals	
Natural Medicines	Subscription-based drug compendia Monographs of dietary supplements Drug interaction tools
Natural Products Database	Subscription-based drug compendia Available through Lexicomp Monographs of dietary supplements Drug interaction tools
Dietary Supplements on PubMed	Search engine Access journal article citations related to vitamin, mineral, and herbal supplements
CAM on PubMed	Search engine Access journal article citations related to CAM therapies, including herbal supplements

NCCIH, National Center for Complementary and Integrative Health; NIH, National Institutes of Health; CAM, complementary and alternative medicine.

Alpha Lipoic Acid

Alpha lipoic acid (ALA) is an antioxidant that can prevent hyperglycemia-induced oxidative stress and damage found in diabetic peripheral neuropathy. Numerous studies have evaluated ALA doses ranging 600 to 1,800

TABLE 16.2 Supplements with possible effectiveness for common pain conditions

Pain condition	Supplement
Arthritis	Capsaicin Comfrey Glucosamine and chondroitin Omega-3 supplements
Back pain	Comfrey Willow bark
Fibromyalgia	5-Hydroxytryptophan Magnesium
Headache	Butterbur Feverfew Magnesium Vitamin B_2
Neuropathy	Alpha lipoic acid Capsaicin Vitamin B_{12}

mg/day administered orally and intravenously. Much of the evidence involving dietary supplements is comprised of short-term clinical trials. Conversely, ALA has been evaluated in a 4-year randomized placebo-controlled study. The growing body of evidence is promising that ALA can increase insulin sensitivity, improve pinprick and touch pressure sensations, and reduce paresthesia and pain. The efficacy of ALA has does not appear to be dose-dependent with 600 mg/day showing consistent effects. It is unclear if short-term treatment with daily infusions followed by oral therapy provides added benefit over orally administered ALA alone. The most commonly cited adverse effect is nausea and is likely to be mild if daily doses of ALA do not exceed 600 mg.

Butterbur

Extracts from the leaves and roots of the butterbur plant have inhibitory effects on L-type voltage-gated calcium channels resulting in decreased neuronal excitability and vasoconstriction, and butterbur demonstrates anti-inflammatory effects through cyclo-oxygenase 2 inhibition. The efficacy of butterbur for migraine headache prophylaxis has been evaluated in randomized placebo-controlled trials. Studies in adult and pediatric patients observed a dose-related reduction in monthly migraine attacks with maximal response to butterbur taking up to 3–4 months. The butterbur plant contains pyrrolizidine alkaloids (PA) that are known to cause liver damage and serious illness in humans and are carcinogenic in rodents. Only processed butterbur formulations that have removed PAs and are certified as PA-free should be used. Cases of hepatotoxicity associated with butterbur use have been reported by the World Health Organization. It is unclear if alkaloids were in the preparations ingested. In 2015, the American Academy of Neurology withdrew the recommendation for butterbur as a migraine preventative due to serious safety concerns over hepatotoxicity.

Capsaicin

Capsaicin exerts analgesic effects as a transient receptor potential vanilloid 1 (TRPV1) receptor agonist that, after repeated contact or exposure to high concentrations, results in desensitization of the nociceptive nerve fibers that express TRPV1. Topical formulations of capsaicin are widely available over-the-counter in creams, lotions, gels, liquids, and patches for pain associated with diabetic peripheral neuropathy, arthritis, and acute back pain. Many studies demonstrating the efficacy of capsaicin are limited by small effect size, large placebo effects, difficulty with double blinding, and a high use of unauthorized medications. The American College of Rheumatology (ACR) provides a conditional recommendation for capsaicin use in knee osteoarthritis. Patients with localized neuropathic pain may benefit from capsaicin cream if an alternative to oral therapies is preferred. A prescription topical patch containing 8% capsaicin is available in the United States for the treatment of neuropathic pain secondary to postherpetic neuralgia or diabetic peripheral neuropathy of the feet and is considered after other therapies have failed due to its high cost and requirement to be administered in a healthcare setting under physician supervision. Capsaicin causes a characteristic burning, stinging, and redness at the application site that may lessen or dissipate after 2 weeks of treatment. Caution should be used to avoid exposing the eyes, mouth, and other mucous membranes to capsaicin.

Comfrey

The root extract of comfrey, known to have anti-inflammatory properties and analgesic effects, has been used in topical preparations to alleviate painful muscles and joints. Randomized, controlled trials of topical comfrey have demonstrated efficacy in reducing upper and lower back pain, decreasing knee osteoarthritis pain, and improving pain, tenderness, and swelling due to ankle sprains. Comfrey applied three to four times daily has only been studied as a short-term treatment—5 days for back pain, 21 days for knee osteoarthritis, and up to 14 days for ankle injuries. Comfrey contains hepatotoxic pyrrolizidine alkaloids; therefore, it should never be ingested and patients should be advised to use topical formulations that are PA-free.

Feverfew

Feverfew leaves contain active constituents that have anti-inflammatory effects. However, the plant's inhibition of serotonin release from platelets and white blood cells is thought to be the anti-migraine mechanism. Findings from clinical studies of feverfew for migraine prevention have been mixed. A Cochrane review determined the evidence for feverfew in the prevention of migraines was inconclusive. In an updated review, results from a more recent study were included in the analysis. While this study showed a greater reduction in migraine attacks after 2–3 months of treatment with feverfew compared to placebo (difference of 0.6 attacks per month), the effects of feverfew need to be confirmed in larger scale trials using more rigorous designs. Feverfew is well-tolerated but has the potential to cause mild nausea and bloating. Mouth ulcers may occur if the plant leaves are chewed or a formula powdered with feverfew is administered and can be avoided by using tablet or encapsulated preparations. Avoid abrupt discontinuation of feverfew to prevent rebound headaches and other withdrawal symptoms including sleep disturbances, anxiety, and muscle soreness. Feverfew can induce uterine contractions and is contraindicated in pregnant women. Avoid concomitant use with antiplatelet agents, anticoagulants, or other substances that increase bleeding risk as feverfew may inhibit platelet activity.

Glucosamine and Chondroitin

Glucosamine is a highly utilized dietary supplement and often taken in combination with chondroitin for osteoarthritis. Both are naturally occurring components of cartilage and exert protective chondrocyte effects within articular joints. The clinical effects of glucosamine and chondroitin supplementation have been evaluated in numerous randomized controlled trials, meta-analyses, and Cochrane reviews with conflicting results. Additionally, reports of efficacy in certain industry-sponsored trials have raised concerns for publication bias. Overall, the evidence indicates a lack of efficacy for the treatment of knee osteoarthritis and large placebo effects. A subset of patients with moderate to severe knee osteoarthritis may experience analgesic efficacy with glucosamine and chondroitin; however, this benefit was not found to persist beyond 6 months of treatment. The ACR recommends against the use of glucosamine and/or chondroitin in the treatment of hip and knee osteoarthritis and conditionally recommends chondroitin as an option for hand osteoarthritis based on a single study showing a reduction in pain. Glucosamine sulfate was evaluated in chronic low back pain and did not show evidence of efficacy. Few adverse effects have been reported and include gastrointestinal disturbances. There are conflicting reports of glucosamine increasing glucose levels in people with diabetes. Increased glucose monitoring may be advisable in that patient population. Glucosamine and chondroitin, individually or in combination, may increase the effects of warfarin and should be avoided in patients treated with the anticoagulant.

Magnesium

Magnesium deficiency appears to be more common in patients with fibromyalgia and migraine headaches. Supplementation with magnesium has been shown to reduce the intensity of fibromyalgia symptoms and number of tender points. Magnesium supplementation initiated at ovulation and continued until the first day of menses benefited female subjects with menstrual migraines, as evidenced by a reduced number of days with migraine, decreased pain, and improved menstrual distress questionnaire scores. Studies assessing supplemental magnesium in adults with migraines showed 5–12 weeks of therapy reduced attack frequency and severity and, in one study, decreased the use of acute medications. Magnesium administered intravenously as an abortive migraine treatment and as a preventive agent has demonstrated conflicting results and may be better for patients not responding to oral magnesium, in those who have migraine with aura, or in people with low magnesium levels. It should be noted that varying formulations and doses of magnesium were utilized in individual clinical studies, and it is unclear if any one formula is superior. Magnesium supplementation is generally well-tolerated, although diarrhea may be experienced. People with kidney disease are at risk of excessive magnesium accumulation and toxicity. Toxic effects are rare and can include muscle weakness, respiratory paralysis, cardiac dysrhythmias, and hypotension.

Omega-3 Supplements

Omega-3 fatty acids have anti-inflammatory properties at high doses. Preparations containing eicosapentaenoic acid (EPA) and docosahexanoic acid (DHA) in combined doses of 2.7 g/day or more have been evaluated for efficacy in the treatment of rheumatoid arthritis. After 12–14 weeks of therapy, omega-3s improved the number of tender joints, the duration of morning stiffness, pain scores, and consumption of nonsteroidal anti-inflammatory drugs (NSAIDs). Evidence also suggests that 5.5 g/day of omega-3s for 1 year may slow the time to medication failure and decrease the time to remission in people with early-onset rheumatoid arthritis who are initiating oral disease-modifying antirheumatic drugs. Research suggests that omega-3 fatty acid doses exceeding 3 g/day can inhibit blood coagulation. The potential of high-dose omega-3s to increase the risk of bleeding should be considered in patients who take antiplatelet medications, anticoagulants, or other therapies that enhance bleed risk.

Vitamin B$_2$

Treatment with vitamin B$_2$ (riboflavin) may have a role in migraine prophylaxis due to its ability to improve mitochondrial metabolism because abnormalities in brain energy metabolism are suspected in some patients with migraine headache. Small-scale studies in adult patients demonstrated that riboflavin 400 mg/day in divided doses was better than placebo in reducing the frequency of migraines after 1–3 months of therapy and showed similar benefits with better tolerability compared to propranolol and valproate.

Vitamin B$_{12}$

Vitamin B$_{12}$ plays a role in nerve regeneration and nerve conduction velocity, and may have anti-inflammatory effects. Vitamin B$_{12}$ supplementation has been studied as a treatment in nerve crush injuries, back pain, and neuralgias. While treatment with vitamin B$_{12}$ has shown to reduce pain related to diabetic neuropathy, herpetic neuralgia, low back pain, nerve crush injuries, and chemotherapy-induced neuralgia, placebo-controlled studies are lacking. Vitamin B$_{12}$ is generally well-tolerated with few reported adverse events. Anaphylactic reactions have occurred with injectable vitamin B$_{12}$ formulations.

Willow Bark

Willow bark has been studied in the treatment of low back pain, joint pain, and arthritis. Salicin, a precursor to acetylsalicylic acid or aspirin, is one of the active constituents in willow bark; however, phenolic acids, flavonoids, and tannins are the components responsible for the anti-inflammatory and analgesic properties of the herb. Willow bark 120–240 mg/day for 4 weeks has shown to have dose-dependent effects in reducing lower back pain and the need for rescue medication. Early research indicates that willow bark is not effective for rheumatoid arthritis, is likely not effective for improving joint stiffness and function, and has conflicting results of efficacy for osteoarthritis pain. It is unknown if willow bark increases the risk of gastrointestinal bleeding or has antiplatelet effects in humans. People who are allergic to salicylates should not take willow bark.

CONCLUSION

Alpha lipoic acid could be recommended for this patient in combination with conventional glucose-lowering treatment as evidence suggests efficacy of the supplement in improving the many symptoms of diabetic neuropathy she is experiencing. Topical capsaicin can generally be considered as an adjunctive treatment in neuropathy; however, it will likely provide little benefit in this case because the symptoms are not localized.

We should recommend she purchase an ALA product with a verification symbol, such as USP Verified, on the label, indicating that quality criteria have been met. Reputable information about dietary supplements can be found on the National Center for Complementary and Integrative Health (NCCIH) Herbs at a Glance website or on the NCCIH mobile application HerbList. Monographs of dietary supplements can be searched in the

Natural Products Database of Lexicomp or through the Natural Medicines compendium.

Further Reading

MedlinePlus. Herbs and supplements. https://medlineplus.gov/druginfo/herb_All.html.

Memorial Sloan Kettering Cancer Center. About herbs, botanicals & other products. https://www.mskcc.org/cancer-care/diagnosis-treatment/symptom-management/integrative-medicine/herbs.

National Center for Complementary and Integrative Health. https://www.nccih.nih.gov/.

National Center for Complimentary and Integrative Health. Evidence-based medicine: Literature reviews. https://www.nccih.nih.gov/health/providers/litreviews.

US Pharmacopeial Convention. USP global public policy position ensuring the quality of dietary supplements. https://www.usp.org/sites/default/files/usp/document/about/public-policy/public-policy-dietary-supplements.pdf

US Food and Drug Administration. MedWatch online voluntary reporting form. https://www.accessdata.fda.gov/scripts/medwatch/index.cfm

17 Choosing the Opioid

Michelle Krichbaum and Neil Miransky

Case Study

FB is a 53-year-old woman with a 6-year history
of neuroendocrine pancreatic cancer. FB initially
presented with epigastric pain radiating posteriorly
to the back, uncontrolled on controlled-release (CR)
oral oxycodone 80 mg every 12 hours and immediate-
release oral oxycodone 30 mg four times daily as
needed for breakthrough pain. She describes the
pain as a severe, constant stabbing and aching. The
patient was initiated on oral methadone 5 mg every 12
hours, while continuing CR oxycodone. Her analgesic
regimen also includes oral gabapentin 600 mg every 8
hours. This was an effective technique for many years,
however FB had disease progression, including a
partial pancreatectomy, metastases to liver, and biliary
stenting secondary to full biliary obstruction. Due to
an increase in nociceptive pain, CR oxycodone 80 mg
was increased to every 8 hours. She was admitted for
uncontrolled emesis, which caused severe pernicious
anemia, weight loss, abdominal pain, and weakness.

What Do I Do Now?

When used appropriately, opioids are integral drugs in the palliative setting for pharmacological management of moderate to severe pain, dyspnea, diarrhea, as well as producing sedation. Rational selection includes not just the pharmacokinetic profile of the opioid, but character, intensity, and timing of the pain being treated. There may also need to be considerations for opioid conversion/rotation if administration routes change or safety and efficacy become a concern.

INDICATIONS

Opioids work primarily by agonizing mu opioid receptors in the central nervous system (CNS), gastrointestinal tract, and immune cells. This agonism at receptors throughout the body accounts for their side-effect profile, including sedation, constipation, endocrine dysfunction, immunosuppression, and respiratory depression that can lead to death.

Pain is the most common reason for initiating an opioid. While much concern regarding their overprescribing has dominated the healthcare landscape, opioids have an established role in the management of acute pain, cancer pain, postoperative pain, and in certain recurring acute on chronic pain conditions like sickle cell disease. Their mechanism of action in pain is by partial or full agonism of the mu opioid receptors in the CNS, leading to inactivation of the ascending and activation of the descending pain pathways.

While opioid overdose can lead to respiratory depression, low doses can be used to manage refractory shortness of breath and are the recommended first line in nearly all guidelines for end-stage management of dyspnea. Opioids decrease the sensitivity to carbon dioxide by agonism of mu and delta opioid receptors in the brainstem, and they also reduce the perception of dyspnea and its subsequent anxiety by mu opioid agonism in the limbic system.[1] While morphine has been considered the drug of choice to treat end-stage dyspnea, there is a paucity of evidence to state that it is superior to any other full mu agonist opioid.

Acute and chronic diarrhea can also be managed with opioids as mu agonism in the gut reduces motility. First-line therapy is the peripheral-acting opioid loperamide that also acts as an antisecretory. At therapeutic doses, loperamide does not cross the blood–brain barrier, but it can cause euphoria and severe cardiac symptoms at supratherapeutic doses. An additional first-line therapy is diphenoxylate/atropine, a combination centrally acting opioid with an anticholinergic to reduce its abuse potential. A second-line option is tincture of opium, which should be used cautiously as it contains morphine and alcohol.

Although the mechanism of the antitussive effects of opioids has been called into question, codeine and hydrocodone are commonly used agents for cough suppression because they are available in a liquid formulation. While the over-the-counter agent dextromethorphan is structurally related to codeine, it does not act on opioid receptors at therapeutic doses.

TYPE OF PAIN

The first consideration for using an opioid is assessment of the type of pain. Since most clinically utilized opioids have mu receptor agonism they can be used for nociceptive pain. Usually arising from tissue damage and often with an inflammatory component, the patient will complain of pain that is aching, dull, throbbing, or sharp.

Neuropathic pain results from damage to the peripheral or central nervous system and will be described as shooting stabbing, radiating, burning, or numbness. While opioids are often used to treat neuropathic pain, their efficacy is mixed.[2] Methadone, tapentadol, tramadol, and levorphanol have varying multimodal analgesic activity including N-methyl-D-aspartate (NMDA) receptor antagonism and norepinephrine reuptake inhibition in addition to mu opioid agonism, making them a potentially better choice if the patient has mixed characteristics of pain. Initially, when FB presented with epigastric pain radiating to her back, methadone was chosen for its neuropathic pain benefit. Increasing oxycodone would have been of limited benefit and may have incurred increased side effects. As she was using 120 mg of oxycodone for rescue throughout the day, this gave us a safe margin to initiate the methadone at a low dose.

Visceral pain is one of the most difficult types of pain to treat. It is a diffuse and poorly localized pain produced by disease of internal organs. It is often referred to other locations and accompanied by nausea and vomiting. Opioids can be used as part of a multidrug regimen to treat visceral pain, but they can cause hyperalgesia in this population, and initiating or increasing other adjuvants may provide better relief.[3]

TEMPORAL CONSIDERATIONS

While timing of medication administration is imperative to ensure pain control, the timing of the pain is equally vital to ensure dosage forms and formulations are selected appropriately. Considerations include if the pain is intermittent versus chronic, the expected duration of pain and if it will change in the near future (e.g., surgery), or if there are acute expected episodes of pain (e.g., wound care or physical therapy). Onset of action for oral opioids is 30–60 minutes, which may be too long to wait for severe acute pain, and a parenteral formulation may be chosen instead. Oral administration can be used for acute episodic pain secondary to procedures with proper education on the timing of the pretreatment of the analgesic. Long-acting oral formulations can be initiated in patients with chronic pain with limited expectation of improvement, such as cancer or sickle cell disease. When ordering opioids for breakthrough pain, it is important to remember the duration of action for most short-acting opioids is 3–5 hours, except for IV fentanyl which is only 30–60 minutes. Ordering as-needed opioids every 4–6 hours often leaves patients with uneven pain control.

ROUTE OF ADMINISTRATION

While most opioids are available in an oral dosage form, alternative administration may be preferred if there is severe emesis or dysphagia, an acute pain crisis, absorption issues secondary to short bowel syndrome, rapid onset of action is needed, or the oral route is unavailable.

In the case of FB, suffering from severe emesis with an increased intensity of pain, a continuous IV infusion of hydromorphone was initiated with a twice daily dose of methadone IV. Dose conversion from oral oxycodone to IV hydromorphone was initiated at 0.6 mg/hr with a dose reduction of approximately 25% due to incomplete cross-tolerance but the patient reporting uncontrolled pain. Methadone was administered at 2.5 mg IV every 12 hours based on an oral-to-parenteral ratio of 2:1. We based their opioid conversions on recommendations from *Demystifying Opioid*

Conversion Calculations: A Guide for Effective Dosing.[4] FB was also provided rescue doses of hydromorphone 1 mg as needed for moderate pain and 2 mg as needed for severe pain every 3 hours.

Subcutaneous administration can also be used in the palliative setting if the patient does not have intravenous access, and this is a less painful administration than intramuscular injections. One drawback is the limited volume that can be injected at one time with 1.5–2 mL recommended as the maximum due to increased pain. A subcutaneous continuous infusion can also be set up for patients to provide smoother pain control. Morphine, hydromorphone, and fentanyl can all be used subcutaneously, although, as increased doses are needed, hydromorphone has more concentrated doses allowing for less volume administered than fentanyl or morphine. Intramuscular injections should be avoided in the palliative setting due to pain and lack of pharmacokinetic advantage over other parenteral routes.

Sublingual and buccal routes avoid first-pass metabolism and have a theoretically faster onset of analgesia than oral administration; however, medications can be unpalatable or the patient may be unable to retain the drug in the mouth for several minutes. Hydrophilic drugs such as morphine, oxycodone, hydrocodone, and hydromorphone are poorly absorbed sublingually or buccally, and the actual benefit is likely due to the drug going down the back of the throat (i.e., "slow swallow"). Lipophilic drugs like fentanyl and methadone are better options sublingual or buccal administration due to superior absorption in the oral mucosa. Buprenorphine is commercially available in a buccal and sublingual dosage form.

Transdermal patches currently available include buprenorphine and fentanyl. They are best used for patients with continuous stable pain along with rescue short-acting opioids especially during the initial titration period. Fevers and heating pads/blankets increase skin temperature and therefore absorption, which may lead to toxic effects. These patches should be removed prior to magnetic resonance imaging. Direct heat (i.e., heating pad or electric blankets) should never be placed over opioid-containing transdermal patches.

The rectal route may also be considered with patients having bowel obstruction, malabsorption issues, or in patients with impaired neuromuscular function. Administration in the lower rectum bypasses first-pass metabolism, but there is considerable variation in bioavailability. The rectal route is not preferred for repeated dosing and may not be feasible if the patient is not admitted to a healthcare facility.

SPECIAL CONSIDERATIONS

Age: Tramadol and codeine are contraindicated in children younger than 12 years and tramadol is contraindicated in children younger than 18 years who have undergone tonsillectomy and/or adenoidectomy. Tramadol and codeine have active metabolites via the liver enzyme CYP2D6, and respiratory failure has occurred in children who were later found to be rapid metabolizers. Hydrocodone is a safer choice in children who need oral pain control.

Renal failure: Opioids of choice in renal failure are fentanyl, methadone, and buprenorphine. Tramadol and oxycodone can also be used with dose reductions once creatinine clearance (CrCl) is less than 30 mL/min and 60 mL/min, respectively. Morphine and hydromorphone have glucuronidated metabolites that are toxic in renal failure. There are limited data to give a renal dysfunction cutoff, but we prefer to dose reduce at CrCl less than 60 mL/min and avoid use once CrCl is less than 30 mL/min. Codeine and meperidine are not recommended.

Allergy: Most common adverse reactions to opioids are nausea, vomiting, or itching, which some patients may believe to be allergies. Codeine and its active metabolite morphine are the most notorious for these "reactions," which may be in part due to an excess of histamine release. If a true allergic reaction, such as a rash or anaphylaxis, occurs, knowing the chemical classes helps in picking alternate therapy. The phenanthrene group includes codeine, morphine, hydrocodone, hydromorphone, oxycodone, and oxymorphone so tolerability is likely similar for these drugs. If allergy occurs within this group, choosing from a different chemical class including phenylpiperidines (fentanyl, diphenoxylate, loperamide), diphenylheptanes (methadone), or phenylpropylamines (tramadol, tapentadol) has a low risk of cross-sensitivity.[5]

QTc prolongation: Methadone has dose-related QT prolongation, and an electrocardiogram is recommended before initiation and periodically for the duration of therapy. Buprenorphine has been thought to have cardiac risk, but a recent literature review suggests that buprenorphine, in the absence of other QT prolonging medications, does not produce a clinically significant prolonged QT interval. There has been concern with tramadol and possible QT prolongation, however this effect has mainly been found with IV doses (currently unavailable in the United States), supratherapeutic doses (>400 mg/day), or in patients with renal insufficiency. More recent data suggest tramadol has little risk for cardiac issues, but it should not be used in patients with a history of seizures.

SUBSTANCE ABUSE

Clinicians continue to have concerns about how to treat pain in patients with current or previous substance abuse. While some recommendations are for the partial agonist buprenorphine exclusively in the face of previous or suspected substance abuse, we disagree with this idea for those receiving palliative care. Buprenorphine has only partial mu opioid agonism and is unlikely to provide analgesic benefit in severe pain. Full mu opioid agonist should be used for the patient with severe pain, with risk mitigation strategies in place, including multidisciplinary care including an addiction specialist or psychiatrist. One risk mitigation strategy may be to use an opioid with a lower "likeability," such as short-acting morphine or hydrocodone. While there does not exist one single source for likeability ratings for the various opioid formulations, in trying to create an Opioid Attractiveness Technology Scale, Butler and colleagues found that subjective ratings of likeability and usability were highest with fentanyl patches, hydromorphone, and oxycodone ER.

> **KEY POINTS TO REMEMBER**
> - Selection of opioids should be based on character and timing of pain in addition to pharmacokinetic profiles.
> - Timing of rescue medications is important to prevent gaps in analgesia.

- All patients need to be risk-stratified when prescribing opioids.
- Naloxone should be made available by prescription or order set when prescribing opioids.

References

1. Mahler DA. Opioids for refractory dyspnea. *Exp Rev Respir Med.* 2013;7(2):123–135.
2. McNicol ED, Midbari A, Eisenberg E. Opioids for neuropathic pain. *Cochrane Database Systematic Rev.* 2013(8):CD006146. doi:10.1002/14651858.CD006146.pub2
3. Davis M. Drug management of visceral pain: concepts from basic research. *Pain Res Treat.* 2012;2012:265605. doi:10.1155/2012/265605. Epub 2012 Apr 24.
4. McPherson ML. *Demystifying Opioid Conversion Calculations: A Guide for Effective Dosing.* Bethesda: ASHP; 2014.
5. Fudin J. Chemical classes of opioids. Updated October 1, 2018. https://paindr.com/wp-content/uploads/2018/10/Opioid-Structural-Classes-Figure_-updated-2018Oct.pdf

Further Reading

Behzadi M, Joukar S, Beik A. Opioids and cardiac arrhythmia: a literature review. *Med Principles Pract.* 2018;27(5):401–414.

Butler SF, Butler SF, Fernandez KC, Benoit C, et al. Measuring attractiveness for abuse of prescription opioids. *Pain Med.* 2010;11(1):67–80.

Dean M. Opioids in renal failure and dialysis patients. *J Pain Sympt Manage.* 2004;28(5):497–504.

Keller GA, Etchegoyen MCV, Fernandez N, et al. Tramadol induced QTc-interval prolongation: Prevalence, clinical factors and correlation to plasma concentrations. *Curr Drug Safe.* 2016;11(3):206–214.

Law PY, Loh HH. Opioid receptors. In WJ. Lennarz, M. Daniel Lane (eds.). *Encyclopedia of Biological Chemistry.* New York: Elsevier: 2004; 167–171.

Lexicomp. Opium tincture. Lexi-Drugs. Lexicomp. Wolters Kluwer Health, Inc. Riverwoods, IL. http://online.lexi.com

Massarella J, Ariyawansa J, Natarajan J, et al. Tramadol hydrochloride at steady state lacks clinically relevant QTc interval increases in healthy adults. *Clin Pharmacol Drug Dev.* 2019;8(1):95–106.

Mercadante S, Fulfaro F. Alternatives to oral opioids for cancer pain. *Palliat Support Care.* 1999;13(2).

Reisfield GM, Wilson GR. Rational use of sublingual opioids in palliative medicine, *J Palliat Med.* 2007;10(2):465–475.

Usach I, Martinez R, Festini T, et al. Subcutaneous injection of drugs: Literature review of factors influencing pain sensation at the injection site. *Adv Ther.* 2019;36 (11):2986–2996.

Wightman R, Perrone J, Portelli I, et al. Likeability and abuse liability of commonly prescribed opioids. *J Med Toxicol.* 2012;8(4):335–340.

18 Methadone and Levorphanol

Amelia L. Persico, Erica L. Wegrzyn, and Jeffrey Fudin

Case Study

A 66-year-old man presents with chronic pain radiating from his lumbar spine through his right buttocks and to his toes bilaterally. He describes aching in his low back, burning and tingling in his right foot. A magnetic resonance imaging (MRI) study shows multilevel severe degenerative disc disease and foraminal stenosis. He states that he cannot stand for greater than 1 minute without the aid of his walker due to severe pain. All physical activities and sitting for extended periods of time exacerbate the pain. The patient has actively participated in physical therapy for chronic pain, utilizes a TENS unit three times per week with some benefit, and uses a heating pad nightly. His pharmacologic pain regimen is oral methadone 10 mg three times a day, oral gabapentin 300 mg three times a day, a lidocaine 5% patch applied to the low back every 12 hours, and oral acetaminophen 1,000 mg three times a day as needed. On chart review you note significant polypharmacy and multiple medical comorbidities including type 2 diabetes and stage 2 chronic kidney disease. His recent electrocardiogram showed a normal rhythm, with a QTc of 496 ms.

What Do I Do Now?

This patient's complaints are consistent with neuropathic and nociceptive pain. Reviewing his medication list, we see that he is on pain therapies that could manage both types of pain. For neuropathic pain, he is prescribed lidocaine patches and gabapentin. For both nociceptive and neuropathic pain he is prescribed methadone. Recall that methadone is unique among opioids due to its efficacy as a mu opioid receptor agonist, a norepinephrine and serotonin reuptake inhibitor, and an N-methyl-D-aspartate (NMDA) receptor antagonist. However, his pain remains uncontrolled. In this type of situation, we can consider dose titrations or therapy changes. Before approaching potential therapy changes or dose titrations, however, a significant safety concern is noted in this patient's chart that needs to be addressed. His QTc interval is nearing 500 ms. Current guidance recommends using a QTc interval of 450 ms as a cutoff for the safe use of methadone. Alternative therapy should be considered in patients with a prior QTc greater than 450 ms.

The relationship between methadone and prolonged QTc interval has been well described in the literature since the 1970s. Methadone (and the majority of other drug-induced causes of long QTc) causes a delay in cardiac myocyte action potential via inhibition of the cardiac ion channel KCNH2. The extended cardiac repolarization period is caused by electrolyte imbalances across cardiac myocyte membranes and can lead to torsade de pointes (TdP), polymorphic ventricular tachycardia, and sudden death. Furthermore, methadone serves as a negative chronotrope due to its anticholinergic properties, and bradycardia is an additional risk factor for prolonged QT interval. In addition to the risks of QTc interval prolongation, methadone has multiple drug-drug interactions owing to its metabolism through the cytochrome P450 enzyme system. In this patient with polypharmacy, transition to a therapy with fewer risks of pharmacokinetic interactions could be of benefit.

It is clear that it would be inappropriate to titrate this patient's dose of methadone given risk of TdP. However, he is experiencing loss of functionality and poor pain control, thus pharmacologic management of his neuropathic and nociceptive pain is clearly indicated. At this time cross-titration from methadone to levorphanol would be appropriate. Levorphanol is a frequently "forgotten opioid" with multiple safety advantages over methadone (see Table 18.1 for thorough comparison of levorphanol and methadone).

Levorphanol and methadone share the unique pharmacology of potent, full mu-opioid receptor agonism combined with inhibition of the reuptake of norepinephrine and serotonin as well as NMDA receptor blockade. Of note, methadone is a more potent serotonin reuptake inhibitor than levorphanol, and serotonin does not contribute to its antinociceptive activity. In addition to their overlapping pharmacology levorphanol is also a kappa opioid and delta opioid receptor agonist. Given their shared activity as mu opioid agonists, NMDA antagonists, and noradrenergic activity, both therapies reduce the perception of nociceptive and neuropathic pain; NMDA antagonism blocks the flood of glutamate associated with neuropathic pain from binding to NMDA receptors thus reducing neuropathic pain experience, and inhibiting the reuptake of norepinephrine leaves more norepinephrine available in neuronal synapses to bind alpha-2-adrenergic receptors. This has downstream effects of hyperpolarizing cell membranes and reducing excitability associated with neuropathic pain and hyperalgesia.

Despite their pharmacologic similarities there are significant pharmacokinetic and pharmacodynamic differences that make levorphanol a safer alternative to methadone for this patient (and many others). Levorphanol is metabolized via phase II metabolism, bypassing phase I, and thus is not subject to the significant pharmacokinetic drug interactions via cytochrome P450 metabolism as is methadone. For example, patients concomitantly prescribed methadone and an inducer of CYP2C19, 3A4, or 2D6 will exhibit decreased serum levels of methadone. Some studies have found evidence of methadone withdrawal in patients initiated on a potent inducer of these enzymes in the setting of ongoing methadone therapy. For this reason levorphanol is preferable in patients with polypharmacy on multiple medications that impact the cytochrome P450 system. Importantly, despite bypassing phase I metabolism, levorphanol is impacted by hepatic impairment because it is subject to glucuronidation (and then excreted renally). Thus, the product labeling recommends that caution is warranted in patients with severe hepatic insufficiency; increasing the dosing interval has also been suggested as a means of safely initiating levorphanol in patients with renal or hepatic impairment. Levorphanol is also not a substrate of P-glycoprotein (PgP), does not have a large and variable volume of distribution, and does not cause QTc prolongation, all significant attributes when considering opioid selection.

When transitioning this patient from methadone to levorphanol keep in mind that levorphanol has a half-life of 11–16 hours (analgesic duration of 6–15 hours), and methadone has a long and variable half life, with serum levels subject to variability based on genetic polymorphisms. Cross-titration should occur gradually and with regard to the prolonged half-life of methadone.

In regards to potential genetic polymorphisms, methadone is metabolized primarily by cytochrome P450 2C19, 2B6, and 2D6 in a stereospecific manner. 2C19 preferentially metabolizes the R-enantiomer, and 2B6 and 2D6 preferentially metabolize the S-enantiomer. S-methadone has a shorter half-life than R-methadone. CYP 3A4 also plays a role in methadone metabolism but demonstrates significantly less stereoselectivity.

This is of significant importance when considering risks of QTc interval prolongation that are attributable to accumulation of the S-enantiomer. S-methadone is cardiotoxic via blockage of the voltage-gated potassium channel of the human ether-a-go-go related gene (hERG). Notably, the R-enantiomer also blocks the voltage-gated potassium channel of hERG but is 2.5 times less potent than the S-enantiomer. This risk is present even in the absence of prolonged QTc interval at baseline. For example, if pharmacogenomic screening is available and a patient is found to be a poor metabolizer of 2B6, this would lead to accumulation of the S-enantiomer of methadone and increased risk of QTc interval prolongation and TdP. Although pharmacogenomic screening is not currently the standard of care prior to initiation of methadone, it is an important consideration in the setting of unexpected serum levels, cardiac risk, and multiple medication failures/intolerances.

A comparison of levorphanol and methadone is shown in the figure.

	Levorphanol	Methadone
Pharmacocolgy		
Opiod agonist activity	μ, δ, κ1, κ3] κ2	μ
NE reuptake inhibition	Weak	Weak
NMDA inhibition	Strong	Weak
Pharmacokinetics		
Bioavailability, Oral	Unknown	35–100%
Duration of action	6–15 hours	4–8 hours
Half-life	11–16 hours	15–60 hours
Metabolic pathway	Phase II glucuronidation to levorphanol-3-glucuronide	3A4-, 2B6-, 2C19-mediated N-demethylation to EDDP
Opioid chemistry	Dehydroxylated Phenanthrane	Diphenylheptane
Dosing		
Oral MED of 30 mg/day	4 mg	7.5 mg
Suggested starting dose in opioid naïve patients	1 mg (1/2 X 2-mg tablet) PO 3 or 4 times daily (maximum daily starting dose, 4 mg); titrate up by up to 25% weekly, i.e., if starting at 1mg PO 4 times daily in the first week, increase to 1 mg PO 5 times daily at second week	2.5 mg (1/2 X 5-mg tablet) PO three times daily (maximum daily starting dose, 7.5 mg); titrate up by upto 25% weekly, i.e., if starting at 2.5 mg PO 3 times daily first week, increase to 2.5 mg PO 4 or 5 times daily at second week (note: as the dose increases, percentage of upward titration decreases due to complex pharmacokinetics)
Routine monitoring	N/A	QTc (ECG preformed at least annually or as clinically indicated)

MOR, DOR, KOR = μ, δ, κ opioid receptor type, respectively; EEDDP = 2-ethylidene-1,5-methyl-3,3-diphenylpyrrolidene; NMDA = N-methy-D-asaparate; MED = morphine-equivalent dose; ECG = electrocardiogram. Refs. [15,19,20].

KEY POINTS TO REMEMBER

- Medication-related QTc prolongation is a cumulative risk. Multiple QTc prolonging agents in a medication regimen pharmacodynamically increase the risk of QTc prolongation.
- Methadone increases QTc interval in a dose-dependent manner.
- Preexisting electrolyte abnormalities increase the risk of QTc prolongation.
- Levorphanol is a mu opioid agonist, NMDA receptor antagonist, and reuptake inhibitor of norepinephrine with no known effect

on cardiac QT interval or enzymatic drug-drug interactions, limited if any risks of variable kinetics due to polymorphism, and absorption is not affected by P-glycoprotein inhibitors or inducers.

Further Reading

Ahmad T, Valentovic MA, Rankin GO. Effects of cytochrome P450 single nucleotide polymorphisms on methadone metabolism and pharmacodynamics. *Biochem Pharmacol*. 2018 July;153:196–204.

Gudin J, Fudin G, Nalamachu S. (2016) Levorphanol use: Past, present and future. *Postgrad Med*. 2016;128:1.

Gupta A, Lawrence AT, Krishnan K, Kavinsky CJ, Trohman RG Current concepts in the mechanisms and management of drug-induced QT prolongation and torsade de pointes. *Am Heart J*. 2007;153:891–899.

Nguyen U, Sparkes S. Unique levorphanol dodges move from forgotten to vanished. November 17th, 2015.PainDr. http://paindr.com/unique-levorphanol-dodges-move-from-forgotten-to-vanished

Pham TC, Fudin J, Raffa RB. Is levorphanol a better option than methadone? *Pain Med* September 2015;15(9):1673–1679.

Woosley RL, Heise CW, Gallo T, Tate J, Woosley D, Romero KA, www.CredibleMeds.org, QTdrugs List, [Accessed November 9, 2021], AZCERT, Inc. 1457 E. Desert Garden Dr., Tucson, AZ 85718.

Stimmel B, Lipski J, Swartz M, Donoso E. Electrocardiographic changes in heroins, methadone and multiple drug abuse: A postulated mechanism of sudden death in narcotic addicts. *Proc Natl Conf Methadone Treat*. 1973;1:706–710.

19 Mixed Agonist/Antagonist Opioids in the Treatment of Pain

Amanda Mullins

Case Study

A 65-year-old White man presents to the emergency department via ambulance after his wife found him on the kitchen floor with decreased consciousness and shallow breathing. He has a history of chronic obstructive pulmonary disease (COPD), and metastatic lung cancer diagnosed 5 years ago, with metastases to his spine and requires 3L of oxygen at home. He recently decided to forego chemotherapy and other curative treatment options and established care with an outpatient palliative care provider, but pain control has been difficult. He was admitted 2 months ago for intractable pain and methadone was started. His home medications include oral methadone 5 mg three times daily and oral dexamethasone 4 mg once daily. He was given intranasal naloxone in the ambulance, and his consciousness and breathing improved immediately; however, he is now with severe pain and rates his pain as a 10 out of 10 using the numeric rating scale. After regaining consciousness, he admits to taking an extra methadone tab because he was in such excruciating pain.

What Do I Do Now?

When considering your next step with regards to this patient case, it's important to consider why this overdose occurred in the first place. His methadone dose is fairly low, and he is on no other interacting medications that can easily explain his central nervous system (CNS) depression. However, he does have a history of chronic obstructive pulmonary disease (COPD), lung cancer, and requires baseline oxygen, which puts him at an increased risk of respiratory depression in combination with opioid therapy. Additionally, he was prescribed methadone for pain, a full mu opioid receptor (MOR) agonist. Full MOR agonists, such as methadone, morphine, and hydrocodone, are commonly used for pain management in palliative care and carry a theoretical increased risk of opioid-induced respiratory depression and other systemic side effects when compared with some other opioids, such as mixed agonist/antagonists.

Mixed agonist/antagonist opioid medications are those that have varying degrees of activity depending on which opioid receptor they are acting on. The four commonly thought of mixed agonist/antagonists are buprenorphine, pentazocine, butorphanol, and nalbuphine. While not available in the United States or Canada, dezocine is still frequently used in other countries for acute pain. Buprenorphine has partial agonist properties at the MOR and antagonist properties at both the kappa (KOR) and delta (DOR) opioid receptors. Pentazocine has partial agonist activity at the mu opioid receptor and full agonist activity at the kappa opioid receptor. Butorphanol has antagonist properties at the mu opioid receptor and partial agonist activity at the kappa opioid receptor. Finally, nalbuphine has antagonist properties at the mu opioid receptor and agonist properties at the kappa opioid receptor. In addition to being classified as mixed agonist/antagonist opioids, buprenorphine, pentazocine, and butorphanol are also classified as partial agonists. These characteristics are summarized in Table 19.1. Partial agonists can exhibit pain relief similar to full mu opioid receptor agonists, but have a lower risk of causing adverse effects, such as respiratory depression. Furthermore, these agents also carry a concern for a dose-related ceiling effect for pain relief, often limiting the ability to continuously up-titrate doses, but data supporting this phenomenon are controversial. Even so, mixed agonists/antagonists probably have a specific niche in pain management and should not be initiated without regards to these concerns.

TABLE 19.1 **Properties of mixed agonist/antagonists**

Mixed agonist/ antagonist	Mu opioid receptor	Kappa opioid receptor	Delta opioid receptor
Buprenorphine*	Partial agonist	Antagonist	Antagonist
Pentazocine*	Partial agonist	Agonist	N/A
Butorphanol*	Antagonist	Partial agonist	N/A
Nalbuphine	Antagonist	Agonist	N/A

*Also considered a partial agonist.

At this point, you may be ready to give this patient a partial agonist, such as buprenorphine, and send him on his way, but it's possible he would return to the hospital complaining of diarrhea, rhinorrhea, and a collection of other potential symptoms as you may have caused him to experience precipitated withdrawal. Timing of administration of mixed agonist/antagonists is crucial in providing a smooth transition of therapy for these patients. If given too soon after a full agonist, a mixed agonist/antagonist has the potential to cause the full MOR agonist to dissociate from the opioid receptor, causing a sudden and uncomfortable shift in pain and onset of withdrawal symptoms.

In order to appropriately transition an individual between full agonists, such as methadone in our patient's case, to a mixed agonist/antagonist, we must consider the patient's current state of withdrawal along with the pharmacodynamic properties of the mixed agonist/antagonist being started. If a mixed agonist/antagonist is warranted, careful consideration must be given to each agent with regards to effectiveness, tolerability, drug interactions, cost, drug delivery systems, and formulary availability, especially if the patient is enrolled in hospice services. A brief review of each of these agents will help to appropriately transition this patient. Table 19.2 demonstrates rudimentary information for consideration for each of these drugs.

Buprenorphine, perhaps the most commonly prescribed mixed agonist/antagonist, has very high binding affinity for the mu opioid receptor. It also displays high binding affinity for the delta and kappa opioid receptors, where it acts as an antagonist. Buprenorphine also exhibits agonist properties with low binding affinity at the opioid receptor-like 1 receptor, a receptor

TABLE 19.2 **Characteristics of mixed agonists/antagonists**

Mixed agonist/antagonist	Available formulations	Control schedule
Buprenorphine	IV, IM, TD, Buccal film	CIII
Pentazocine[a]	IV, IM, SUBQ, PO	CIV[b]
Butorphanol	IV, IM, Nasal	CIV
Nalbuphine	IV, IM, SUBQ	N/A[c]

TD, transdermal; IV, intravenous; IM, intramuscular; SUBQ, subcutaneous

[a]Pentazocine is also available as three separate tablet products, one in combination with acetaminophen, one with aspirin, and the other with naloxone.

[b]Some states, including Illinois and South Carolina (injectable only), classify pentazocine as a CII. Kentucky classifies pentazocine as a CIII.

[c]Kentucky classifies nalbuphine as a CIV.

thought to be responsible for attenuating the effect of buprenorphine on the mu opioid receptor. What does this all mean? Buprenorphine's very high binding affinity at the MOR will likely displace any other opioid currently occupying those receptors, assuming a lower binding affinity, and may precipitate withdrawal if you're not careful.

In our case, buprenorphine may be a good choice to transition to because of the lower risk of respiratory depression, especially coupled with this patient's COPD and lung cancer. Additionally, we know that increasing this patient's methadone dose may cause him to experience another unintentional overdose, as witnessed by his wife earlier. This risk would remain constant with any other full MOR agonist as well. Buprenorphine will also provide substantial pain relief and is available as a patch, sublingual (SL) film, SL tablet, and injection, contributing to its ease of use in the community and will avoid any potential swallowing issues in the future. Furthermore, we may be able to initiate buprenorphine more easily at this time as the patient was already given naloxone in the ambulance. Although this may benefit our ability to transition this patient to buprenorphine, it will not always make transitioning to a mixed agonist/antagonist more straightforward. While the naloxone has displaced methadone from the mu receptors, as evidenced by this patient's return to consciousness, we must act quickly and administer buprenorphine as soon as possible should this be the intended direction of therapy. If we wait too long, the methadone in the patient's system may have the opportunity to rebind to the mu opioid receptors, leading to one of two potential outcomes. First, the patient may return to an overdosed state as before. Second, we will likely precipitate withdrawal if we give him buprenorphine after the methadone rebinds.

WHY DOES METHADONE REBIND TO OPIOID RECEPTORS AFTER NALOXONE IS GIVEN?

One critical component to keep in mind is which medication the patient is being transitioned from. For example, our patient was on methadone prior to his presentation to the emergency department. Even though he was given naloxone in the ambulance, we must consider methadone's pharmacokinetic properties and predict the next 24 hours of this patient's course. While our patient is currently conscious and breathing on his own, it is quite possible that he may fall back into an overdosed state as soon as the naloxone wears off and the methadone still in his system rebinds to his opioid receptors. The ability of an opioid to rebind to the opioid receptors after the naloxone dissociates *mainly* depends on its half-life and most often will be a problem with methadone and long-acting or controlled-release formulations of opioids. Phillips et al. describes a case of initiating buprenorphine therapy after elective naloxone-induced opioid withdrawal.

WHY DOES ADMINISTERING BUPRENORPHINE PRECIPITATE WITHDRAWAL IF THE METHADONE IS ABLE TO REBIND TO THE OPIOID RECEPTORS?

As previously mentioned, another concern for predicting a patient's course after naloxone administration is binding affinity. Binding affinity can be described as the attraction between a drug and the receptor and is frequently denoted as the dissociation constant, or "K_i." Those with higher binding affinities will create a stronger bond with its receptor, and those with lower binding affinities will be left waiting for those drugs with higher affinities to dissociate. Table 19.3 demonstrates the binding affinity of each of the mixed agonist/antagonists discussed here, along with opioid antagonists,

TABLE 19.3 **Relative affinity of select opioid agonists and antagonists to the mu opioid receptor**

Medication	Ki (nM) Value
Buprenorphine	0.216
Butorphanol	0.762
Naltrexone	1
Fentanyl	1.346
Methadone	3.378
Naloxone	1.1
Morphine	1.168
Nalbuphine	2.118
Pentazocine	117.8

Drugs listed in boldface are mixed agonist/antagonists; italicized drugs are opioid antagonists.

such as naloxone, and full MOR agonists, such as methadone. In general, the lower the K_i value a drug possesses, the stronger receptor affinity it displays. Drugs with a higher binding affinity will displace drugs with a lower binding affinity from the receptors. If a drug with a higher binding affinity is not a full opioid agonist, it may precipitate withdrawal if given after full MOR agonists. Pay careful attention to which medications are likely to displace others, as this concept is imperative when timing the initial administration of these medications.

Pentazocine, butorphanol, and nalbuphine may all be reasonable options for this patient in the emergency department setting, but would be less than ideal once he leaves the hospital and transitions care back to his community providers. If choosing to use one of these medications, then consideration regarding timing of administration is still critical. The same thought process that was outlined for buprenorphine administration should be followed for pentazocine, butorphanol, and nalbuphine.

In our patient case example, now would be a perfect time to initiate buprenorphine for pain management. He has already been given naloxone in the ambulance and is still in precipitated withdrawal, evidenced by his consciousness and severe pain. For ease of transition of care back to the community after discharge from the emergency department, I recommend ordering a sublingual or buccal formulation. Administering buprenorphine via one of these routes should provide pain relief within 30–60 minutes, if not sooner. A typical starting dose of the sublingual tablet is 2–4 mg. If after about 60 minutes his pain is not well controlled, he can be redosed if needed with another 2 mg. This process can be repeated until a dose sufficient to control his pain is reached. Total daily doses ranging from 4 to 16 mg, given in 3–4 divided doses, have been described in the literature.

Choosing to initiate medication therapy with a mixed agonist/antagonist can be a difficult and frightening task for those not familiar with certain pharmacokinetic and pharmacodynamic concepts. This chapter is meant to supply you with the foundational knowledge necessary to make the transition from full mu opioid receptor agonists to mixed agonist/antagonists as easily and smoothly as possible. Mixed agonist/antagonists are appropriate options for pain management in a palliative care population, specifically for those with substantial risk factors for unintentional overdoses, such as coexisting pulmonary disease, drug interactions, or other general intolerability of full mu opioid receptor agonists. All palliative care providers should be aware of these concepts to best assist their patients when there seems to be no other option for pain relief.

KEY POINTS TO REMEMBER

- Full agonists carry a higher risk of respiratory depression compared with partial agonists.
- Buprenorphine, pentazocine, butorphanol, and nalbuphine are all classified as mixed agonists/antagonists.
- Buprenorphine, pentazocine, and butorphanol are further classified as partial agonists.
- If a mixed agonist/antagonist has a higher binding affinity than a full agonist, it will cause the full agonist to disassociate from the opioid receptor and can cause precipitated withdrawal.

- Naloxone may not reverse opioid-induced respiratory depression if the opioid has a higher binding affinity (lower K$_i$ value) than naloxone.
- Route of administration is important when choosing a mixed agonist/antagonist for pain management.

Further Reading

Buprenorphine (Butrans) [Prescribing Information]. Stamford, CT: Purdue Pharma L.P.; 2014.

Butorphanol [Prescribing Information]. Bedford, OH: Bedford Laboratories; 2001.

DEA Diversion Control Division. Controlled Substance Schedules. https://www.deadiversion.usdoj.gov/schedules/orangebook/c_cs_alpha.pdf

Gudin J, Fudin J. A narrative pharmacological review on buprenorphine: A unique opioid for the treatment of chronic pain. *Pain Therapeutics*. 2020;9(1):41–54.

Herndon CM, Arnstein P, Darnall B, et al. *Principles of Analgesic Use*. 7th ed. Glenville, IL: American Pain Society. 2016.

Jones KF. Buprenorphine use in palliative care. J Hospice Palliat Nurs. 2019;21(6):540–547.

Nalbuphine [Prescribing Information]. Chestnut Ridge, NY: Par Pharmaceutical; 2016.

Pentazocine-naloxone [Prescribing Information]. Bridgewater, NJ: Sanofi-aventis U.S. LLC; 2011.

Phillips RH, Salzman M, Haroz R, et al. Elective naloxone-induced opioid withdrawal for rapid initiation of medication-assisted treatment of opioid use disorder. *Ann Emerg Med*. 2019 September;74(3):430–432.

Quill TE, Bower KA, Holloway RG, et al. *Primer of Palliative Care*. 7th ed. Chicago: American Academy of Hospice and Palliative Medicine. 2019.

Raynor K, Kong H, Chen Y, et al. Pharmacological characterization of the cloned kappa-, delta-, and mu- opioid receptors. *Mol Pharmacol*. February 1994;45(2):330–334.

Tam SW. (+)-[³H]SKF 10,047, (+)-[³H]ethylketocyclazocine, μ, κ, δ and phencyclidine binding sites in guinea pig brain membranes. *Eur J Pharmacol*. February 1985;109(1):33–41.

Volpe DA, Tobin GAM, Mellon RD, et al. Uniform assessment and ranking of opioid mu receptor binding constants for selected opioid drugs. *Regulatory Toxicol Pharmacol*. 2011;59:385–390.

20 Opioid-Induced Constipation

Jayne Pawasauskas

Case Study

MJ is a 56-year-old white woman who has been referred to the palliative care clinic for continuing management of her chronic pain and symptoms resulting from an automobile accident approximately 3 years ago. She presently describes the pain as being sufficiently controlled (pain ratings of 4 out of 10) by her regimen of extended-release oral morphine 60 mg twice daily, as-needed oxycodone 5 mg, and oral ibuprofen 400 mg three times daily. She currently reports signs and symptoms of constipation, which have occurred since starting her opioid regimen approximately 2 years ago. MJ reports difficulty and straining during defecation and dry, hard feces but denies any blood in the stool. She states that she has approximately one spontaneous bowel movement (BM) per week and must use laxatives to induce a BM. She currently takes oral bisacodyl 5 mg daily and oral polyethylene glycol 17 g daily. Previously she tried psyllium fiber (Metamucil), lactulose, and linaclotide.

What Do I Do Now?

Opioid-induced constipation (OIC) is a common occurrence in patients who use opioids regularly or chronically and should therefore be considered whenever a patient is given a prescription for an opioid analgesic. OIC is more common in women, older patients, and those with longer durations of opioid use.[1] Opioid analgesics are known to exert beneficial effects on different opioid receptors, namely the mu, kappa, and delta receptors, in terms of providing analgesic relief. However, these receptors are also known to have sites within the gastrointestinal (GI) system, and opioid analgesic binding at these sites creates unwanted adverse effects. Physiologically, the binding of opioid agonist analgesics to these receptor sites within the GI tract causes impairments in motility of intestinal contents, increased fluid absorption from bowel contents, increased nonpropulsive intestinal contractions, and increased anal sphincter tone.[2,3] *Opioid bowel dysfunction* is a term that describes a larger set of GI symptoms that may result from opioid use, including gastroesophageal reflux, nausea, vomiting, bloating, abdominal pain, and constipation. However, constipation is the most commonly reported GI effect of opioids. When assessing for constipation clinically, most methods subjectively measure number of bowel movements and associated symptoms (i.e., straining), or the quality of stool produced. The latter is often assessed by use of the Bristol Stool Form.[4]

DIAGNOSIS

To aid in correct diagnosis of OIC, the Rome criteria was revised in 2016 to address constipation that is specifically caused by the use of opioid analgesic medications.[5] In this scenario, the patient must have new or worsening constipation following the start or alteration of opioid therapy which includes at least two of the following findings: at least 25% of BMs associated with symptoms of straining, lumpy or hard stools (indicated by a score of 1–2 on the Bristol Stool Form), sensation of incomplete evacuation, sensation of obstruction or blockage, use of manual maneuvers to aid evacuation, or fewer than three spontaneous BMs per week. Loose stools should only be noted when laxatives are used.

MANAGEMENT

Most patients whose pain management regimen includes opioid analgesics should be counseled about the likelihood of developing constipation. Patients may attempt lifestyle modifications to manage their constipation, including increased fluid and dietary fiber intake or exercise. However, these approaches are not proved to be as effective for OIC, and increased exercise may not be possible for many patients with chronic pain. Patients may consider switching to a different opioid or a different route of administration. For example, transdermal opioids have been associated with lower rates of constipation compared to those administered orally.[2,3]

LAXATIVES

Laxatives are recommended for initial prevention of OIC, with either increasing doses or use of alternate bowel agents upon OIC occurrence.[3] The term "laxative" is used in a general sense to refer to any medication that assists with passage of a BM and typically refers to stimulants, stool softeners, lubricants, and osmotic agents. These are largely available without prescription, are generally considered safe, and are less expensive than prescription options.

The stool softener docusate is commonly used for constipation, although there is little evidence of its efficacy as a monotherapy approach. The drug's surfactant properties lower the surface tension of feces, thereby allowing water and lipids to penetrate the stool. This softens the stool contents and aims to enhance spontaneous defecation. Docusate can require up to 3 days of use before an effect is seen and should therefore not be used as monotherapy if rapid passage of a BM is desired. Senna and bisacodyl exert their effects by irritating nerve endings within the intestinal lumen, causing a stimulation of colonic motility. Both of these are expected to produce a BM within 6–12 hours, and patients may report abdominal pain, cramping, or discomfort.

Polyethylene glycol, magnesium salts (hydroxide or citrate), and lactulose are osmotic laxatives that improve stool fluid absorption. These may be especially helpful for patients reporting lower scores on the Bristol Stool

Form. Up to 4 days of use of polyethylene glycol may be required before improvement is seen, whereas magnesium salts often produce an effect within a few hours. Lactulose typically produces an effect within 1–2 days, and should be used cautiously in patients with diabetes due to lactose and galactose contents. Last, mineral oil is a lubricant that will soften the stool when used orally and lubricate the lower intestinal lining when administered rectally. Rectal enema formulations of mineral oil have been shown to produce a BM within minutes after administration.

MJ is currently using a combination of stool softener and stimulant laxatives, which is a common approach to preventing OIC. Her history indicates that she has also tried other approaches, including linaclotide. Unfortunately, linaclotide is used for management of chronic idiopathic constipation (CIC) or irritable bowel syndrome with constipation (IBS-C). Although it acts on intestinal luminal surface epithelium to stimulate secretion of chloride and bicarbonate into the intestinal lumen, it is not recommended for management of OIC, and its use should be restricted to CIC or IBS-C. Similarly, the use of psyllium or fiber-based laxatives is not supported in OIC based on the pathophysiologic mechanisms by which opioid analgesics produce constipation.

There are no compelling data to show superiority of a particular laxative over another; however, stimulant and osmotic-type laxatives have the most evidence of efficacy in studies of OIC. Patients should have tried a combination regimen of laxatives before escalation of therapy. It has also been suggested in the most recent guidelines that at least one of the laxative doses be taken in a scheduled manner, rather than used as needed, for at least 2 to 3 weeks.[3] For patients whose OIC persists despite these laxative recommendations, escalation to prescription therapies may be needed. The Bowel Function Index (BFI) is a validated, three-question tool that assesses the patient's severity of symptoms.[1] Using this tool, patients provide a numeric score on a 0–100 scale in response to three questions about their bowel function. The questions ask about ease of defecation, feeling of incomplete bowel evacuation, and overall self-assessed constipation rating. The response scores are averaged to generate a total score. Previous utilization and evaluation of this tool has considered a score of 30 or more to indicate inadequate response to laxatives and likelihood of benefitting from prescription therapy. This tool is simple and brief and may be utilized in various settings.

PRESCRIPTION THERAPIES FOR OIC

Prescription therapies may include lubiprostone (Amitiza), methylnaltrexone (Relistor), naloxegol (Movantik), or naldemedine (Symproic). Lubiprostone acts as an activator of epithelial CIC-2 chloride channels, which increases transport of fluid to the intestinal lumen. Initially this medication was used for CIC or IBS-C; however, it later gained approval of the US Food and Drug Administration (FDA) for use in OIC associated with chronic, non-cancer pain. The drug shows modest improvement in OIC symptoms compared with placebo, with more patients producing a BM within 24 hours after administration of lubiprostone. Across studies, patients reported improvements in OIC symptoms such as straining, discomfort, overall symptom severity, and consistency of the stool. This medication should be dosed as 24 µg orally twice daily and taken with food. The dose of lubiprostone should be adjusted for patients with hepatic dysfunction, and its effectiveness when administered to patients also taking diphenylheptane opioids (i.e., methadone) is diminished. In addition to common adverse effects that are gastrointestinal in nature (i.e., nausea, diarrhea, abdominal pain), lubiprostone may cause a syndrome of dyspnea and chest tightness. This typically occurs 30–60 minutes after the first dose and may recur with subsequent doses. Patients should be informed about these symptoms, and some will discontinue therapy as a result. The current guidelines make no recommendation for the use of lubiprostone in OIC, citing low-quality evidence to support its use.[3]

PERIPHERALLY ACTING MU RECEPTOR ANTAGONISTS

A class of medications referred to as PAMORAs, or peripherally acting mu receptor antagonists, has demonstrated efficacy in treating OIC that is refractory to laxative use. PAMORAs are medications that will bind to mu opioid receptors located within the GI tract to inhibit their ability to affect GI function. Each of the medications within this class has a unique chemical structure that impairs its absorption or transport into the central nervous system (CNS), as distribution of an opioid receptor antagonist to the CNS could reverse analgesic effects of opioid analgesics and precipitate withdrawal. When used as recommended, PAMORAs will remain within the GI tract and exert their opioid antagonistic effects locally. In general, PAMORAs should not be used for any patient with a known or suspected bowel obstruction. Their adverse-effect profile includes discomfort, diarrhea, flatulence, nausea, or abdominal pain, which may be severe.

The first of this class to become available was a subcutaneous injection of methylnaltrexone for use in patients with advanced illness and OIC. Dosing for this indication is weight-based, with administration every other day. This is a notable clinical finding, as most of the prescription therapies for OIC have been mostly evaluated (and FDA-approved) for use in patients with chronic, non-cancer pain (CNCP). In addition, methylnaltrexone is the only PAMORA currently available in an injectable formulation, which may be an advantage for some patients. Studies of the subcutaneous formulation found a significant number of patients who could produce a BM within 4 hours after administration. Later, methylnaltrexone acquired an indication for CNCP, which utilizes a daily subcutaneous regimen of 12 mg. More recently, an oral formulation of this medication for CNCP became available. Recommended dosing is 450 mg orally once daily, to be taken in the morning approximately 30 minutes before the first meal of the day. The dose should be reduced for patients with reduced creatinine clearance (≤60 mL/min) or moderate to severe hepatic impairment.

Naloxegol is a derivative of the opioid receptor antagonist naloxone and utilizes a pegylated structure to prevent crossing the blood–brain barrier. Current guidelines give a strong recommendation for naloxegol based on available evidence. The typical dose of naloxegol is 25 mg orally daily, and it should be taken 1 hour before the first meal of the day or 2 hours afterward. For patients with intolerable adverse effects (abdominal pain, nausea, diarrhea), a lower dose of 12.5 mg is recommended. This lower dose should also be used in patients with creatinine clearance of less than 60 mL/min. A potential factor limiting the use of naloxegol is its drug interaction profile. As a substrate of the P450 enzyme 3A4, concurrent use with 3A4 inhibitors should be evaluated: its use concurrently with strong 3A4 inhibitors or inducers is not recommended. For patients taking moderate 3A4 inhibitors (i.e., diltiazem, verapamil, erythromycin) who are deemed to benefit from naloxegol, a reduced daily dosage of 12.5 mg is recommended. Patients should be instructed not to consume grapefruits or grapefruit juice while taking naloxegol.

Naldemedine is the final medication in the class of PAMORAs and has a strong recommendation for use in refractory OIC in current guidelines. The recommendation is based on the quantity and quality of studies evaluating its use in CNCP. Naldemedine should be dosed as 0.2 mg once daily and may be administered without regard to food. It should not be used in patients with severe hepatic impairment or those taking strong 3A4 inhibitors as naldemedine is a substrate of this P450 metabolic pathway. Patients taking moderate 3A4 or P-glycoprotein inhibitors should be monitored for adverse effects.

In general it is recommended to discontinue laxatives prior to the start of lubiprostone or a PAMORA to be able to best evaluate the effectiveness of the prescription therapy and limit adverse effects. Once a patient begins OIC management with a prescription therapy, they may begin to add back laxatives. All of the prescription therapies should be avoided in any patient with known or suspected bowel obstruction due to the risk for perforation. Cost will be an issue with prescription therapies and clinical decisions should take into account the affordability for patients in the outpatient setting. There are no strong data comparing efficacy of the prescription therapies for OIC against each other. Furthermore, most of the studies of prescription therapies which showed efficacy required patients to be stable on their pain regimens, and this should be a consideration when beginning therapy with one of these more expensive approaches.

The patient MJ has used laxative approaches, including combinations, and continues to experience signs and symptoms consistent with OIC. She should discontinue use of laxatives and begin a trial period with a PAMORA. Naloxegol or naldemedine would be recommended initially, due to the strength of literature support.[3] However, if MJ was concurrently taking a strong 3A4 inhibitor medication or was to begin on in the future, these medications would be contraindicated for her. Her progress can be assessed utilizing the BFI and self-reported symptoms.

KEY POINTS TO REMEMBER

- Opioids cause constipation, and patients should take medications to prevent and treat its occurrence.

- Laxatives are first-line recommendations for opioid-induced constipation.
- Of the PAMORAs, naloxegol and naldemedine have the strongest recommendations for use from the American Gastrointestinal Association guidelines.
- Drug-drug interactions should be taken into account when prescribing therapies for OIC.
- Patients should assess their constipation symptoms by use of the Bristol Stool Form and Bowel Function Index.

References
1. Argoff CE, Brennan MJ, Camilleri M, et al. Consensus recommendations on initiating prescription therapies for opioid-induced constipation. *Pain Med.* 2015;16:2324–2337.
2. Muller-Lissner S, Bassotti G, Coffin B, et al. Opioid-induced constipation and bowel dysfunction: a clinical guideline. *Pain Med.* 2017;18:1838–1863.
3. Crockett SD, Greer KB, Heidelbaugh JJ, Falck-Ytter Y, Hanson BJ, Sultan S on behalf of the American Gastroenterological Association Institute Clinical Guidelines Committee. American Gastroenterological Association Institute guideline on the medical management of opioid-induced constipation. *Gastroenterology.* 2019;156:218–226.
4. Lewis SJ, Heaton KW. Stool form scale used as a useful guide to intestinal transit time. *Scand J Gastroenterol.* 1997 September;32(9):920–924.
5. Lacy BE, Mearin F, Chang L, Chey WD, Lembo AJ, Simren M, Spiller R. Bowel disorders. *Gastroenterology.* 2016;150:1393–1407.

21 Opioid Side Effects: Central Nervous System

Elise Fazio and Dominic Moore

Case Study

AS is a 36-year-old man with extensive squamous cell carcinoma of his face. By the time he was diagnosed, the cancer had eroded through much of his facial soft tissue and had destroyed his facial bones. As a result of the destruction, he required a tracheostomy and a percutaneous endoscopic gastrostomy (PEG) tube for administration of artificial nutrition. Palliative treatment with cemiplimab-rwlc was initiated as he was no longer a candidate for curative surgery or radiation. A few days after his most recent discharge, his family found him unresponsive at home and called 911. He was found to be somnolent and hypoxic by the emergency medical crew and was started on supplemental oxygen. In the emergency department, he required spontaneous pressure support with supplemental oxygen. Urine toxicology was positive for opioids. A computed tomography scan of his head and chest x-ray did not show any acute findings. On exam, he does not arouse to voice or sternal rub. He is saturating at 95% on the ventilator using an FIO_2 of 30%. Blood pressure is 100/60. Heart rate is 75, and respiratory rate is 10. You are asked to see him in the ER to make further recommendations to his treatment plan as you are his palliative care provider.

What Do I Do Now?

Recognizing and managing the side effects of opioids can be a challenging task in palliative care. Patients often carry complex diagnoses with complicated treatment plans and have frequently changing health status. In addition, prescribers face intense scrutiny when prescribing opiates in the midst of an opioid crisis. The goal of this chapter is to help providers recognize and treat the central nervous system (CNS) side effects of opioids. We will review the basic pharmacology of opioids, explore the various CNS side effects, and discuss a management plan for the patient listed in the example case scenario. Although there is rarely a single right or wrong answer, the fundamentals presented in this chapter can guide you in creating an appropriate treatment plan.

Opioids are a powerful tool to manage a variety of symptoms: dyspnea, acute/post-op/traumatic pain, cancer related pain, diarrhea suppression, and cough suppression. The benefits and side effects of opioids are directly related to the various opioid receptors. This section will mention the most clinically relevant receptors. The mu opioid receptors are most responsible for the analgesic effects of opioids. These receptors are located within the CNS and peripheral nervous system (PNS) in differing concentrations. Also called OP3 or MOR (morphine opioid receptors), the Mu-1 receptor is located within the forebrain, midbrain, brainstem, and spinal cord and is responsible for the analgesic and euphoric effects. The M2 receptor is in the same location and is responsible for additional effects, including respiratory depression, physical dependence, anorexia, and sedation. The second opioid receptor, kappa, also called OP2 or KOR (kappa opioid receptor), is located within the brainstem and spinal cord as well as the limbic system. It is therefore involved with the dysphoric effects of opioids, including hallucinations. It also has a role in facilitating respiratory depression, sedation, and dependence. Last, the delta receptor, also called OP1 or DOR (delta opioid receptor) is located throughout the CNS and PNS and is most closely related to cardiovascular and respiratory depression.

With the basic pharmacology of opioids in mind, providers can anticipate the intended therapeutic effects as well as the unintended, undesired effects. Knowledge of these central side effects of opioids is essential in the care of palliative patients. They range from common, less severe symptoms such as drowsiness and sedation to rare, more severe effects such as neurotoxicity and respiratory depression. When appropriate dosing is followed, providers will often see that the severe effects are usually preceded by the less severe ones. For example, patients often note that hyperreflexia precedes myoclonus and sedation precedes respiratory depression. When more mild adverse effects manifest, prescribers should modify a treatment plan in order to avoid development of more serious effects.

General approaches to the management of adverse effects of opioids should guide providers working through CNS issues. These include dose reduction, symptomatic management with additional medications, opioid rotation, and cessation of opioid administration. The development of adverse effects from opioids should always guide clinicians to weigh the treatment risks against the expected benefits. Tolerance to most of the CNS side effects develops within a few days to a week after starting an opioid. The most important exception to this rule is respiratory depression, which is dose related (i.e., the higher the opioid dose, the more likely it is to illicit respiratory depression) and may increase with time on the medication. A prescriber can avoid this risk by instituting the "start low and go slow" rule when initiating an opioid prescription. After initiation, the clinician must monitor the patient closely for development of side effects.

The incidence of the most common CNS side effects is in the range of 15–25%. These include impacts on sleep, executive functioning, and mood. Sedation, drowsiness, and sleep disturbance usually subside within a few days of starting opioids. Make sure opioids are administered at the suggested starting doses, with lower doses for the elderly or compromised patients, and then increase the opioid as necessary. As a last resort, psychostimulants are useful for the treatment of opioid-induced sedation and include caffeine, modafinil, dextroamphetamine, and methylphenidate. These carry their own side effects, so it is imperative to discuss the reasons for initiating these additional drugs (opioid-induced sedation) and reasons for stopping them (appetite suppression associated with weight loss). Providers should assess for other causes of sedation, including the concomitant use of other sedating medications, sleep deprivation, systemic illness, metabolic disturbance, and CNS pathology.

Dysphoria, delirium, confusion, hallucinations, and restlessness can also be reported by patients. Overall, they can cause cognitive impairment, interfering with the thinking process and ability to react. These symptoms will usually abate after a reduction of the dose or switching to another opioid. It is useful to distinguish mental clouding caused by opioid-induced sedation from mental clouding caused by delirium. Always remember that psychostimulants will improve these symptoms in the former case but will worsen them in the latter.

The most severe adverse effects are also the rarest, occurring at an incidence of about 1%. These include the direct toxic effects of opioids on neurons including hyperalgesia, opioid-induced neurotoxicity (OIN), and, most importantly, overdose and death. Because of the severity of these effects, we will discuss recognition and management in detail.

Hyperalgesia is defined as increased sensitivity to a painful stimulus and should be considered when paradoxical pain increases with increased dose. This results in a lowering of pain threshold, clinically manifested as apparent opioid tolerance, worsening pain despite accelerating opioid doses, and abnormal pain symptoms, such as allodynia. A patient may report that the specific region of pain initially described becomes a more generalized pain and hurts "everywhere." Even light touch may elicit pain. This symptom, like many other CNS side effects of opioid use, usually improves with a dose reduction or opioid rotation.

Hyperalgesia can be part of a constellation of symptoms present in OIN. This is a CNS excitation syndrome with neuropsychiatric effects including hyperreflexia, myoclonus, cognitive impairment, hyperalgesia, agitation, delirium, and tonic-clonic seizures. These effects can exist independently or in combination. OIN may occur due toxic metabolite accumulation, which increases with higher doses or renal failure. Morphine is the most common culprit, followed by hydromorphone. The first sign is usually myoclonus and can be detected by regular monitoring of deep tendon reflexes as hyperreflexia precedes myoclonus. Be aware that this can be confused with "benign nocturnal myoclonus," a normal phenomenon consisting of a sudden jumping of seemingly the whole body during periods of drowsiness. This may be reported by family observing the active dying of a loved one. Gentle reassurance of family, after ruling out OIN, is always recommended.

Predisposing factors to the development of OIN include high doses, rapid escalation of dose, extended treatment, reduction in analgesic need, dehydration, renal failure, infection, preexisting cognitive impairment, older age, other psychoactive drugs (benzodiazepines), and metabolic abnormality. One objective way to assess for risk of developing OIN is to monitor urine output as most neurotoxic opioid metabolites are renally excreted. Fentanyl and methadone are unique in this respect, since their renally cleared metabolites tend to be non-neurotoxic.

If OIN is suspected, the fundamentals of management include quick recognition, treatment of any reversible contributing causes, dose reduction, discontinuation of long-acting medication and continuing short-acting only, discontinuing the opioid altogether, and opioid rotation. When renal failure is present, opioid rotation, dose reduction, and discontinuation of long-acting medication often resolve OIN. Rotation to an N-methyl-D-aspartate (NMDA) antagonist for pain management, such as ketamine or methadone, is another specific option. For mild opioid-induced myoclonus symptoms, you can explain the phenomenon to the patient and carefully monitor for worsening. If the myoclonus does worsen and there is concern for inadequate pain management if the opioid is reduced or discontinued, addition of a benzodiazepine (first line) or alternatives (gabapentin, baclofen) has proved effective. Last, non-opioid analgesics should be utilized effectively in order to reduce the amount of opioid required. Even nonpharmacologic methods such as nerve block or intrathecal delivery of an opioid can be warranted in severe cases of OIN.

Overdose is the most important and serious adverse effect of opioids. Respiratory depression, bradycardia, and hypotension make up the triad in an overdose. This is important to distinguish from the isolated effect of *somnolence*, a nonlethal side effect. Somnolence is managed with close observation and does not require intervention with a reversal agent such as naloxone. Only once the patient has low oxygen saturation, hypotension, and respiratory depression should it be treated as an overdose. According to various studies, overdose occurs at an incidence ranging from less than 1% to 5% per year for those on chronic opioids. Of note, these statistics do not differentiate between overdose due to illicit opioids versus prescription opioids or a combination of both. This risk is greatly lowered when the prescriber and patient follow standard dosing guidelines. Adverse CNS effects of opioids appear to occur in a dose-dependent fashion. There are differing estimates of this risk, but recent literature has demonstrated an 8.9-fold increase among patients prescribed more than 100 morphine milliequivalents (MME)/day (relative to patients on opioid regimens of less than 20 mg) and a 3.7-fold increase among patients prescribed more than 50 MMEs/day.

Management of overdose is simple but requires clear thinking on the part of providers and patients. First, stop further opioid administration temporarily and review all medications given. Overdose related to benzodiazepines will not respond to naloxone. Second, administer naloxone and continue administration with repeated doses until stabilized. Observation should be for 4 hours, at least. Once the patient is stable and alert, a thorough evaluation should be undertaken before resuming opioids. Of note, this process is different for the imminently dying patient. Providers should be aware that they will likely create more distress for patients, families, and staff with overly aggressive administration of naloxone to a terminal patient resulting in a withdrawal syndrome. Watchful waiting is often all that is warranted in the actively dying patient.

The recommended dose of naloxone differs for treatment of overdose depending on the opiates. Overdose from full agonists like fentanyl and morphine (fast dissociation kinetics) can reverse with a single dose of naloxone, while overdose involving partial agonists such as buprenorphine (slow dissociation kinetics) often requires a naloxone infusion. Most palliative patients do not receive buprenorphine for pain management, but some may use buprenorphine for medication-assisted treatment. Therefore, it is still important to know the different management strategies of specific opioid overdose.

Diluted naloxone for suspected overdose should be administered to avoid a withdrawal syndrome, at a concentration of 0.4 mg in 10 mL of saline given as 1 mL boluses every 1–2 minutes until the patient is breathing appropriately. Due to the short half-life of naloxone in comparison to most opioids, a repeated dose may be needed. Once the patient is stable and alert, the provider and team need to determine what led to the overdose and make necessary adjustments before resuming opioids, if that is deemed appropriate.

The problem of overdose exists in the context of the current opioid crisis and the general "opi-phobia" that both prescribers and patients exhibit. Prescribers should keep a few key points in mind when prescribing opioids for the palliative care patient population. First, malignant pain and dyspnea secondary to advanced cardiorespiratory illness are well studied and appropriate indications for the use of opioids. Second, it is important to follow guidelines for initiating an opioid and for the subsequent monitoring of its effectiveness as well as side effects. Finally, use of proper and clear terminology is crucial when using these medications. Opiates are naturally occurring alkaloids, such as morphine or codeine. "Opioid" is the term used broadly to describe all compounds that work at the opioid receptor. "Narcotic" is a term originally used to describe medications for sleep and is now used to describe drugs that are abused. *Tolerance* and *dependence* are expected physiologic responses following initiation of an opioid. *Addiction* is the persistent misuse of opioids for their nontherapeutic effects. Describing medications using their appropriate names rather than "narcotic" will help reassure our patients about the safety and appropriateness of prescribing practices.

It's time to revisit AS, the patient in our case study. The palliative care team, who had been seeing him for months, was asked to come to the bedside to discuss goals of care with the family. Upon arrival to the bedside, the patient was somnolent, lacked capacity, and was dependent on a ventilator. The medical team had no reason yet to explain his altered mental status and respiratory depression based on his laboratory and diagnostic studies. He had no evidence of metastases to his lung or brain, intracranial hemorrhage, pneumonia, seizures, or sepsis. Suspecting a possible overdose, 0.4 mg of diluted naloxone was ordered. His symptoms improved after the entire bolus (10 mL) had been administered, and he no longer required any respiratory support. He was admitted to the ICU for close monitoring. Overdose was initially overlooked, and his clinical presentation was attributed to his end-stage cancer diagnosis. This case highlights the importance of evaluating every possible differential diagnosis when treating the palliative care patient.

The patient later disclosed that his pain had spiked after a recent washout of an oral abscess. He had made the decision to take 16 mg of short-acting hydromorphone rather than 4 mg. He denied suicidal ideation, stating he still had a relatively good quality of life. He thought it was safe to take more than the recommended dose of hydromorphone without consulting his prescribing physician. A frank discussion followed, along with a revision of his medication regimen and follow-up plan. His pain and clinical status both improved with close follow-up over the next several weeks.

In summary, clinicians are responsible for discussing potential risks of chronic opioid therapy with patients considering this treatment option. Despite increased use of opioids for management of pain, there remain large gaps in understanding the basic physiology, efficacy, and side effects of opioid medications, particularly when used over long periods of times. By observing the fundamentals of opioid prescribing and management of the CNS side effects, providers can empower patients to live as comfortably as possible so that they do not have to struggle with the challenges of serious illness.

KEY POINTS TO REMEMBER

- Opioids are a powerful tool to manage a variety of symptoms related to advanced illness, such as dyspnea and cancer-related pain.
- Opioid receptors are located throughout the CNS and, as such, carry a wide range of side effects.
- Common side effects include drowsiness, sleep disturbance, and sedation.
- Rare effects include hyperalgesia, opioid-induced neurotoxicity, and overdose.
- Management of CNS side effects include dose reduction, symptomatic management with additional medications, opioid rotation, and cessation of opioid administration.
- Suspected overdose demonstrated by bradycardia, hypotension, and hypoxia is treated with naloxone.
- The development of adverse effects from opioids should always guide clinicians to weigh the treatment risks against the expected benefits.

Further Reading

Alford D, Compton P, Samet J. Acute pain management for patients receiving maintenance methadone or buprenorphine therapy. *Ann Intern Med.* 2006;144:127–134.

Baldini A, Von Korff M, Lin EHB. A review of potential adverse effects of long-term opioid therapy: A practitioner's guide. *Primary Care Companion for CNS Disorders.* 2012;14(3):PCC.11m01326.

Bodtke S, Ligon K. *Hospice and Palliative Medicine Handbook: A Clinical Guide.* Seattle: CreatSpace Independent Publishing; 2/24/16.

Boom M, Niesters M, Sarton E. Non-analgesic effects of opioids: Opioid induced respiratory depression. *Curr Pharmaceuti Design.* 18(37):5994–6004.

Chen Q, Larochelle MR, Weaver DT. Prevention of prescription opioid misuse and projected overdose deaths in the United States. *JAMA Network Open.* 2019;2(2):e187621. doi:10.1001/jamanetworkopen.2018.7621

Trescot A, Datta S, Lee M, Hansen H. Opioid pharmacology. *Pain Physician J.* 2008;Opioid Special Issue 11:S133–S153.

Vella-Brincat J, MacLeod AD. Adverse effects of opioids on the central nervous systems of palliative care patients. *J Pain Palliat Care Pharmacother.* 2007;21(1):15–25.

Zacharoff KL, Pujol LM, Corsini E. *A Pocket Guide to Pain Management*, 4th ed. Irvine: Inflexion; 2010.

22 Non-Gastrointestinal/Central Nervous System Side Effects of Opioid Analgesics

Gary Houchard and Justin Kullgren

Case Study

HK is a 52-year-old man recently diagnosed with stage II colon cancer. He is reporting moderate to severe upper quadrant pain for which he was started on hydromorphone 2 mg by mouth every 4 hours as needed after failing a trial of over-the-counter analgesics. This is HK's first time using an opioid. Although his pain has improved from an 8/10 to a 4/10 with hydromorphone, HK is now describing intense itching on his face and arms. No other signs or symptoms occur along with the itching. HK is reporting occasional nausea, loss of appetite, and a 15-pound weight loss over 2 months. His last bowel movement was 2 days ago. Other medical problems include hypertension and type 2 diabetes, and he currently takes hydrochlorothiazide, sennosides, lisinopril, atorvastatin, metformin, and metoprolol. HK endorses 3–4 doses of hydromorphone daily.

What Do I Do Now?

PRURITUS

Pruritus is commonly defined as an unpleasant sensation resulting in the need to scratch. Pruritus has many causes, one of which is opioids. Pruritus occurs in approximately 10–50% of patients administered systemic opioids, though is much more common with neuraxial administration (20–100%). Opioid-induced pruritus (OIP) is commonly recognized in acute pain, such as surgery or childbirth, and can contribute to the patient's overall symptom burden. Although OIP is less common than other opioid side effects, it is still critical for the palliative care clinician to have a framework with which to approach treating a patient with OIP.

The itch associated with OIP is believed to primarily be a result of a centrally produced event that results in the need to scratch. Several mechanisms for OIP have been proposed. Animal models and increasing data point to a central mu opioid receptor (MOR)-mediated process. In addition to the MOR, central serotonin 5-HT$_3$ receptors have been implicated in OIP. Mast cell destabilization leading to histamine release from systemically administered codeine or morphine is proposed to contribute to a possible peripheral component of OIP. Histamine's role in OIP has not been well substantiated in studies or clinical practice. Dopamine D$_2$ receptors, prostaglandins, and gamma-aminobutyric acid (GABA) receptors have also been studied as potential causes of or contributing factors to OIP.

Management of OIP can be separated into two categories—treatment and prevention. Most available data are on prevention of OIP in patients receiving neuraxial opioids for either surgery or obstetrics. These clinical scenarios are less likely to be managed by palliative care clinicians and thus will only be briefly discussed. The opioid antagonists (naloxone) or mixed opioid agonists-antagonists (nalbuphine) appear to be the most effective agents at preventing OIP from neuraxial opioids. Utilization of an opioid antagonist or mixed opioid agonist-antagonist warrants close monitoring for worsening pain as well as opioid withdrawal. Ondansetron, a 5-HT$_3$ receptor antagonist, has also shown promise for decreasing the incidence of OIP from neuraxial opioids.

Medications studied for the treatment of documented OIP include propofol, nalbuphine, ondansetron, naloxone, and rifampicin. Of these medications, nalbuphine, naloxone, and ondansetron have been most studied.

Nalbuphine was found to be effective and well tolerated in doses ranging from 2 to 4 mg, with doses at or higher than 4–5 mg risking decreased analgesia. Ondansetron in doses ranging from 4 to 8 mg have shown positive results for managing OIP associated with intrathecal morphine. Since much of the positive data for nalbuphine and ondansetron was seen in post-caesarean or surgical patients receiving intrathecal morphine, caution is warranted when extrapolating to patients with life-limiting illness taking systemic opioids. Robust data supporting the use of antihistamines for OIP are lacking, yet this practice remains common. Uncertainty remains if the benefit of first-generation antihistamines results from direct effects on histamine or as a result of sedation. The risk of additive sedation must be considered when using antihistamines and opioids concomitantly. Though data are difficult to find to support the following approach, either lowering the dose or rotating to a different opioid is a treatment option for OIP and may benefit our patient, HK.

OIP is an adverse effect that more commonly occurs with either intrathecal or epidural opioids compared to systemic opioid administration. OIP is likely caused by a central effect on the MOR, with other possible contributing factors including central serotoninergic receptors and a peripheral histamine pathway. Utilization of naloxone or nalbuphine for the prevention and/or treatment of intraspinal morphine has shown the most promise. Treatment of OIP caused by systemically administered opioids is less straightforward. Naloxone and nalbuphine may be beneficial, though their use is limited by their mode of administration. Ondansetron is a consideration, particularly in patients with concomitant nausea or vomiting. Antihistamines have long been taught as a viable treatment option, though data and experience do not support this approach as being consistently effective. HK presents with significant pruritus following initiation of oral hydromorphone. Based on HK's medical history and the timing of the symptoms he is very likely experiencing OIP. In this scenario, since an opioid (hydromorphone) has proved effective yet is causing significant OIP, the authors would recommend an opioid rotation to oxycodone.

IMMUNOSUPPRESSION

The role of opioids in human immune functioning has long been an area of interest for researchers. As early as the late nineteenth century, experimental studies established an inhibitory effect of opium administration on phagocyte activity both in vivo and in vitro. Following these initial findings, significant research has demonstrated the inhibition of various human immune pathways in vitro, and in vivo in animals as well. Still, the impact of this immunomodulation in humans remains uncertain and will require more robust investigations to determine the clinical implications of long-term opioids' effects on the immune system.

The immunomodulating effect of exogenous opioids stems from the role of endogenous opioids in normal human immune functioning. Endogenous opioid peptides, including beta-endorphin, met- and leu-enkephalins, and dynorphins, are active regulators of immune homeostasis. This is evidenced by the presence of opioid receptors on various immune cells, including macrophages and T cells. While the exact mechanism has not been fully elucidated, the role of endogenous opioids in maintaining immune homeostasis via both the innate and adaptive immune systems has been demonstrated in numerous studies.

Exogenous opioids can modulate the innate immune system through various mechanisms. Each component of the innate immune response, including macrophages, neutrophils, natural killer cells, mast cells, and dendritic cells, can be impaired to some degree by opioids. For example, morphine exhibits an inhibitory effect on macrophage proliferation, chemotaxis, and phagocytosis. In addition to its effect on macrophages, morphine causes immune dysfunction in numerous other areas, including inhibition of cytokine production, mucosal barrier integrity, and antigen presentation.

Exogenous opioids also appear to have a deleterious effect on the cells of the adaptive immune system, potentially reducing its ability to respond to previously encountered antigens. T lymphocytes, the primary component of the adaptive immune system, express all three types of opioid receptors (mu, kappa, and delta), with prolonged opioid exposure shown to upregulate the expression of these receptors on the cell surface.[13] The pharmacodynamic differences between mu, kappa, and delta binding remains unclear, so opioids may have variable effects based on receptor binding properties and activity.

Despite the evidence suggesting a significant role for opioids in human immunology, the clinical impact of chronic use remains unclear. While a correlation between opportunistic infections and chronic opioid use has been established, significant confounders exist in the study population, primarily composed of patients with opioid use disorder. A causative relationship is difficult to establish in a population where poverty, needle sharing, and other factors known to increase the incidence of infection are so pervasive. Consequently, further research is needed to examine the effect of opioid selection, dose, duration, and indication on rates of infection in this population; thus, the clinical implications and treatment of opioid-induced immunosuppression remain unclear.

ENDOCRINE

Opioid-induced hypogonadism remains one of the most common adverse effects associated with long-term opioid use. With many factors influencing the degree of endocrine dysfunction, including dose and duration of use, the prevalence of hypogonadism reportedly ranges from 21% to 86% in patients on chronic opioids. This disruption can result in numerous distressing adverse effects for patients, including fatigue, depression, infertility, and erectile dysfunction in men, with reduced libido and amenorrhea occurring in women. Although symptoms become more pronounced with long-term opioid use, hormonal disturbances have been shown to occur following a single dose. While hormonal dysregulation may occur with relatively little opioid exposure, a heightened risk of clinical hypogonadism has been associated with daily doses of morphine exceeding 100 mg.

Both endogenous and exogenous opioids can directly regulate human endocrine function via opioid receptors on the hypothalamus and pituitary gland. Downstream effects include modulation of both the hypothalamic-pituitary-adrenal (HPA) and hypothalamic-pituitary-gonadal (HPG) axes. Opioid-induced dysregulation of the HPG axis inhibits the production of luteinizing hormone, follicle stimulating hormone, and testosterone, whereas HPA dysregulation reduces cortisol levels and impairs the adrenal response to corticotrophin releasing hormone (CRH).

Studies investigating the long-term effects of opioids on thyroid function have been conflicting. Although exogenous opioids can suppress hypothalamic release of thyroid releasing hormone (TRH), which consequently results in decreased production of thyroid stimulating hormone (TSH), the clinical significance of this appears to be minimal. In one study of 50 opioid-addicted patients, there was no difference in serum T4 and TSH concentrations compared to control, although a slight but significant increase in T3 was observed. However, a second study of patients receiving intrathecal opioids for an average duration of 3.6 years found no such aberrations. Based on current evidence, thyroid function testing should only be recommended if otherwise clinically indicated.

Testosterone replacement therapy has shown benefit in men experiencing intolerable adverse effects related to opioid-induced hypogonadism. Testosterone supplementation was associated with significant improvement in libido and mood among 90 patients on chronic opioid therapy. Furthermore, a large cohort study of more than 21,000 patients found a significant reduction in all-cause mortality as well as reduced incidence of major cardiovascular events, anemia, and femoral and hip fracture among chronic opioid users receiving testosterone replacement. While this may be a reasonable treatment approach for patients with opioid-induced hypogonadism, randomized controlled trials are needed to further elucidate the long-term risks and benefits of testosterone replacement in this population. Increased monitoring of free testosterone levels may be reasonable in patients receiving long-term opioids in excess of 100 morphine milligram equivalents (MME) due to the increased prevalence of hypogonadism observed at these doses.

BONE MINERAL DENSITY

An increased risk of bone fracture has been associated with chronic opioid exposure. While this correlation has historically been attributed to cognitive and psychomotor disturbances leading to increased fall risk, increased bone fragility may also play a large role. Research into males receiving chronic opioid therapy has identified a significant reduction in bone mineral density in this population, thought to be related to opioid-induced androgen deficiency interfering with normal bone remodeling processes. One study examining 140 patients on long-term opioid replacement therapy (ORT) found that approximately 75% of patients had clinical osteoporosis or osteopenia. Although age was positively correlated with low bone density, subgroup analysis of patients under the age of 40 showed an uncharacteristically high prevalence of osteoporosis and osteopenia compared to controls (65.8% vs. 41.7%).

While there is a lack of guidance for bone density monitoring in patients on long-term opioids, it may be reasonable to follow the recommended monitoring parameters for patients with clinical hypogonadism. Guidelines released by the National Osteoporosis Foundation (NOF) identify hypogonadism as a risk factor for osteoporosis, suggesting bone density testing every 2 years in this population. Given the high prevalence of hypogonadism associated with chronic opioid use, particularly with doses exceeding 100 MME, biannual screenings in these patients is also advised. Testosterone replacement therapy has been shown to reduce the incidence of hip and femur fracture in chronic opioid users and may be an effective risk reduction strategy in male patients, although long-term data are lacking and risks versus benefits must be carefully weighed. Although estrogen has shown benefit in treatment of postmenopausal osteoporosis, serious cardiovascular adverse effects have limited its use in this population and may show a similarly unacceptable risk-benefit profile in opioid-induced osteoporosis. Pharmacologic intervention with other treatments of osteoporosis approved by the US Food and Drug Administration (FDA), such as bisphosphonates and calcitonin, may be reasonable alternatives in the appropriate clinical setting.

HK returns to clinic with well-controlled pain after rotation from hydromorphone to oxycodone. The pruritus has improved, though HK is now reporting worsening energy and libido over the past 3 months. HK asks about potential causes and how to treat it.

While reduced energy and libido may be related to HK's advanced disease, it may also be a sign of opioid-induced hypogonadism, which can be determined via a serum free testosterone level. If results indicate low testosterone, HK may see symptomatic improvement with testosterone replacement therapy. Testosterone replacement therapy has been shown to increase mood and libido for patients on long-term opioids while also reducing the risk of fracture. Prior to treatment initiation, it is important to discuss the potential risks and benefits of treatment in the context of HK's individual prognosis.

KEY POINTS TO REMEMBER

- Opioid-induced pruritus (OIP) is a poorly understood adverse effect that may significantly impact patient quality of life.
- OIP can be either treated or prevented with a number of treatment modalities, including opioid antagonists, partial agonists, and serotonin antagonists.
- Opioid modulation of the endocrine symptom is complex, and symptoms of hypogonadism should be judiciously monitored.
- Opioids may contribute to immunosuppression, although data from well controlled studies are largely lacking.

References

1. Gozashti MH, Mohammadzadeh E, Divsalar K, et al. The effect of opium addiction on thyroid function tests. *J Diabetes Metab Dis.* 2014;13(1):1–5.
2. Jannuzzi RG. Nalbuphine for treatment of opioid-induced pruritus: A systematic review of literature. *Clin J Pain.* 2016 January; 32(1):87–93
3. Blick G, Khera M, Bhattacharya RK, et al. Testosterone replacement therapy outcomes among opioid users: The Testim Registry in the United States (TRiUS). *Pain Med.* 2012;13(5): 688–698.
4. Gotthardt F, Huber C, Thierfelder C, et al. Bone mineral density and its determinants in men with opioid dependence. *J Bone Mineral Metab.* 2017;35(1):99–107.
5. Palm S, Moenig H, Maier C. Effects of oral treatment with sustained release morphine tablets on hypothalamic-pituitary-adrenal axis. *Methods Findings Exp Clin Pharmacol.* 1997;19(4):269–273.

Further Reading

Ganesh A, Maxwell LG. Pathophysiology and management of opioid-induced pruritus. *Drugs.* 2007;67(16):2323–2333.

Kumar K, Sing SI. Neuraxial opioid-induced pruritus: An update. *J Anaesthesiol Clin Pharmacol.* 2013 July;29(3):303–307.

Roy S, Ninkovic J, Banerjee S, et al. Opioid drug abuse and modulation of immune function: consequences in the susceptibility to opportunistic infections. *J Neuroimmune Pharmacol.* 2011;6(4):442–465.

Jasuja GK Ameli O, Reisman JI, et al. Health outcomes among long-term opioid users with testosterone prescription in the Veterans Health Administration. *JAMA Network Open*. 2019;2(12):e1917141–e1917141.

Watts NB, Lewiecki EM, Miller PD, et al. National Osteoporosis Foundation 2008 Clinician's Guide to Prevention and Treatment of Osteoporosis and the World Health Organization Fracture Risk Assessment Tool (FRAX): What they mean to the bone densitometrist and bone technologist. *J Clin Densitometry*. 2008;11(4):473–477.

23 Opioid Tolerance and Hyperalgesia

Sandra DiScala and Christine M. Vartan

Case Study

TJ is a 67-year-old Hispanic man who presented to the ED with uncontrolled back pain radiating to buttocks and hips, worsening for several weeks. Work-up revealed multiple metastatic lesions in his lumbar spine, pelvis region, and brain area with a primary cancer site being the lung. His other past medical history is significant for chronic kidney disease stage IV, type 2 diabetes, hyperlipidemia, insomnia, post-laminectomy syndrome of lumbar spine, hypertension, anemia, falls, and prior marijuana smoker. Goals were to stabilize pain and then be discharged to home hospice. TJ was admitted to the hospice unit on controlled-release morphine, which was titrated for pain control. The patient had immediate-release morphine as needed for pain. Sustained-release morphine was steadily increased over a 2-week period to a total daily dose of 400 mg, with improvement in pain. Several days later, nursing reports hallucinations, myoclonic jerking, and uncontrolled pain. Additionally, TJ reports that his legs are very painful even to the slightest touch during daily care.

What Do I Do Now?

As a hospice clinician contributing to the care of this case, the urgency to control and manage the recent development of myoclonus and uncontrolled pain is a priority. The comorbid brain metastases cannot be ruled out as a reason for the recent jerking activity, but comorbid chronic kidney disease (CKD), along with scheduled morphine sulfate also is to a causality risk factor to consider as well. Morphine sulfate SA was dosed at 45 mg orally twice daily on admission, and, over the course of 2 weeks, was increased to 200 mg orally twice daily with improved pain control. No further labs were desired per hospice goals of care, therefore recent renal function was not available to the clinician. Upper and lower extremity twitching and jerking similar to myoclonus was observed during hospice rounds. Opioid use is intended to result in an analgesic effect, however there is also a potential for tolerance or even opioid-induced hyperalgesia (OIH) to occur. It is important to distinguish that tolerance and OIH are different. *Tolerance* is a decreased response to the effect of the opioid over time without a change in the underlying cause of pain.[1] OIH is a pro-nociceptive process that leads to an increased sensitization resulting in more pain related to opioid treatment or increased opioid dosage.[1–3] Opioid metabolites can also contribute to hyperalgesia, and having a keen sense of observation to identify physical manifestations that display hyperalgesia is crucial to the hospice clinician. Morphine is primarily metabolized by glucuronidation in the liver that is catalyzed by UDP-glucuronosyltransferase (UGT) 2B7 resulting in an approximate ratio of 5:1 morphine-3-glucuronide (M3G) to morphine-6-glucuronide (M6G) metabolites.[4] The M3G metabolite is the morphine metabolite which does not contribute to analgesia but does have adverse effects such as myoclonus, seizures, and allodynia.[4] The M6G is a metabolite that displays more potent analgesia in comparison to the parent drug morphine.[4]

While the exact mechanism of OIH is not known, there are several theories regarding its development. One theory is the activation of the central glutaminergic system, in which N-methyl-D-aspartate (NMDA) receptors activate. In this theory, the glutamate transport system becomes inhibited, resulting in more glutamate availability; with the continued administration of morphine, this can result in neurotoxicity.[5] Morphine has also been described through a cross-talk mechanism in which b-arrestin2 is dissociated from the transient receptor potential family V1 channel (TRPV1), leading to increased thermal sensitivity of the receptor and a potential pathway for OIH.[1] Another theory is the spinal dynorphin mechanism, in which an increase in spinal dynorphin levels occurs with continued use of mu opioid agonists, resulting in more spinal excitatory neuropeptides and therefore increased nociception.[5] Descending facilitation is one theory where activity by some neurons in the rostral ventromedial medulla may result in nociception. While mammalian target of rapamycin (mTOR) is usually found to be inactive, another theory illustrates that continued use of morphine activates mu opioid receptors, resulting in mTOR activation. This leads to protein translation and thereby nociception, OIH, and tolerance.[6] Genetic influence may play a role in OIH as well. In this theory, the enzyme catechol-o-methyltransferase (COMT) may have three genotypes of polymorphism which may affect central pain modulation.[2] Additionally, the glial cell theory indicates that when opioids are given, this activates glial cells (particularly microglia and astrocytes), which results in pro-inflammation and, ultimately, an increase in neuronal excitability leading to increased nociception.[7]

There is no formal diagnostic criteria for OIH. Instead, clinicians can assess the patient in other ways to determine if OIH is occurring. First, it is important to determine if other factors may be contributing to the patient's worsening pain, such as whether the patient is having progression of their condition or if the pain is a result of an injury. The invasiveness of an evaluation would depend on the patient's preference for care and must be in line with their goals of care. One key point is that OIH may present as a more generalized pain (compared to the patient's original condition) that cannot be explained by other causes. Patients may experience *allodynia*, which is pain from a typically nonpainful stimulus. Additionally, while tolerance can be managed with an opioid dose increase, patients with OIH may actually experience worsening pain with an increase in opioid dose.[1,3,8,9] In the case of TJ, his pain was originally located in the back, and, although his pain was managed initially, the increase in the morphine dose resulted in the patient developing allodynia (which was located in his legs, not the area of his original pain report) and his current pain regimen was inadequate to control his pain. Given that the opioid was ineffective at a higher dose, this would not indicate tolerance, but rather OIH.

Methods to manage OIH include opioid dose reduction, opioid tapering to discontinuation, addition of non-opioid medication(s) that may result in an opioid-sparing effect, or opioid rotation. Methadone specifically has been shown to be helpful in OIH, likely due to its antagonism at the NMDA receptor. Examples of adjuvant agents that may help mitigate OIH include use of acetaminophen, dexmedetomidine, clonidine, gabapentinoids, intravenous lidocaine, NMDA receptor antagonists, nonsteroidal anti-inflammatory drugs (NSAIDs), or steroids.[1-3,9] Choice of agent may depend on patient acceptance, institutional formulary, product availability, clinician comfort and/or experience with prescribing, and institutional restrictions on appropriate setting for medication administration. In this case, an opioid rotation to methadone was selected to eliminate the issue with concerns for accumulation of morphine metabolites resulting in toxic effects (myoclonus, seizures, and hallucinations) given the setting of CKD and also to abate OIH and allodynia. The patient had developed dysphagia; however, nursing confirmed the patient's ability to swallow and therefore a concentrated liquid formulation of methadone was selected to allow a sublingual (SL) route of administration. The patient continued to be monitored for myoclonus, seizures, and hallucinations as well as pain control. Methadone was dosed at a range of 7% of prior morphine sulfate dosage at 10 mg SL three times daily, clonazepam 1 mg orally twice daily for myoclonus, and oxycodone immediate-release was initiated for breakthrough pain. Seven days later the methadone was titrated to 12.5 mg orally three times daily with down-titration of clonazepam to 0.5 mg orally twice daily as improvement in myoclonus was reported. The following week, the methadone was titrated to 15 mg orally three times daily and changed to tablet formulation per patient request as dysphagia improved. Two weeks after his opioid was converted to methadone, the patient found his pain under satisfactory control and was tolerating his pain regimen well. He was discharged to home hospice care on a pain regimen of methadone 15 mg orally three times daily and oxycodone immediate release for breakthrough pain.

KEY POINTS TO REMEMBER

- Tolerance can be mitigated through an opioid dose increase to provide similar analgesic relief.

- Several ways to identify hyperalgesia are through observation of opioid toxicity, worsening of pain after opioid dosage increase, pain complaint may occur at a new location and be more widespread, or pain may have a character similar to neuropathy.
- Opioid changes to mitigate OIH include dose reduction, tapering to discontinuation, or opioid rotation.
- Remember, opioid metabolites can also contribute to the development of OIH.
- Alternative analgesic additions and/or substitution of analgesics in the treatment of OIH are NSAID medications, NMDA receptor antagonists, gabapentinoids, dexmedetomidine, clonidine, steroids, intravenous lidocaine, and acetaminophen.

References

1. Calvin L, Bull F, Hales T. Perioperative opioid analgesia—when is enough too much? A review of opioid-induced tolerance and hyperalgesia. *Lancet*. 2019;393:1558–1568.
2. Lee M, Silverman SM, Hansen H, Patel VB, Manchikanti L. A comprehensive review of opioid-induced hyperalgesia. *Pain Physician*. 2011;14(2):145–161.
3. Yi P, Pryzbylkowski P. Opioid induced hyperalgesia. *Pain Med*. 2015;16 Suppl 1:S32–36.
4. De Gregori S, De Gregori M, Ranzani GN, et al. Morphine metabolism, transport and brain disposition. *Metab Brain Dis*. 2012;27:1–5.
5. Silverman SM. Opioid induced hyperalgesia: Clinical implications for the pain practitioner. *Pain Physician*. 2009;12(3):679–684.
6. Lutz BM, Nia S, Xiong M, Tao YX, Bekker A. mTOR, a new potential target for chronic pain and opioid-induced tolerance and hyperalgesia. *Mol Pain*. 2015;11:32.
7. Watkins LR, Hutchinson MR, Rice KC, Maier SF. The "toll" of opioid-induced glial activation: improving the clinical efficacy or opioids by targeting glia. *Trends Pharmacol Sci*. 2009;30(11):581–591.
8. Roeckel L, Le Coz G, Gaveriaux-Ruff C, et al. Opioid-induced hyperalgesia: cellular and molecular mechanisms. *Neuroscience*. 2016;338:160–182.
9. Arout CA, Edens E, Petrakis IL, Sofuoglu M. Targeting opioid-induced hyperalgesia in clinical treatment: Neurobiological considerations. *CNS Drugs*. 2015;29(6):465–486.

24 Opioid Conversion Calculations

Mary Lynn McPherson

Case Study

JR is a 48-year-old woman with stage 4 breast cancer. She complains of several types of pain, starting with numbness in her left axilla that is present constantly (rates as a 5/10 on average); episodically, she experiences a shooting, electrical pain that travels from her left axilla to her hand, with the pain shooting out of her thumb and index finger (rates as a 10+). She also complains of chest wall pain on the left side of her chest (rates as an 8). Last, she has been diagnosed with painful metastatic bone pain in her left ribs (rates as a 5–10). JR is in the hospital for poorly controlled pain and has opted for hospice care, awaiting transfer to the inpatient hospice unit. The patient is 5'7", and her weight fluctuates between 90 and 95 pounds. On admission to the hospice unit she is receiving transdermal fentanyl 50 µg/hr (which she says has never really helped) and oxycodone 5 mg/acetaminophen 325, 1–2 tablets every 4 hours as needed (takes about 8 per day). The hospice attending would like to switch JR to IV hydromorphone.

What Do I Do Now?

There are many reasons why a practitioner may need to switch a patient from one opioid regimen to a different opioid regimen. In the case of JR, her pain is not controlled, and, in fact, she is experiencing a pain crisis, requiring not only switching opioids, but changing the route of administration as well. Other reasons include the development of adverse effects that are not easily managed or resolve with time. A patient's status may change, such as experiencing a pain crisis (such as with JR), or a patient transitioning out of the hospital to home or a facility and preferring the oral route of administration. At some point patients with a serious illness may have difficulty swallowing, necessitating a switch to either an oral concentrated solution or a transdermal, rectal, or parenteral opioid. Other reasons may include patient/family health beliefs, opioid shortages, or a need to switch to a less abusable opioid drug delivery system.

Regardless of the reason that we need to switch the opioid regimen, we can use a five-step process that is designed to complete the switch safely and effectively. The steps follow and will be applied to the case of JR.[1]

1. Assess the patient's complaint of pain, preferably using a multidimensional pain assessment.
2. Calculate the patient's average daily use of opioid; consider use of "as needed" doses and adherence.
3. Use an equianalgesic chart to set up a ratio to determine the equivalent of the new regimen.
4. Individualize the new opioid dose you calculated based on assessment data (e.g., is the pain well controlled, or is the patient in pain).
5. Monitor the patient carefully and adjust the regimen as needed.

Let's apply all five steps to the case of JR.

Step 1. A multidimensional pain assessment will allow us to more effectively assess JR's pain situation. There are several validated instruments available, but one easy-to-use model is the PQRSTU mnemonic: precipitating events, palliating events, previous treatment or therapy, quality of pain, region/radiation, severity (at rest, with movement, best, worst, average), temporal aspects of pain, and how the pain affects you (U). JR is describing pain in four different areas—numbness/pain in left axilla, shooting pain down her arm to thumb and index finger, chest wall pain on her left side of chest, and metastatic bone pain in her ribs. Each pain should be assessed separately, collecting 32 pieces of information. Clearly she is experiencing pain of mixed pathology. The axilla pain and shooting pain is likely neuropathic. The chest wall pain is likely nociceptive, and the rib pain is likely nociceptive somatic pain. An important part of this step is identifying the most likely pathogenesis of the pain. Often, on further assessment, we realize that perhaps adding an adjunctive analgesic such as a nonsteroidal anti-inflammatory drug (NSAID) or corticosteroid for the metastatic rib pain may be preferable to simply switching opioids. JR has such a complicated presentation that it would be reasonable, however, to switch to a parenteral infusion with bolus to see how she responds (and we can still add on the NSAID or steroid).

Step 2. In this step we calculate the patient's total daily average use of opioids. We confirm that she has been on a transdermal fentanyl patch 50 µg/hr for 2 weeks and has been consistently taking 8 tablets per day of oxycodone 5 mg/acetaminophen 325 mg. She states she has been consistently adherent to her analgesic regimen.

Step 3. We have already been asked by the hospice inpatient unit attending physician to calculate an appropriate IV hydromorphone regimen for JR. We must now consider how to convert from transdermal fentanyl and from oral oxycodone/acetaminophen to parenteral hydromorphone. This is where a practitioner would consult an equianalgesic opioid chart; an adapted sample is shown in Table 24.1.[2] The theory behind an equianalgesic opioid chart is that all the milligram amounts shown will provide approximately equivalent pain relief. For example, 10 mg of parenteral morphine (IV, IM, or SQ) will provide about the same degree of pain relief as 25 mg oral morphine (with chronic dosing). Similarly, 25 mg of oral morphine will give approximately the same amount of pain relief as 2 mg of parenteral hydromorphone (again, with chronic dosing). When using a chart such as this, we generally work in total daily doses (not single doses). Also, even though this chart is created using the very best data available, there are still flaws to using this approach. Where did the data come from? Some data are from single-dose cross-over studies, but increasingly the chart is informed from chronic, steady-state conversion trials. No matter how accurate an equianalgesic chart is, none of them considers patient-specific variables such as age, size, gender, polymorphism, organ function, and so

TABLE 24.1 **Equianalgesic opioid chart**

Opioid	Equianalgesic equivalence	
	Parenteral	Oral
Morphine	10	25
Hydromorphone	2	5
Oxycodone	NA	20

Adapted with permission from: McPherson ML. *Demystifying Opioid Conversion Calculations: A Guide for Effective Dosing*, 2nd ed. Bethesda, MD: American Society of Health-System Pharmacists; 2018. The reader is strongly encouraged to review the original publication source.

forth. Also, there is no guarantee that the data are bidirectional. Despite these drawbacks, this is the best we have at this time, but use should be tempered with a large dose of common sense and "does that *look* right?"

Let's consider the oxycodone/acetaminophen and transdermal fentanyl separately. First, when converting from a combination analgesic containing acetaminophen, I do not consider the impact of the non-opioid; we can always give that separately if appropriate with the newly calculated regimen. Looking at the equianalgesic opioid chart, we see that 20 mg of oral oxycodone gives approximately the same effect as 2 mg parenteral hydromorphone. Working with the patient's total daily dose of 40 mg oral oxycodone, let's set up a conversion calculation based on this equivalency:

$$\frac{\text{"x" mg IV hydromorphone}}{40 \text{ mg oral oxycodone}} = \frac{2 \text{ mg IV hydromorphone}}{20 \text{ mg oral oxycodone}}$$

Cross multiply and solve for x:

(x)(20) = (40)(2)

x = 4 mg IV hydromorphone per day (equivalent to 40 mg oral oxycodone).

On to the transdermal fentanyl: How do we determine what dose of IV hydromorphone is equivalent to transdermal fentanyl 50 µg/hr? You notice that transdermal fentanyl isn't represented on the equianalgesic opioid chart. There are several proposed methods for converting to and from transdermal fentanyl; one popular method is the 2:1 ratio. For every 2 mg oral morphine per day, that is approximately equivalent to 1 µg/hr of transdermal fentanyl (and vice versa).[3] Based on that assumption, a 50 μg/hr transdermal fentanyl patch would be approximately equal to 100 mg oral morphine. How much IV hydromorphone per day is approximately equivalent to 100 mg oral morphine per day? If we set up our equation, we can figure it out:

$$\frac{\text{"x" mg IV hydromorphone}}{100 \text{ mg oral morphine}} = \frac{2 \text{ mg IV hydromorphone}}{25 \text{ mg oral morphine}}$$

Cross multiply and solve for x:

$(x)(25) = (2)(100)$

x = 8 mg IV hydromorphone per day (equivalent to 100 mg oral morphine per day, which is approximately equivalent to transdermal fentanyl 50 μg/hr).

Theoretically, the patient is receiving the equivalent of 4 mg IV hydromorphone per day from the oxycodone/acetaminophen and 8 mg IV hydromorphone per day from the transdermal fentanyl. But should we *really* go with 12 mg IV hydromorphone/24 hrs? Maybe we should go on to Step 4 before making any hasty decisions!

Step 4. This step is a critical thinking step, where you individualize the dose for the patient, adjusting what you calculated based on your knowledge of the situation. Let's consider the oxycodone first. When you switch from one opioid to a different opioid, we generally reduce the calculated dose by 25–50% because the patient will not have complete cross-tolerance to the new opioid. Before you pull the trigger on that, let's also recall that this patient is having uncontrolled pain, so do we *really* want to reduce the dose? Let's assume those two facts are a wash, and we'll consider the oxycodone equivalent to 4 mg IV hydromorphone per day.

What about the transdermal fentanyl? JR has already shared that she doesn't believe the transdermal fentanyl was doing much to control her pain. She may, in fact, be telling you true when you consider her body mass index (BMI). She is 5'7" tall, weighs between 90 and 95 pounds, and is very cachectic in appearance. Heiskanen and colleagues demonstrated lower fentanyl serum concentrations in patients with cancer with a BMI of less than 16 kg/m².[4] JR's BMI is in the 14–15 kg/m² range so she may not be getting the expected response from the transdermal fentanyl. The problem is how do we factor this in? Do we completely disregard the contribution of the transdermal fentanyl, or perhaps give 50% credit? This is purely a judgment call, but, based on her cachexia and her complaint that the transdermal fentanyl patch didn't seem to help her pain, at the most I would count the transdermal fentanyl as equivalent to 2 mg/day of IV hydromorphone (a 75% reduction from what we calculated). If we're considering her oral oxycodone per day to be equivalent to 4 mg IV hydromorphone per day and the transdermal fentanyl to be equivalent to approximately 2 mg IV hydromorphone per day, that's a total of 6 mg/day IV hydromorphone. We've made a *lot* of assumptions in this case! Remember our goal: to achieve safe and effective pain control as quickly as possible. We don't want to overdose the patient, but we want her to achieve pain relief as soon as we can. First, let's calculate the continuous infusion of IV hydromorphone. Six milligrams over 24 hours would be 0.25 mg IV hydromorphone as a continuous infusion. I know in the back of your head you're wondering "what about the residual fentanyl still being absorbed (if any) even though we're removing the patch?" We know that in a normal body habitus it takes about 17 hours after patch removal to eliminate about 50% of the fentanyl. But, again, she is very cachectic and may not have much fentanyl on board, *and* she's in quite a bit of pain right now. Based on those variables, I'm comfortable starting at 0.25 mg/hr IV hydromorphone. What if we've low-balled it, and she is still experiencing pain? It's important that we provide a patient-demand bolus dose as well. The patient-demand bolus dose on top of a continuous infusion in an opioid-tolerant patient with an advanced illness ranges anywhere from 50% to 150% of the hourly infusion rate.[5] I generally recommend the bolus dose be available every 15 minutes if given IV, or every 30 minutes if given SQ. In this case, let's recommend IV hydromorphone 0.25 mg every 15 minutes as needed for additional pain. One last thing to consider is a clinician bolus that may be administered at the discretion of the nurse in the hospice inpatient unit. The nurse will of course evaluate the patient's pain complaint and determine if the patient is experiencing an opioid-related toxicity or overdose. Let's recommend a clinician bolus of an additional 0.5 mg hourly per nursing judgment. If after three boluses the patient's pain is not responding, the nurse should contact the prescriber. The last consideration is when can the continuous infusion rate be increased? In healthy adults, the half-life of hydromorphone is 2–3 hours, therefore it would take 10–15 hours to get to pseudo-steady state (assuming JR does not have renal impairment). The soonest we should increase the continuous infusion would be 12 hours; 24 hours is even better!

Let's recap our order for JR as follows. Remove transdermal fentanyl patch and discontinue oxycodone/acetaminophen. Administer a clinician loading bolus dose of 0.5 mg IV hydromorphone and begin a continuous infusion of IV hydromorphone 0.25 mg/hr, with patient-demand dosing of 0.25 mg every 15 minutes as needed for additional pain. If pain is not improved after three clinician boluses, contact prescriber. Do not increase the continuous infusion before 12 hours.

Step 5. Just when you think the hard work is over, here comes step 5—monitoring your patient! The medical staff will monitor JR's response to this new regimen, determining if she has met her therapeutic goal and avoided toxicity. For example, after 24 hours JR reports her average pain rating is between a 4 and 6 (average for all her pain complaints). She feels like she is definitely making progress, but a lower pain rating and enhanced mobility would be welcome. Over the past 24 hours, JR has received the 0.25 mg/hr hydromorphone by continuous infusion, and an additional 7.2 mg IV hydromorphone between patient-demand doses and nurse clinician boluses. The prescriber increases the continuous infusion to IV hydromorphone 0.5 mg/hr by continuous infusion and keeps the patient-demand bolus and clinician bolus as originally prescribed. One week later, JR's pain is fairly well controlled on 0.7 mg/hr IV hydromorphone by continuous infusion and an average of 3.2 mg by patient demand and clinician bolus per 24 hours. Her metastatic bone pain has responded well to dexamethasone, but she did not tolerate gabapentin during her inpatient stay and she still complains of neuropathic pain. The attending asks you to calculate an appropriate dose of methadone in hopes of better controlling the neuropathic pain, and the patient would rather not go home on an IV infusion. More math!

Conversion to oral methadone. JR's total daily dose of IV hydromorphone on average is 20 mg. When converting to oral methadone, the first step is to convert to oral morphine. Looking at our equianalgesic chart, we set up our ratio as follows:

$$\frac{\text{"x" mg oral morphine}}{\text{20 mg IV hydromorphone}} = \frac{\text{25 mg oral morphine}}{\text{2 mg IV hydromorphone}}$$

Cross multiply and solve for "x" as follows:

$$(x)(2) = (25)(20)$$
$$x = 250 \text{ oral morphine equivalents per day}$$

There are numerous recommended methods for switching from other opioids to methadone. The recommended conversion by a consensus panel for methadone in hospice and palliative care recommends the following[6]:

Total daily dose oral morphine equivalent (OME)	Conversion ratio to oral methadone
0–59 mg	Follow opioid-naïve dosing (2–7.5 mg methadone per day)
60–199 OME *and* <65 years of age	10 mg OME: 1 mg oral methadone
>200 mg OME *and/or* >65 years old	20 mg OME: 1 mg oral methadone

After calculating the methadone dose, reduce the calculated dose by 25–30% if the patient is receiving strong enzyme inhibitors of methadone. In JR's case, she is older than 65 years but receiving >200 mg OME (her OME is 250 mg), which would be a 20:1 (OME:methadone) conversion, or 12.5 mg oral methadone per day. Based on clinical experience, she's actually fairly young, and 250 mg OME isn't *that* much over 200 mg OME, so let's recommend oral methadone 5 mg every 8 hours or 7.5 mg orally every 12 hours. It is preferred that we do *not* use methadone for breakthrough pain, so let's recommend one oral morphine 15 mg tablet as needed for moderate pain *or* two oral morphine 15 mg tablets every 2 hours as needed for severe pain. We will ask the patient to keep a pain diary documenting use of the oral morphine and her pain ratings. The home hospice nurse will visit daily for the next 5 days to assess the patient, and we will not increase the methadone before 5 days, and by no more than 5 mg per day in total.

This conversion can be carried out by stopping the continuous infusion of IV hydromorphone and continuing the bolus options (patient-demand and clinician bolus) for another 24–48 hours while starting oral methadone or switching entirely to the oral methadone and morphine regimen. It would be preferred to make the switch while the patient was still in the hospice inpatient unit for closer monitoring if possible. JR was discharged to home hospice after 36 hours, and within 3–4 days her pain control had improved, she was meeting her goals, and not experiencing toxicity.

KEY POINTS TO REMEMBER

- It is not uncommon for patients with a serious or advanced illness to require switching from one opioid regimen to a different opioid regimen.
- Use the recommended five-step process that includes a multidimensional pain assessment, accurate accounting for 24-hour opioid use, opioid conversion calculation, adjustment of calculated dose based on patient's presentation, and monitoring.
- Do not increase a continuous opioid infusion before a minimum of 12, preferably 24 hours.
- When switching to oral methadone, use a 10:1 (morphine:methadone) or 20:1 (morphine:methadone) conversion.
- Do not increase a methadone dose before 5 days, and do not increase the total daily methadone dose by more than 5 mg/day (until you get to 30 mg a day of oral methadone, then you can increase by up to 10 mg/day in total).

References

1. Gammaitoni AR, Fine P, Alvarez N, et al. Clinical application of opioid equianalgesic data. *Clin J Pain*. 2003;19:286-297.
2. McPherson ML. *Demystifying Opioid Conversion Calculations: A Guide for Effective Dosing*. 2nd ed. Bethesda, MD: American Society of Health-System Pharmacists; 2018.
3. Breitbart W, Chandler S, Eagle B, et al. An alternative algorithm for dosing transdermal fentanyl for cancer-related pain. *Oncology*. 2000;14:695–705.
4. Heiskanen T, Matzke S, Haakana S, et al. Transdermal fentanyl in cachectic cancer patients. *Pain*. 2009;144:218–222.

5. Weinstein E, Arnold R. Weissman De. *Fast Facts and Concepts #54: Opioid Infusions in the Imminently Dying Patient.* 3rd ed. Appleton, WI: PC Now Palliative Care Network of Wisconsin; 2015.
6. McPherson ML, Walker KA, Davis MP, et al. Safe and appropriate use of methadone in hospice and palliative care: Expert consensus white paper. *J Pain Symptom Manage.* 2019;57(3):635–645.

Further Reading
Corli O, Roberto A, Corsi N, et al. Opioid switching and variability in response in pain cancer patients. *Support Care Cancer.* 2019;27:2321–2327.
Reddy A, Vidal M, Stephen S, et al. The conversion ratio from intravenous hydromorphone to oral opioids in cancer patients. *J Pain Symptom Manage.* 2017;54(3):280–288.
Treillet E, Laurent S, Hadjiat Y. Practical management of opioid rotation and equianalgesia. *J Pain Research.* 2018;11:2587–2601.

25 Treatment of Pain in Palliative Care with Co-Occurring Opioid Use Disorder

Amanda Mullins

Case Study

A 75-year-old African American man was admitted to a home hospice program for metastatic prostate cancer (T3b, N1, M1b, Gleason Score 9). He also has a history of opioid use disorder, diagnosed 10 years ago, and has reservations about stopping his buprenorphine/naloxone therapy. He was on buprenorphine/naloxone 8 mg once daily for 9 years and reported little to no cravings until he relapsed about 1 year ago and started using heroin secondary to increasing amounts of pain. His buprenorphine/naloxone dose was subsequently increased to 16 mg sublingually once daily by his provider in response. He states this has been doing well for his cravings, however, he feels the naloxone is preventing him from achieving any pain relief, and he is now complaining of increasing widespread pain, currently rated a 9 out of 10, specifically localized to the right hip, thoracic spine, and sternum. Other home medications include oral dexamethasone 4 mg twice daily.

What Do I Do Now?

Substance use disorders in hospice and palliative care can be expected to increase in frequency given the rise of opioid use in the community. Managing patients with both diagnosed opioid use disorder (OUD) and opioid dependence can present many challenges for these clinicians. Pain is often undertreated in this patient population, most frequently due to a provider's unfamiliarity with medication-assisted treatment (MAT) and opioid use disorder as a whole, along with stigmatization. In order to appropriately treat our patient's acute, increasing pain in the case study, we must first acquaint ourselves with basic pharmacokinetic and pharmacodynamic properties of the two most common medication options for MAT, buprenorphine and methadone. The availability of both buprenorphine and methadone for pain contributes to the complexity and legality of using them for pain management in palliative care, particularly in those with OUD. Naltrexone, an opioid antagonist, is also approved for use in OUD and will be discussed briefly.

Use of buprenorphine for MAT has increased in recent years due to its lessened restrictions from the Drug Enforcement Agency (DEA), specifically since the Drug Addiction Treatment Act (DATA) was passed by Congress in 2000, known as the DATA 2000 law. This law permits qualified providers to treat opioid dependence with schedules III–V controlled substances that have been approved by the Food and Drug Administration (FDA) for OUD. Qualified providers are those who have completed the MAT certification and have been granted their DATA-waiver, or X-waiver, by Substance Abuse and Mental Health Services Administration (SAMHSA). MAT with buprenorphine has substantially increased access to treatment, particularly in the primary care setting. Buprenorphine, a mixed agonist/antagonist opioid, displays partial agonist properties at the mu opioid receptor, antagonist properties at the kappa and delta opioid receptors, and agonist properties at the opioid receptor-like 1 receptor. It is estimated that buprenorphine is approximately 25–115 times more potent than morphine. Its half-life is approximately 24–48 hours, and it dissociates slowly from the opioid receptors, thus contributing to its effectiveness in treating OUD.

However, while buprenorphine binds to the receptors for an extended period of time, it has been documented that the pain relief associated with buprenorphine is severely shortened, at about 6 hours. This is a common clinical complaint of many patients on buprenorphine for OUD and is usually quite fixable if providers are familiar with buprenorphine. Buprenorphine is typically administered once daily for OUD, although it can be split into twice daily or even three to four times daily dosing for those patients with coexisting pain. In our patient case, we know he is experiencing increasing pain and is on buprenorphine/naloxone 16 mg sublingually once daily. An appropriate next step would be to either split his dose to 8 mg twice daily or increase his total daily dose to 16 mg twice daily, depending on his reported pain relief and expected trajectory of pain over the next couple of days. While it has been documented that buprenorphine displays a ceiling effect for analgesia, data are conflicting on whether or not this is true. Should the patient in our case need more pain relief after a buprenorphine dose increase, it may be wise to transition him to methadone because there is no ceiling effect associated with its use. It is important to note that different formulations of buprenorphine products have specific FDA approvals, as outlined in Table 25.1, and that only those with FDA-approved indications of OUD may be used for those patients. Conversely, many clinicians use those same products off-label for pain, and no special credentialing is required for providers to use buprenorphine formulations for pain.

We just discussed why continuing this patient's buprenorphine/naloxone therapy for pain may be a decent option for immediate pain relief; however, he still has the concern that the naloxone in his buprenorphine formulation is preventing him from receiving any further pain relief. This is an extremely common misunderstanding surrounding the purpose of naloxone in these combination products. Naloxone in combination with buprenorphine is formulated to prevent any misuse of the products, such as crushing the tablets to be administered nasally or intravenously, although this has started to cause some controversy. Naloxone's oral bioavailability was previously documented as severely low, implying that is has little absorption when used appropriately in combination buprenorphine products. However, as use of these products has increased, so have patient complaints of side effects. In fact, naloxone's sublingual absorption may be great enough to be detected on a urine drug screen. For patients presenting with complaints of side effects, most commonly headaches, fatigue, and gastrointestinal upset, rotating to a single-ingredient buprenorphine product may be beneficial.

The other medication used for MAT in OUD is methadone. Methadone has been around since the late 1940s and has been used to treat OUD for many years. Many providers are uncomfortable with methadone, particularly because of its extremely variable half-life (from 8 to 59 hours) and bioavailability (anywhere from 36% to 100%). It is a full mu opioid receptor agonist with no action on the kappa and delta opioid receptors and no action on the opioid receptor-like 1 receptor. Similar to buprenorphine, methadone's duration of pain relief is about 8 hours, even though it binds to the receptors for a prolonged amount of time. Methadone for OUD has started falling to the wayside since buprenorphine was approved, and it has found a new niche population in those individuals uncontrolled on MAT with buprenorphine. One major restriction governing the use of methadone for those with OUD is that use of methadone is majorly limited to federally certified opioid treatment programs, often referred to as "methadone clinics." Additionally, methadone may be dispensed or administered in these programs, but not prescribed. I highly recommend reaching out to a patient's methadone provider if someone on methadone for OUD is admitted to palliative care or hospice services to continue appropriate care. As with buprenorphine, no special credentialing is required for providers using methadone for pain.

Naltrexone, an antagonist at the mu opioid receptor, is available in both oral and injectable formulations and is used for OUD and alcohol use disorder. Since administration of naltrexone blocks the effects of opioid agonists, it offers very little to no pain relief. As such, we will not dive into naltrexone therapy; however, it is important to know how to treat these individuals should the situation arise. If a patient presents to your service on naltrexone for OUD, particularly the depot injectable form, its antagonist effects may be overcome by administering exogenous opioids, such as morphine or methadone, for pain. The general rule of thumb for achieving pain relief is to "start low and go slow" although higher doses will often be needed. Be sure to monitor for signs and symptoms of opioid overdose, especially if continuously increasing the dose of the opioid agonist.

At this point you may be wondering what to do for pain relief in our patient case. After all of the information you just received on buprenorphine and methadone in OUD and pain management, you may feel a bit confused as to where to go next. The best approach to take in cases like these,

TABLE 25.1 US Food and Drug Administration (FDA)-approved indications of different buprenorphine products

Buprenorphine product	FDA-approved indication
Transdermal system (Butrans)	Pain
Sublingual tablet	OUD
with naloxone (Zubsolv[a], Suboxone)	Pain
without naloxone (Subutex)[b]	
Sublingual film	OUD
with naloxone	Pain
without naloxone	
Buccal film	OUD
with naloxone (Bunavail)[a]	Pain
without naloxone (Belbuca)	
Solution for injection	Pain
Depot injection (Sublocade)	OUD
Implant (Probuphine)	OUD

[a]Dose is more potent than other buprenorphine products and cannot be used interchangeably.

[b]Now available solely as a generic product.

where questions of legality and difficult pharmacokinetics prevail, is to ask what you are treating. Table 25.2 provides best approaches for varying patient presentations. If ever in doubt or in an uncomfortable situation, reach out to the patient's OUD provider to determine if they will continue to treat the patient while enrolled in palliative care and hospice services. If this approach is used, you may still give the patient opioid therapy for pain management. Non-opioid pharmacologic alternatives should also be considered if clinically appropriate, such as non-steroidal anti-inflammatories (NSAIDs), acetaminophen, skeletal muscle relaxants, antidepressants, and anticonvulsants. Additionally, nonpharmacologic modalities, such as acupuncture, cognitive-behavioral therapy, and physical therapy, among others, may be appropriate choices to augment this patient's pain management care.

MAT in palliative care is an extremely gray area that requires familiarity with both legal aspects and pharmacokinetic and pharmacodynamic

TABLE 25.2 **What to do when encountering a patient on medication-assisted therapy for opioid use disorder (OUD) with coexisting pain**

If you have your DATA waiver (X-waiver) and the patient presents on

Buprenorphine/naloxone therapy:	Option 1: Split/increase the dose. There is no concern for legality.	Option 2: Provide additional opioid and non-opioid analgesia	
Methadone therapy:	Option 1: Collaborate with OUD provider: they may be willing to split the dose	Option 2: Provide additional opioid and non-opioid analgesic	

If you do NOT have your DATA waiver (X-waiver) and the patient presents on:

Buprenorphine/naloxone therapy:	Option 1: Collaborate with OUD provider: they may be willing to split the dose.	Option 2: Provide buprenorphine for pain. There is some concern for legality.	Option 3: Provide additional opioid and non-opioid analgesia
Methadone therapy:	Option 1: Collaborate with OUD provider: they may be willing to split the dose	Option 2: Provide additional opioid and non-opioid analgesic	

parameters of the agent being used. If there is ever any doubt regarding the best next step, I recommend collaborating with the patient's OUD provider because they are likely much more familiar with any legal concerns and may continue to follow the patient while enrolled in palliative care or hospice services. If you have your DATA waiver and are comfortable assuming responsibility of the patient's buprenorphine therapy, this is certainly an option. I recommend reading the chapter on buprenorphine and other mixed agonist/antagonists as this will provide some insight on more in-depth concerns regarding buprenorphine's characteristics.

- Buprenorphine, methadone, and naltrexone are all used as MAT in OUD.
- A DATA waiver, commonly referred to as an X waiver, is required to prescribe buprenorphine for OUD in the United States. Prescribing methadone for OUD requires different credentialing and is typically done in methadone clinics.
- If prescribing buprenorphine for OUD, the product formulation you use must have an FDA-approved indication for OUD.
- If prescribing buprenorphine and methadone for pain, you do not need any extra credentialing. This can be done with your normal DEA number.
- When increasing doses of buprenorphine are not adequately controlling pain, it may be time to switch to a full mu agonist for pain, such as methadone or morphine.
- Prescribing opioids for pain while the patient is on methadone, buprenorphine, or naltrexone for OUD is an option. "Start low and go slow."

Further Reading

Alford DP, Compton P, Samet JH. Acute pain management for patients receiving maintenance methadone or buprenorphine therapy. *Ann Intern Med*. 2006 March 21;144(6):460.

Jones KF. Buprenorphine use in palliative care. *J Hospice Palliat Nurs*. 2019 December;21(6):540–547.

Quill TE, Bower KA, Holloway RG, et al. *Primer of Palliative Care*. 7th ed. Chicago: American Academy of Hospice and Palliative Medicine. 2019.

Reisfield GM, Paulian GD, Wilson GR. Substance use disorders in the palliative care patient. Fast Facts and Concepts #127. Palliative Care Network of Wisconsin. https://www.mypcnow.org/wp-content/uploads/2019/02/FF-127-substance-abuse.-3rd-edition.pdf

Sager ZS, Buss MK, Hill KP, et al. Managing opioid use disorder in the setting of a terminal disease: Opportunities and challenges. *J Palliat Med*. 2020;23(2):296–299.

Substance Abuse and Mental Health Services Administration (SAMHSA). Medications for opioid use disorder: For healthcare and addiction professionals, policymakers, patients, and families. (Treatment Improvement Protocol [TIP] Series, No. 63, Chapter 3D: Buprenorphine). Rockville, MD: Substance Abuse and Mental Health Services Administration; 2018. https://www.ncbi.nlm.nih.gov/books/NBK535267/

Substance Abuse and Mental Health Services Administration (SAMHSA). Clinical guidelines for the use of buprenorphine in the treatment of opioid addiction. (TIP No. 40). 2004. https://www.ncbi.nlm.nih.gov/books/NBK64245/pdf/Bookshelf_NBK64245.pdf

Volpe KD. Managing opioid use disorders and chronic pain. *Practical Pain Manage.* 2017;17(2).

26 Radiopharmaceuticals in the Treatment of Pain in Palliative Care

Tanya J. Uritsky and Erin McMenamin

Case Study

GJ is a 36-year-old White man who presented to the ED 9 months ago with a history of diarrhea for several weeks, decreased appetite, and flushing. Physical examination revealed a pale, thin man. Laboratory values, including a complete blood count, electrolytes, liver function tests, urinalysis, and an abdominal obstruction series and a chest x-ray were unremarkable. A computed tomography (CT) scan demonstrated a 4 cm mass in the small intestine, and a subsequent biopsy demonstrated a well-differentiated neuroendocrine neoplasm (NEN). A positron emission tomography (PET) scan revealed local lymph node involvement. The patient began treatment with octreotide long-acting repeatable (LAR) intramuscularly every 4 weeks. GJ's symptoms subsided after the initiation of treatment. One year later, GJ returns to the ED with abdominal pain, diarrhea, and flushing. A CT scan of the abdomen is highly suspicious for progression of his disease to regional lymph nodes and several small nodules in the liver.

What Do I Do Now?

Neuroendocrine neoplasms (NENs) can occur in most organs in the body. In the gastrointestinal tract, they may occur in the stomach, small and large intestine, pancreas, appendix, and rectum. Neuroendocrine NENs are epithelial cancers with neuroendocrine features. Approximately 20% of tumors secrete large amounts of serotonin and polypeptides resulting in carcinoid syndrome (CS). The overall average survival for NENs is 9.3 years and varies based on classification, the presence of carcinoid syndrome, and location of the tumor. Metastasis to the liver occurs in 50–95% of NENs. Patients with metastatic disease have an average overall survival (OS) of 5 years.

Neuroendocrine tumors are divided into three types. Well-differentiated tumors (NENs) have historically been referred to as *carcinoid tumors* and classified as grade 1. They have a 5-year survival of approximately 67%. Poorly differentiated neuroendocrine cancers (NECs) are high-grade cancers that resemble small or large cell cancers of the lung and are classified as grade 2. High-grade NENs are associated with a more rapid progression of disease and shorter length of survival.

NENs that secrete excess hormones (such as insulin, glucagon, somatostatin, vasoactive intestinal peptide [VIP], serotonin, gastrin, etc.) based on the presence of clinical symptoms are referred to as *functioning tumors*. The presence of functioning tumors impacts prognosis; however, the behavior of the tumor is classified by the grade and stage of the cancer. Other factors assessed for NENs include mitotic rate and Ki-67 labeling index, but clear guidelines to differentiate between low-, intermediate-, and high-grade NENs are inconsistent in the literature and vary based on the site of the tumor.

Surgical resection is the treatment of choice when feasible, although GJ has been deemed a nonsurgical candidate. Somatostatins, such as octreotide, have been the primary treatment to control the symptoms associated with the hypersecretions of hormones associated with NENs. They may also control tumor growth in 40–60% of NENs. It is unclear whether somatostatins increase survival of patients with NENs.

Since this patient has progressed on octreotide, another option may be treatment with radionuclide therapy. Peptide receptor radionuclide therapy (PRRT) is a form of systemic radiotherapy that delivers targeted radionuclides to tumor cells expressing high levels of the somatostatin receptor. In patients with progressive metastatic NEN of the midgut, ^{177}Lu-dotatate has been used for more than 10 years, and studies of patients diagnosed with gastrointestinal NENs demonstrate exceptional tolerability and efficacy in comparison with high-dose octreotide.

PRRTs work on the somatostatin receptor, which is commonly expressed in high density in NENs. Lower grade tumors have a higher expression of somatostatin receptors compared to high-grade tumors. Once PRRTs bind to the receptor, they are internalized through the usual cell breakdown cycle, and the breakdown products are then stored in lysosomes that bring the radiolabeled peptides into the interior of the tumor cell. PRRTs consist of the radionuclide isotope, a carrier molecule derivative of octreotide, and a chelator that serves to stabilize the complex. Chelators are either tetrazacyclododecane-tetra-acetic acid (DOTA) or diethylenetriamine penta-acetic acid (DTPA) and radionuclides can be either ^{111}In, ^{90}Y, or ^{177}Lu. ^{111}In may not effectively penetrate large tumors, but ^{90}Y and ^{177}Lu emit higher energy beta particles that give them greater therapeutic potential. ^{177}Lu can also be used for dosimetry and tumor response monitoring.

The one requirement for treatment with a PRRT is the expression of the somatostatin receptor. The higher the expression of this receptor on tumor cells, the greater the predicted response. For patients with grade 4 uptake on octreoscans, an overall response rate (ORR) of about 60% has been reported. ^{68}Ga-DOTATOC PET/CT scans with a maximum standard uptake value (SUV) of greater than 16 will predict tumor response with a 95% sensitivity and 60% specificity. Additional consideration should be given to the primary tumor site and the tumor burden. Pancreatic NENs seem to respond well but tend to relapse quickly. Patients with large lesions or high hepatic tumor burden are generally less responsive to PRRT. Su et al. also reported long-term liver toxicity associated with Yttrium-90 radioembolization of the liver.[1] Long-term follow-up of these patients revealed a cirrhosis-like morphology in 26.7%, ascites in 13.3%, varices in 6.7%, and enlarged spleen in 21.9%.

^{177}Lu-dotatate is the most commonly used radiopeptide. Of the available PRRTs, this has demonstrated the most efficacy with the best tolerability profile and the least hematologic toxicity, which tends to limit application of this therapeutic modality. The ORR in the treatment of gastrointestinal NEN has been reported at 30%, with a median OS of 46 months.

For patients who did not progress while on treatment, the median time to eventual progression was 40 months. Poorer outcomes have been associated with a poor performance status, extensive liver involvement, and high tumor burden. There does not appear to be a benefit to treating with PRRTs as first-line compared to later in the treatment course. A more recent study demonstrated objective response rates between 18% and 44%, with an average disease control rate of 81%. There are also associated significant improvements in quality of life after ^{177}Lu-dotatate therapy.

In considering our patient, studies support a progression free survival (PFS) interval of 33–36 months in patients with advanced NEN of the small bowel with documented disease progression or uncontrolled carcinoid symptoms (reference high-dose octreotide). ^{177}Lu-dotatate was compared to high-dose octreotide (60 mg/month) in patients who had progressed on standard dose of octreotide. ^{177}Lu-dotatate was associated with a 79% risk reduction of progression or death versus high-dose octreotide, although it did not meet median PFS compared to the high dose-octreotide group (8.4 months). Subgroup analyses showed consistent benefit, and ^{177}Lu-dotatate had an ORR of 18% compared to 3% with high-dose octreotide. Interim results are in favor of a significant improvement in OS as well, but long-term follow-up is needed. Combination therapies with standard chemotherapy such as everolimus or capecitabine and temozolamide, demonstrate promising improvements in ORR ranging from 24% to 44%. It is unclear if giving these simultaneously versus in succession offers any clear benefits although there does not seem to be a significant increase in toxicity profile with the combination. Combinations of radionuclides may also offer some benefit. The combination of 90Y-DOTATOC with ^{177}Lu-dotatate yielded a reduction in the risk of progression or death of 36%, and prospective studies are needed to investigate this more thoroughly.

Safety considerations with these agents include acute nausea and vomiting, which are attributable to the amino acid infusion used with treatment and are generally mild and self-limiting. Fatigue and abdominal pain may also be reported. A small percentage of patients (1%) may develop carcinoid syndrome within 48 hours of the infusion. Myelosuppression is a toxicity caused by irradiation to the bone marrow and generally occurs about 4–6 weeks after the infusion. The myelosuppression is generally mild and reversible. Grade 3 or 4 hematologic toxicity may occur, with lymphopenia being the most severe. However, PRRT administration is generally not associated with the development of opportunistic infections. There is a theoretical risk of hepatic injury in patients with a high burden of hepatic disease, although there is no documented evidence of this risk. Long term, PRRTs may cause renal failure due to accumulation of radiopeptides in the renal interstitium leading to inflammation and kidney damage, but overall this is a rare occurrence (1.5%). Administration of PRRTs may also lead to secondary leukemia/myelodysplastic syndromes (MDS). Risk factors for development of leukemia or MDS include age older than 70 years, baseline cytopenia, presence of bone metastases, high number of prior therapies, prior treatment with alkylating agents, and prior radiotherapy.

Our patient seems to be the perfect candidate for treatment with ^{177}Lu-dotatate. Having progressed through treatment with octreotide and having an advanced NEN of the small intestine, it would be best to start ^{177}Lu-dotatate before the tumor burden gets too large to perceive any benefit from the radionuclide therapy. His labs do not demonstrate cytopenias that could be exacerbated by the radionuclide therapy, and liver disease burden is not extensive. The octreotide uptake scans should be reviewed to determine the likelihood of response to ^{177}Lu-dotatate. It is essential to explain the palliative intent of this therapy to the patient and his loved ones. It is not likely that the disease will yield a complete response, but the treatment is generally well tolerated and may delay further disease progression. An additional goal of the therapy is to improve his quality of life and decrease his symptom burden. Additional focus should be on setting the expectation that he may experience some nausea, abdominal pain, and fatigue around the time of infusion as well as what to do to prevent them, but also how to intervene if he does experience those adverse effects.

Additional attention should also be given to his symptom burden and providing supportive care. His abdominal pain is likely due to disease progression and inflammation in the regional lymph nodes that have been affected. This inflammatory pain will likely respond best to a course of steroids such as dexamethasone 4–8 mg daily for 5–7 days. A quick taper may help prevent rebound pain symptoms. In this case, tapering the dose over 3–5 days may be considered. Opioids may alleviate the visceral nature of the pain and should be prescribed and titrated to satisfactory relief based on patient response and tolerability. Any cramping pain from the diarrhea can be addressed with an anticholinergic medication, such as dicyclomine or hyoscyamine. While decreasing abdominal cramping, these will also help decrease the secretions and may decrease diarrhea. Opioid derivatives, such as loperamide and atropine-diphenoxylate, may also be considered, although they may offer limited benefit in a patient already on systemic opioids. Bulk-forming agents, such as psyllium or cholestyramine, may be considered but may be hard to tolerate given the significant volume required to ingest these medications.

KEY POINTS TO REMEMBER

- Incidence of advanced NENs is increasing, likely due to increased ability to detect the disease, but still most patients are diagnosed in the advanced stages.
- Initial therapy with octreotide will help many patients, and patients with pancreatic NEN may respond best, but they have a quick relapse rate while patients with NEN of the small intestine may have a lower response rate but also have a more indolent cancer.
- Patients who progress on standard octreotide therapy may benefit from treatment with a radionuclide, such as ^{177}Lu-dotatate versus a trial of high-dose octreotide. Combination therapy with chemotherapy may also confer some benefit, although more studies are needed to determine the best regimens and the true benefits versus risks.
- ^{177}Lu-dotatate is generally well tolerated. It is associated with nausea and vomiting on administration, which should be prophylactically treated, as well as the long-term risks of cytopenias and secondary MDS or leukemia.

References
1. Su YK, Mackey RV, Riaz A, et al. Long-term hepatotoxicity of Yttrium-90 radioembolization as treatment of metastatic neuroendocrine tumor to the liver. *J Vasc Interv Radiol.* 2017;28(11):1520–1526.

2. Khan S, Krenning EP, van Essen M, et al. Quality of life in 265 patients with gastroenteropancreatic or bronchial neuroendocrine tumors treated with [177Lu-DOTAo,Tyr3] octreotate. *J Nucl Med.* 2011;52(9):1361–1368.

Further Reading

Cives M, Strosberg J. Radionuclide therapy for neuroendocrine tumors. *Curr Oncol Rep.* 2017;19:1–9.

Dasari A, Shen C, Halperin D, et al. Trends in the incidence, prevalence, and survival outcomes in patients with neuroendocrine tumors in the United States. *JAMA Oncol.* 2017;3:1335–1342. doi:10.1001/jamaoncol.2017.0589

Ezziddin S, Khalaf F, Vanezi M, et al. Outcome of peptide receptor radionuclide therapy with 177Lu-octreotate in advanced grade 1/2 pancreatic neuroendocrine tumours. *Eur J Nucl Med Mol Imaging.* 2014;41(5):925–933.

Halperin DM, Shen C, Dasari A, et al. (2017). The frequency of carcinoid syndrome at neuroendocrine tumor diagnosis: A large population-based study using SEER-Medicare data. *Lancet Oncol.* 2017;18:525–534. doi:10.1016/S1470-2045(17)30110-9

Kwekkeboom DJ, de Herder WW, Kam BL, et al. Treatment with the radiolabeled somatostatin analog [177 LuDOTA 0, Tyr3] octreotate: Toxicity, efficacy, and survival. *J Clin Oncol.* 2008;26:2124–2130. doi:10.1200/JCO.2007.15.2553

Strosberg J, El-Haddad G, Wolin E, et al. NETTER-1 trial investigators. *N Engl J Med.* 2017;376:125–135. doi:10.1056/NEJMoa1607427

Ter-Minassian M, Zhang S, Brooks NV, et al. Association between tumor progression endpoints and overall survival in patients with advanced neuroendocrine tumors. *Oncologist.* 2017;22:165–172.

27 Rectal Administration of Analgesics

Cara Brock and Patti Murray

Case Study

JD is a 71-year-old Hispanic man with low back pain that did not respond to over-the-counter medication, heat, ice, or physical therapy. His workup revealed aggressive stage IV prostate cancer with a Total Gleason score of $4 + 3 = 7$. The patient chose conservative management of his disease, focusing on functionality and quality of life. Despite disease progression and the need for a diverting colostomy due to carcinomatosis, his pain remained well-controlled on controlled release (CR) oxycodone 20 mg every 12 hours with immediate-release (IR) oxycodone every 4 hours as needed, averaging two doses of breakthrough medication per day. He subsequently declined clinically, and a family conference was held to discuss his clinical condition and explore alternate routes of medication administration that aligned with his wishes to not be connected to machines and to die at home. JD's previous wishes precluded intravenous, subcutaneous, and intramuscular access as viable delivery options. Transmucosal and transdermal delivery of medications are not viable due to his health status.

What Do I Do Now?

When the oral route is no longer viable and other routes are not possible or ideal, the rectal route has been shown in many studies to be an effective and safe route of administration for opioids. Commercially available rectal opioid dosage forms in the United States are morphine, oxycodone, oxymorphone, and hydromorphone suppositories. Additionally, other opioids and/or strengths may be compounded by pharmacies when needed. It is important to assess the patient for a patent anal sphincter if considering the rectal route as this is required for retention of rectally administered drugs (Table 27.1).

TABLE 27.1 **Advantages and disadvantages of rectal administration of opioids**

Advantages	Disadvantages
Ease of administration	Variation in bioavailability amongst individuals
Less invasive and costly then intravenous route	Cannot be used in severely constipated or impacted patients or patients with diarrhea
Good evidence for efficacy and safety	Patients or caregivers may be unwilling or unable to administer medications rectally
Fast onset of immediate release formulations	Should not be used if administration will cause pain— hemorrhoids, fissures, or lesions on the anus or rectum
Longer duration of action for extended-release formulations	Avoid in patients with bleeding disorders
Similar adverse effect profile to oral administration	Loss of dose due to defecation
Useful in patients with nausea, vomiting, dysphagia, GI obstruction, malabsorption, impaired neuromuscular function and in patients who are unconscious	Delayed absorption of extended-release dosage forms
Solid dosage forms can be removed from the rectum if the patient experiences adverse effects	

The HCT and health care power of attorney (HCPOA) agreed that the rectal delivery route was the best option for medication delivery for JD. This aligned with the wishes of the patient, it was cost neutral, and he would be able to go home. Consent was obtained from his partner to administer his oxycodone via per rectal (PR) route. A complication arises for JD since managing his pain around the clock with commercially available rectal suppositories would require frequent dosing, which may cause discomfort and be an inconvenience to caregivers. Fortunately, several studies and case reports have reported both efficacy and safety of rectally administered oral immediate- (IR) and extended-release (ER) opioid formulations. This allows for much more flexibility in initiating and titrating doses along with many options for the rectal use of ER opioids. Compared to solid dosage forms, liquid dosage forms are absorbed more rapidly in the rectum, so a faster onset of pain relief can be expected compared to suppositories and solid dosage forms, which require time for the drug to dissolve before absorption.

Suppositories are compounded in a fatty base meant to melt in the rectum. Absorption depends on the time needed for the suppository to melt and the time for the drug to dissolve in the rectal fluid, resulting in a longer time to onset compared to suspensions or solutions. IR and ER solid dosage forms like tablets and capsules require an aqueous environment to allow dissolution of the drug for absorption in the rectum, so the amount of fluid in the rectum will affect absorption. If the rectum is dry, 10 mL of warm water may be administered before the tablet or capsule.

Commercially available oral opioids may be administered rectally in a variety of ways.

- IR or ER capsules or tablets may be directly administered into the rectum.
- Microenemas (up to 25 mL) of oral or IV solution or suspension may be administered rectally with a syringe or catheter.
- IV or oral solution, suspension, or multiple doses of tablets may be placed in a gelatin capsule for rectal administration.

IV or oral solutions or suspensions may be chosen when strengths not available in a tablet are needed or when a rapid onset is desired. For JD, the HCT and his partner decided to continue his current opioid regimen, administering both CR and IR oxycodone tablets rectally as this is what was most comfortable for his partner who would be providing care when JD returned home.

ABSORPTION AND BIOAVAILABILITY

Although the rectum has a smaller surface area, higher pH, and decreased fluid content compared to the upper gastrointestinal tract, rectally administered opioids are absorbed in a similar manner as in the upper gastrointestinal tract via passive diffusion. The rectum is drained by three venous blood vessels (Figure 27.1).

The superior rectal vein drains the upper rectum to the portal vein, which then directs blood through the liver before returning to systemic circulation, therefore resulting in first-pass metabolism and decreased bioavailability. The inferior and middle rectal veins drain the lower rectum and avoid the portal system by directly draining to the inferior vena cava, which

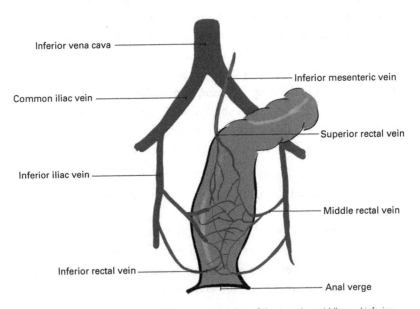

FIGURE 27.1 The venous drainage of the rectum consists of the superior, middle, and inferior rectal veins. The inferior and middle rectal veins flow into the inferior vena cava, thus bypassing first pass. The superior rectal vein flows to the inferior mesenteric vein, which transports blood back through the hepatoportal system.

bypasses the liver and returns to the heart. Any portion of drug absorbed in the lower part of the rectum will bypass first-pass metabolism and have increased bioavailability compared to the oral dose. However, due to varying degrees of anastomoses within the submucosal venous plexus, it is difficult to determine the exact division in the rectum between drainage to portal or systemic circulation and therefore the bioavailability based on drug placement in the rectum. Absorption of rectally administered opioids is also dependent on several other factors: surface area of the rectum, amount of fluid available to dissolve the dosage form, and presence of stool in the rectum. Placement of drug in a rectum filled with stool may decrease drug contact with the mucosa; in constipated patients, the drug may be adsorbed into the feces. Both these situations reduce absorption of the drug.

Available studies comparing rectal and oral opioid pharmacokinetics mainly focus on morphine, however there are data from pharmacokinetic studies to support the absorption of rectally administered hydromorphone, oxycodone, oxymorphone, and methadone as well. Rectally administered ER morphine can provide good pain control with no change in side effects with dosing intervals of 8–12 hours. Peak concentrations are 10–25% less than oral, and the time to peak concentration is delayed by 2–3 hours.

The recommended conversion from oral to rectal opioids is 1:1, with dosing intervals mirroring the oral route; however, the clinician should be aware of the many variables that affect absorption and bioavailability when using the rectal route and be prepared to adjust doses if needed based on pain relief and side effects. Although bioavailability of rectally administered opioids varies among the studies and case reports, studies that assessed adverse effects suggest that the prevalence is similar compared to oral opioids. Large, well-controlled studies are lacking regarding the use of oral opioids administered rectally, and pharmacokinetic data, as well as clinical experience, should be considered when recommending the rectal administration of opioids.

STOMAL ADMINISTRATION

In patients with ostomies, administration of opioids via the stoma is an option as well. Left-sided sigmoid colostomies are ideal for drug administration compared to ostomies of the jejunum, ileum, ascending, transverse, and high descending colon, which are significantly less ideal due to rapid transit times and less formed stools resulting in decreased absorption. Drugs placed into the colon through an ostomy will be absorbed and drained by vessels that drain to the portal circulation, therefore bioavailability would be expected to be reduced due to first-pass metabolism similar to oral absorption.

1. Insert dosage form one finger length into the stoma in the direction of the colon, then
2. You may use a foam colostomy plug to ensure retention if it is a high-functioning ostomy. If not, gauze may be placed over the stoma to keep the suppository in place.
3. Instruct the patient to recline for 15–30 minutes to prevent leakage of drug due to gravity.

ADMINISTRATION OF RECTAL OPIOIDS

CR dosage forms should be inserted intact into the rectum or stoma and should not be crushed or dissolved as this may destroy the CR delivery system and result in a bolus dose of opioid. Although most patients and healthcare professionals insert suppositories apex (top) first, tolerance is the same when the base is inserted first which improves retention. To ensure the appropriate dose, suppositories should not be cut as drug may not be evenly distributed throughout. When administering microenemas the volume inserted should range between 1 and 25 mL to ensure retention and absorption of the entire dose; volumes over 60 mL are not recommended.

1. If possible, have the patient empty the rectum before administration.
2. Position the patient on the left side with the right leg flexed if able.
3. Lubricate the dosage form if needed with water-based lubricant.
4. If the rectum is dry, 10 mL of warm water may be instilled before insertion of the dosage form.
5. Insert the suppository, capsule, tablet, or device delivering liquid drug approximately one finger-length into the rectum.

6. Place the dosage form in contact with the rectal wall to facilitate absorption. If the drug is inserted into stool or not placed against the mucous membrane, absorption may be affected.
7. Once inserted, press the buttocks together until the urge to expel has passed.

JD was discharged to home 1 week ago, and his partner has reported acceptable pain control and no issues with administration of his medications. He expressed his gratitude to the entire HCT for respecting JD's wishes and allowing him to be at home with friends and family without being hooked up to machines.

As we discussed regarding our patient JD, the rectal route is viable and effective for administration of opioids for pain and symptom management. The rectal route may also be considered for other drugs used in palliative care including antiemetics, anxiolytics, non-opioid analgesics, and corticosteroids to name a few.

ADMINISTRATION VIA RECTAL CATHETER

The US Food and Drug Administration (FDA) approved rectal Macy Catheter (Hospi Corporation) is a discrete 14 F silicone catheter shaft with a 15 mL balloon similar to a urinary catheter and a valved medication port that can be easily accessed to administer fluids and medications via the rectal route. The catheter tip is positioned above the rectal sphincter, and position and placement are maintained by inflating the balloon. The patient does not need to be repositioned for medication delivery. Liquid medication and pills may be crushed with the pill pulverizing system provided and mixed with water for ease of delivery via this rectal route. The catheter is then flushed with 3 mL of water to keep it patent. Absorption in the distal third of the rectum eliminates the first-pass effect, thus supporting clinical efficacy of this route of administration. One study found that patients achieved therapeutic response faster with the Macy catheter compared to suppositories. Absorption is not inhibited by stool in the rectum. The catheter may be left in place up to 28 days, and, if expelled during defecation, it may be replaced. The administration port is taped to the patient's leg for ease of medication administration.

- Insert suppositories base first to improve retention.
- Do not cut suppositories as the drug may not be evenly dispersed throughout.
- Consult with your pharmacist to explore which medication may be compounded and given rectally.
- Oral to rectal route conversion is 1:1 and titrated to patient effect.
- Advise the patient and/or caregiver that the empty tablet or capsule casing may be expelled when ER formulations are given rectally.
- The medication will have been absorbed from the pill leaving a remnant carcass and should be disposed of appropriately.

Further Reading

Cole L, Hanning CD Review of the rectal use of opioids. *J Pain Symptom Manage.* 1990;5(2):118–126.

Davis MP, Walsh D, LeGrand SB, Naughton M. Symptom control in cancer patients: The clinical pharmacology and therapeutic role of suppositories and rectal suspensions. *Support Care Cancer.* 2002;10(2):117–138.

Kestenbaum MG, Vilches AO, Messersmith S, et al. Alternative routes to oral opioid administration in palliative care: A review and clinical summary. *Pain Med.* 2014;15(7):1129–1153.

Lam YWF, Lam A, Macy B. Pharmacokinetics of phenobarbital in microenema via Macy catheter vs suppository. *J Pain Symptom Manage.* 2016;51(6): 994–1001.

Latuga NM, Gordon M, Farwell P, Farrell MO. A cost and quality analysis of utilizing a rectal catheter for medication administration in end-of-life symptom management. *J Pain Palliat Care Pharmacother.* 2018. doi:10.1080/15360288.2018.1500509

McCaffery M, Martin L, Ferrell BR. Analgesic administration via rectum or stoma. *J ET Nurs.* 1992;19(4):114–121.

Mercadante SG. When oral morphine fails in cancer pain: The role of the alternative routes. *Am J Hospice Palliat Med.* 1998;15(6):333–342.

Paez K, Gregg M, Massion CT, Macy B. Promoting excellence in symptom management case series. *J Hospice Palliat Nurs.* 2016 December;18(6):498–504.

Ripamonti C, Bruera E. Rectal, buccal, and sublingual narcotics for the management of cancer pain. *J Palliat Care.* 19917(1):30–35.

Warren DE. Practical use of rectal medications in palliative care. *J Pain Symptom Manage.* 1996;11(6):378–387.

28 Epidural and Intrathecal Analgesia in Palliative Care

Theodore Pham Nguyen

Case Study

AA is a 73-year-old man with metastatic colorectal adenocarcinoma who is admitted for a pain crisis. AA was ineligible to receive further chemotherapy because of his lack of response and declining functional status. His daughter has noted his increasing difficulty with taking oral medications. AA reported his rectal and abdominal pain as constant, sharp, and burning, with a severity of 10 out of 10 using a numeric rating scale. AA experienced minimal relief from intravenous (IV) morphine, but he exhibited altered mental status and sedation when exceeding 100 mg oral morphine equivalents per day despite opioid rotation attempts and avoiding all possible offending medications (i.e., benzodiazepines and anticholinergics). AA could not tolerate positioning required for a proposed superior hypogastric plexus block procedure. His pain was refractory to adjuvant analgesics such as low-dose ketamine and lidocaine infusions. AA was in agonizing pain affected by dose-limiting side effects with a likely prognosis of days to weeks.

What Do I Do Now?

This is a challenging pain management case initiated in the late stages of this patient's disease. He had limited viable medication options because of his dysphagia. Several adjuvant agents have been utilized without success at improving his pain, and interventional nerve blocks were not considered an option. Although he could not tolerate placement in the prone position required for an interventional nerve block, further discussion was made with the acute pain service to trial neuraxial analgesics.

PATIENT SELECTION AND ROUTE OF ADMINISTRATION

Epidural (ED) and intrathecal (IT) analgesics are typically not first-line approaches to pain management due to the invasive nature involved. Many factors are taken into consideration when evaluating the potential benefits neuraxial analgesia would provide, including the etiology of pain, location of pain, systemic exposure to opioids, comorbidities, ability to tolerate an implant procedure, coagulation status, and psychosocial support available to the patient.[1-3] Practical barriers of neuraxial analgesics involve the accessibility of community resources to refill and adjust pump settings, the availability of a compounding pharmacy, and insurance coverage for medications and refill procedures. ED and IT analgesics have been found to have an improved side-effect profile because of the substantially reduced opioid doses and systemic exposure.[4] However, patients having a failed response from escalating systemic opioids unrelated to dose-limiting side effects may suggest likely failure with neuraxial administration of opioids.[5] A key detail in AA's case was that his pain responded to opioids, but dose-limiting side effects served as a primary barrier to his pain control.

The decision between using an IT or ED route will depend on different patient factors and individual provider experience or preference. Ultimately, the anticipated duration of use or patient prognosis is an important factor when making this decision. Pump devices can be used in both routes, with adjustable bolus dose and basal rate settings. Compared to the more invasive IT route, ED catheters are subjected to higher incidents of complications with long-term use including obstruction, dislodgement, and leakage.[5] In contrast, the ED route has a lower incidence of acute headaches from dura punctures causing cerebrospinal fluid (CSF) leakages. Lower drug concentrations used in the ED route may allow for more precise and flexible dose titrations compared to the IT route. Smaller doses used in IT therapy may reduce the burden of systemic adverse effects and safety concerns from potentially fatal overdoses from rare ED to IT catheter migrations.[6]

External pump systems may be a suitable choice for refractory pain patients with a limited prognosis, but this requires adequate caregiver education for proper maintenance and monitoring because infection risk increases with duration of use.[2,5] External neuraxial pumps with expected use beyond several days require the use of tunneled catheters to reduce the risk of infections and dislodgement as well as pump support from home care or hospice services. Implanted IT devices are not typically utilized in patients with an expected prognosis of less than 3 months because of the costs associated with the procedure and device.[5] A cost utilization analysis estimated that patients requiring high-cost pain regimens (requiring parenteral therapy, >1,000 mg oral morphine equivalents [OME], and nongeneric opioid products) may achieve a cost benefit within 6 months of implanted IT therapy.[7] This may suggest that providers should consider earlier implementation of IT therapies for patients requiring high-dose opioids or complex systemic therapies. As in AA's case, palliative care clinicians may be consulted only when the patient's condition has reached later stages of progression. This limits patient eligibility and therapeutic options for such interventions. Given AA's very limited prognosis, the anesthesia team opted for an external pump via an ED catheter due to a lower incidence of dural puncture headaches. After discussion with the team, AA and his daughter consented to proceed with the ED analgesia with the understanding of potential side effects and complications.

In contrast, patients who may not be suitable candidates for neuraxial therapies are those with active infections, primary headaches or facial pain, or lack of caregiver support or transportation. Consideration of neuraxial opioid therapy may require cautious evaluation in patients with morbid obesity, advanced age, central or obstructive sleep apnea, pulmonary disease, and cardiac disease.[5] Neuraxial interventions should not be performed in patients with sepsis or actively taking anticoagulation therapies.[2] Recommendations for the management of anticoagulation precautions are well defined within the Polyanalgesic Consensus Conference (PACC) 2017 Guidelines and American Society of Regional Anesthesia Guidelines for Interventional Procedures.[5,8]

NEURAXIAL MEDICATION OPTIONS

The PACC 2017 guidelines recommend the use of morphine or ziconotide monotherapy as first-line intrathecal agents approved by the US Food and Drug Administration (FDA) for nociceptive and neuropathic pain, with a preference for ziconotide in non-cancer pain. Alternatively, the use of bupivacaine in combination with an opioid would be considered a reasonable alternative first-line combination in the setting of cancer-related pain. It is imperative to have adequate resources to review compatibility data before considering the use of any drug combinations or admixtures. Using admixtures or higher drug concentrations may place patients at higher risk to experience neuraxial complications, such as the formation of granulomas or fibrosis.[5] The development of catheter-tip granulomas can lead to loss of drug effect, radicular pain, and spinal cord neurological deficits.[9] In such instances, the provider should evaluate whether the benefits may outweigh the risks. Overall, evidence of the efficacy of different drug combinations for neuraxial administration varies among palliative care settings and should be evaluated on a case-by-case basis.

Ziconotide is FDA indicated for intrathecal use for pain and works on the dorsal horn of the spinal cord by blocking presynaptic N-type calcium channels. Ziconotide is an appealing non-opioid option, but its overall accessibility and cost is a major barrier for its use. When initiating IT ziconotide, it is recommended to complete a single trial dose as it may provide an adequate predicted response.[8] The recommended initial starting dose is 0.5–1.2 µg/day, which is lower than that noted on the package insert.[10] Due to its narrow therapeutic window, slow titrations of ziconotide by increments of 0.05–0.1 µg/hr over 3 weeks reduce the incidence of adverse effects including dizziness, confusion, nystagmus, abnormal gait, and cognitive impairment.[10] IT dosing should not exceed 19.2 µg/day (see Table 28.1). It should be avoided in patients with a history of psychosis. Although rare, there have been case reports of ziconotide causing rhabdomyolysis, which requires routine monitoring of creatinine kinase levels and related symptoms such as muscle weakness, myalgias, and dark-colored urine.[5,10]

IT opioids have been well studied in the setting of chronic pain and cancer pain. The pharmacokinetic properties of IT opioids are directly

TABLE 28.1 **Dose Recommendations for Intrathecal Therapy. Doses of initial intrathecal opioids depend on required systemic therapies. Regardless of opioid tolerance status, bolus dose trials are required to determine effective and safe pump settings**

Drug	Starting Daily Dose Range	Bolus Dose Trials	Maximum Concentration	Maximum Daily Dose
Morphine	0.1–0.5 mg/day	0.1–0.5 mg (0.15 mg)[a]	20 mg/mL	15 mg
Hydromorphone	0.01–0.15 mg/day	0.025–0.1 mg (0.04 mg)[a]	15 mg/mL	10 mg
Fentanyl	25–75 µg/day	15–75 µg (25 µg)[a]	10 mg/mL	1000 µg
Sufentanil	10–20 µg/day	5–20 µg	5 mg/mL	500 µg
Bupivacaine	0.1–4 mg/day	0.5–2.5 mg	30 mg/mL	15–20 mg
Clonidine	20–100 µg/day	5–20 µg	1,000 µg/mL	600 µg
Ziconotide	0.5–1.2 µg/day	1–5 µg	100 µg/mL	19.2 µg

*Recommended maximum initial dose for opioid-naïve patients in an outpatient setting. (Deer, Pope, et al. 2017)

impacted by molecular lipophilicity. Hydrophilic IT opioids (i.e., morphine and hydromorphone) have longer half-lives, smaller volumes of distribution, and wider rostral spread. In contrast, lipophilic agents (i.e., fentanyl and sufentanil) have a smaller rostral spread allowing for a more targeted dermatomal response. Currently, morphine is the only opioid with FDA approval for IT therapy. Despite minimizing opioid doses to limit systemic exposure and toxicity, IT opioids are still subject to similar adverse effects: nausea and vomiting, sedation and somnolence, urinary retention, pruritus, myoclonic activity, and respiratory depression.[2,5,10] On the same note, there needs to be caution with concurrent use of systemic central nervous system (CNS) depressants, which may compound additive risks of respiratory depression. Chronic use of IT opioids faces similar long-term side effects of systemic opioid use such as suppression of the hypothalamic-pituitary-adrenal axis, opioid-induced androgen deficiency (OPIAD), and osteoporosis. In a prospective observational study on cancer patients undergoing IT opioid therapy, it was found that patients undergoing IT opioid therapy required substantial doses (average IT morphine doses of >4.2 mg/day and average IT hydromorphone doses of >6.8 mg/day) to produce detectable opioid serum levels.[4] Patients with undetectable opioids serum levels were not associated with worsened pain reports, suggesting that IT opioid therapy may allow for adequate pain management with reduced systemic adverse effects.[4] Initial IT opioid doses are typically based on the number of systemic opioids required by the patient. A frequently referenced morphine conversion ratio is 300 mg oral = 100 mg IV = 10 mg epidural = 1 mg intrathecal; however, there are reports of successful equianalgesic conversion with varying resulting ratios, especially in the setting of combination therapies.[5,9] Due to the lack of studies to validate neuraxial conversion factors, it is recommended to use conservative dosing in anticipation of the need to titrate doses to effect. Patients and caregivers should be educated on the potential side effects of opioid withdrawals in the event of the dislodgement of the catheter or pump failure.

Bupivacaine is a local anesthetic often used in admixtures or alone in interventional pain management. It is a highly lipophilic amide local anesthetic that inhibits action potentials in the dorsal horn through sodium channel blockade and is frequently used as an off-label IT therapy.[2] IT coadministration of bupivacaine with opioids has been shown to have synergistic pain relief and reduce overall opioids requirements, which was an appealing option for AA. Adverse effects from local anesthetics include sensory deficits, motor weakness, urinary retention, orthostatic hypotension, and possible neurotoxicity. Given the high lipophilicity limiting its intrathecal spread, it is suggested that neuraxial catheter placement be centered in the spinal dermatome associated with the targeted pain.[5] Local anesthetics are unlikely to result in withdrawal symptoms in the event of abrupt discontinuation.

Baclofen can be used intrathecally for chronic pain or intractable spasticity, but it is most commonly used in admixtures to treat pain with spasticity.[5,11,12] Some patients may have suboptimal therapeutic responses to oral baclofen therapy despite titration to the maximum safe dose of

80 mg daily but may still obtain benefits from IT baclofen.[13] Inpatient dose titration recommendations allow for 5–15% daily dose increases in cerebral-origin spasticity and 10–30% daily dose increases in spinal-origin spasticity.[11] In an outpatient setting, titrations are recommended to occur on a weekly or biweekly basis. It is recommended for patients on oral baclofen to begin tapering by as much as 25–50% oral dose reductions at the same time as IT baclofen is titrated.[11] IT baclofen is commonly set as simple continuous infusions, but can be set at various rates throughout the day. In some instances, patients who have limited response despite dose escalations may require periodic bolus settings to facilitate better drug distribution within the CSF.[11] Patients and caregivers will require substantial education on the importance of adherence with pump refills and signs of potentially fatal baclofen withdrawal: increased tonicity, altered mental status, hypotension, paresthesia, and seizures. IT baclofen withdrawal requires admission into a monitored floor. Acute management can include the use of low-dose propofol or IV benzodiazepines in the event IT baclofen administration through lumbar puncture is not possible.[14] Oral baclofen may not achieve sufficient CSF concentrations to be a reliable treatment.[15]

Clonidine is an alpha-2 adrenergic agonist that is commonly used in the setting of neuropathic pain. It is thought that clonidine may inhibit the afferent fibers in the dorsal horn of the spinal cord and reduce activation of glial cells, leading to the inhibited production of proinflammatory cytokines. Currently, it is only FDA-indicated for epidural infusions, but it has been studied via IT administration. It requires close initial monitoring due to its commonly reported adverse effects including sedation, xerostomia, bradycardia, and hypotension.[2,5,9]

AA was placed on a percutaneous ED catheter pump, and his pain responded well to several bolus doses. His pump was configured with a continuous infusion and as-needed demand boluses. After a couple of days, he had substantially reduced systemic opioid requirements, exhibited fewer episodes of delirium, and expressed having little to no pain. Low-dose ED opioid therapy allotted him more meaningful interactions with his daughter without the distress of uncontrolled pain. A few days later, AA died peacefully in the unit in the presence of family.

- Neuraxial analgesia is a viable option for patients with pain refractory to standard therapies or impaired by dose-limiting side effects.
- Neuraxial analgesia should not be limited to last-line therapy and should be considered earlier in patients requiring high OMEs or high-cost regimens.
- Implanted IT devices may attain cost benefits in select patients with a prognosis greater than 6 months.
- Patients and caregivers need to be provided with sufficient education about realistic goals, protocols for pump refills, adverse effects, and signs of withdrawals.

References

1. Ertas IE, Sehirali S, Ocek SO, et al. The effectiveness of subcutaneously implanted epidural ports for relief of severe pain in patients with advanced-stage gynecological cancer: A prospective study. *Ağrı—J Turk Soc Algology.* 2014;26(1):8–14. http://www.journalagent.com/z4/download_fulltext.asp?pdir=agri&plng=tur&un=AGRI-14227

2. Farquhar-Smith P, Chapman S. Neuraxial (epidural and intrathecal) opioids for intractable pain. *Br J Pain.* 2012;6(1):25–35. http://journals.sagepub.com/doi/10.1177/2049463712439256

3. Hawley P, Beddard-Huber E, Grose C, et al. Intrathecal infusions for intractable cancer pain: A qualitative study of the impact on a case series of patients and caregivers. *Pain Res Manage.* 2009;14(5):371–379. http://www.hindawi.com/journals/prm/2009/538675/

4. Brogan SE, Sindt JE, Jackman CM, et al. Prospective association of serum opioid levels and clinical outcomes in patients with cancer pain treated with intrathecal opioid therapy. *Anesthes Analgesia.* 2020;130(4):1035–1044. http://journals.lww.com/10.1213/ANE.0000000000004276

5. Deer TR, Pope JE, Hayek SM, et al. The polyanalgesic consensus conference (PACC): Recommendations on intrathecal drug infusion systems best practices and guidelines. *Neuromodulation.* 2017 May 25;20(2):96–132. http://www.ncbi.nlm.nih.gov/pubmed/28042904

6. Simpson RK. Mechanisms of action of intrathecal medications. *Neurosurg Clin N Am.* 2003;14(3):353–364. https://linkinghub.elsevier.com/retrieve/pii/S1042368003000135

7. Brogan SE, Winter NB, Abiodun A, et al. A cost utilization analysis of intrathecal therapy for refractory cancer pain: Identifying factors associated with cost

benefit. *Pain Med.* 2013;14(4):478–486. https://academic.oup.com/painmedicine/article-lookup/doi/10.1111/pme.12060

8. Deer TR, Hayek SM, Pope JE, et al. The polyanalgesic consensus conference (PACC): Recommendations for trialing of intrathecal drug delivery infusion therapy. *Neuromodulation.* 2017 May 26;20(2):133–54. http://www.ncbi.nlm.nih.gov/pubmed/28042906

9. Ghafoor VL, Epshteyn M, Carlson GH, et al. Intrathecal drug therapy for long-term pain management. *Am J Health-Syst Pharmacy.* 2017;64(23):2447–2461. https://academic.oup.com/ajhp/article/64/23/2447/5135084.

10. Deer TR, Pope JE, Hanes MC, et al. Intrathecal therapy for chronic pain: A review of morphine and ziconotide as firstline options. *Pain Med (US).* 2019;20(4):784–798.

11. Boster AL, Adair RL, Gooch JL, et al. Best practices for intrathecal baclofen therapy: Dosing and long-term management. *Neuromodulation.* 2019;19(6):623–631. http://doi.wiley.com/10.1111/ner.12388

12. Boster AL, Bennett SE, Bilsky GS, et al. Best practices for intrathecal baclofen therapy: screening test. *Neuromodulation.* 2016;19(6):616–622. http://doi.wiley.com/10.1111/ner.12437

13. Saulino M, Ivanhoe CB, McGuire JR, et al. Best practices for intrathecal baclofen therapy: patient selection. *Neuromodulation* 2016;19(6):607–615. http://doi.wiley.com/10.1111/ner.12447

14. Saulino M, Anderson DJ, Doble J, et al. Best practices for intrathecal baclofen therapy: Troubleshooting. *Neuromodulation.* 2016;19(6):632–641. http://doi.wiley.com/10.1111/ner.12388

15. Watve SV, Sivan M, Raza WA, et al. Management of acute overdose or withdrawal state in intrathecal baclofen therapy. *Spinal Cord.* 2012;50(2):107–111. http://www.nature.com/articles/sc2011112

Further Reading

Narouze S, Benzon HT, Provenzano D, et al. Interventional spine and pain procedures in patients on antiplatelet and anticoagulant medications (second edition). *Reg Anesth Pain Med.* 2017;43(3):1.

29 Palliative Sedation as a Means for Pain Control

L. Toledo-Franco, Jane E. Loitman, and Matthew D. Clark

Case Study

CG is a 63-year-old man with adenocarcinoma of the prostate with bone metastases to his ribs, pelvis, femur, and sternum for which he has previously received radiation. His oncologist recently withdrew him from a study protocol, and there are no further oncologic interventions available. CG was given a prognosis of weeks. His goal of care changed to comfort, and, over the past several weeks, he was tried on several adjuvants as well as morphine via patient-controlled anesthesia (PCA) titrated to 400 mg/day. Despite these interventions, his pain remained at 10/10 and he developed myoclonus and confusion. His pain was reduced to 7/10 with a hydromorphone PCA, then to 6/10 with a fentanyl PCA at 4,000 μg/day. The myoclonus improved slightly although his confusion persisted with an increase in his anxiety. CG expressed a desire to stop his suffering.

What Do I Do Now?

This chapter reviews palliative sedation (PS) as a means of relieving suffering in patients like CG. PS is a procedure for the terminal phase of life. It is considered an acceptable treatment option in cases where physical suffering persists despite aggressive symptom strategies, although controversy exists over the use of PS for psychological or existential suffering.

Open discussions regarding alleviating suffering with PS would be an initial step for this patient with uncontrolled pain and suffering. If the patient lacks capacity, conversations with the family and surrogate are appropriate to determine if intolerable physical suffering from pain or other symptoms have reached a level that the patient would consider intolerable.

The goal of PS, namely, to reduce suffering, is often confused with euthanasia, physician-assisted suicide, or the double effect. *Euthanasia* is an act intended to hasten death, as in a doctor who intends to hasten the death of a terminally ill patient by injecting a large dose of morphine. *Physician-assisted suicide* is an act intended to hasten death with medications endorsed by a physician, as in a doctor providing a prescription and instructions on how to use the medications to hasten death. The *doctrine* or *principle of double effect* acknowledges that an act meant to promote a good end may bring about foreseen side effects which may be harmful, wherein analgesics and sedatives may lead to death though the goal is sedation and comfort. PS is appropriate to offer to patients with symptoms at the end of life for whom reasonable alternatives have been exhausted. It is for this reason that this procedure is also called *sedation for the terminally ill* or the *imminently dying*, with usually a prognosis of 2 weeks or less. The descriptor "terminal sedation" is seldom used to avoid the confusion just described.

The consent for PS is incredibly important and includes a discussion of the procedure, the risks, benefits, and limitations, as well as ethical concepts with the patient, family, or both. Here the clinician should explain the variety of PS medications to be used, possible side effects, stages at the end of life, and what to expect. Documentation of the patient/family informed decision is equally paramount. Include the depth and desired length of time (brief, respite sedation, or in an ongoing manner) of sedation, as well as the intended plans to assess comfort. Bear in mind that the decision to use PS is revocable.

It is beyond the scope of this chapter to discuss the ethical concerns and particular distinctions for its use, although many medical and ethical organizations have position statements on PS for reference.

The following steps should act as a guide:

1. Document the decision, consent, and discussion addressed earlier.
2. Make the entire treating team aware of the plan and thoroughly document to avoid any potential misunderstandings, doubts, or disagreements about PS.
3. Document that a palliative care provider with an expertise in symptom management has exhausted less invasive, standard options before initiating PS. (PS is a medical treatment and therefore an experienced provider should lead the procedure.)
4. Support the family and others with the interdisciplinary team.
5. Assure there is a "do not resuscitate order" for the patient.
6. Document discussion and plans to provide comfort in the place of life-prolonging interventions such as dialysis, chemotherapy, or transfusions.
7. Document any decisions about artificial nutrition and hydration (ANH). Patients being lightly sedated may be able to eat or drink as desired with monitoring of aspiration risk. With moderate and deep sedation, patient-controlled intake of food and fluids is unlikely. Additionally, to avoid fluid overload, aspiration, and additional discomfort, it may be wise to discontinue ANH.
8. Establish the medication regimen to be used, the setting where the care will be provided, the titration of sedation, the route of administration, and the methods to assess benefits and side effects. Follow the institution's protocol, if present.
9. Monitor efficacy and symptoms in a noninvasive manner with nonverbal manifestations and body language if the patient is not able to communicate. Frequent testing for signs or response to painful stimuli is not recommended. *There are no specific tools to measure comfort, only level of sedation, so one's evaluation is based on clinical assessment of those at the bedside.*

10. Re-evaluate the patient and the family during this time repeatedly. Prognosis is uncertain, and thus the duration of treatment is uncertain.

11. Maintain team support and ongoing education for all involved in the patient's care, during and after the procedure, to include counseling and debriefing once the patient has died. The feelings associated with this particular procedure can facilitate countertransference and feelings of caregiver helplessness if not addressed adequately and on time.

12. Develop a clinical practice guideline, policy, or order set, if one is not already present, to narrow the variation in practice and thereby improve the quality of care.

MEDICATIONS

Classes of medications typically used for PS symptom management include benzodiazepines, antipsychotics, barbiturates, and general anesthetics. Unfortunately, there are no data supporting the use of one agent over the other. Treatment is usually administered in a continuous intravenous (IV) or subcutaneous (SC) infusion, though oral and rectal routes are also potential options. Following the initial bolus, titration of drug occurs until relief is achieved. In home hospice, SC infusions for PS are feasible, however, suppositories may alternatively be used to achieve target sedation without the technology required for parenteral delivery. It is recommended to use medication(s) that the provider is most familiar and comfortable with, start low, and titrate to desired effect.

Benzodiazepines have anxiolytic and anticonvulsant effects and can cause amnesia. These agents also have synergistic sedative effects with opioids. Midazolam is the most commonly used benzodiazepine for PS owing to its short half-life and rapid onset of action. An initial IV bolus dose should range from 0.5 to 5 mg with a continuous rate of 0.5–1 mg/hr. Subcutaneous doses should start at 1.5–2.5 mg with a 50% increase in dose every 4 hours if given with a bolus of 5 mg. Patients who have previously been on a benzodiazepine may require higher initial doses, such as 1.5–3.5 mg every 5 minutes. Titration should be proportional to symptom severity. In the case of delirium, the administration of benzodiazepines can exacerbate symptoms. Therefore, good alternatives to midazolam include neuroleptics (e.g., haloperidol, chlorpromazine) and barbiturates (e.g., phenobarbital). Chlorpromazine is more sedating than haloperidol and thus may have a preferred pharmacodynamic profile for use in PS. Prochlorperazine has been used for PS due to its neuroleptic properties and ready availability. Propofol, which usually requires administration in a closely monitored environment, is another potential PS sedative which additionally has antiemetic, antipruritic, and bronchodilatory effects.

Combinations of these medication with opioids should be considered as these classes of medications offer little to no analgesic effects. Stopping opioids to administer sedatives for PS should be avoided because this practice could result in severe pain exacerbation and acute opioid withdrawal. Prior opioid doses should be continued for pain and/or dyspnea and continue to be titrated as would be done absent PS. Sedative combinations can be administered in an alternating fashion where the regimen is based on the half-life of the shortest acting agent. For instance, if using a combination of an opioid with a half-life of 4 hours and a benzodiazepine with a half-life of 4 hours, each medication would be dosed every 4 hours, though the patient will receive medications every 2 hours. Medications frequently used in PS are provided in Table 29.1.

CONCLUSION

CG was sedated with chlorpromazine, lorazepam, and methadone for 10 days with his wife by his side. She described her husband's death as peaceful after a prolonged battle with cancer pain.

Patients like CG may experience refractory symptoms during the final moments of their life, and these should be addressed aggressively. PS is a potential treatment option of last resort to reduce suffering from symptoms that are unresponsive to traditional modalities. Unlike euthanasia and physician-assisted suicide, the intent of PS is to relieve refractory symptoms rather than hasten death. The procedure has specific indications and steps which include thorough communication and support for the patient, family, and all team members involved. Sedation should be proportionate to the refractoriness of the experienced symptom(s). In other words, sedative agents

TABLE 29.1 **Agents used for palliative sedation**

Benzodiazepines

Drug	Dose	Clinical pearls
Midazolam	Initial bolus: 0.5–5 mg IV/SQ Continuous infusion: 0.5–1 mg/hr IV/SQ Effective dose: 1–20 mg/hr	Short half-life Rapid onset
Lorazepam	Initial bolus: 1–5 mg IV/SQ Continuous Infusion: 0.5–1 mg/hr IV/SQ Maintenance dose: 4–40 mg/day	Peak effect 30 min after IV administration Elimination is not altered by renal or hepatic insufficiency

Neuroleptics

Drug	Dose	Clinical pearls
Chlorpromazine	Initial bolus: 50 mg IV every 6 hours Continuous infusion: 3–5 mg/hr Effective dose: 37.5–150 mg/day	Widely available Multiple routes of administration (IV/IM/PR) Antipsychotic effects
Haloperidol	Initial bolus: 1–5 mg IV/SQ Continuous infusion: 5 mg/day IV/SQ Maintenance dose: 5–15 mg/day	

Barbiturates

Drug	Dose	Clinical pearls
Phenobarbital	Initial bolus: 100–200 mg IV/SQ/IM Continuous infusion: 600 mg/day Maintenance dose: 600–1,600 mg/day	Prior to infusion: Decrease opioid dose by 50% and discontinuebenzodiazepines
Pentobarbital	Initial bolus: 2–3 mg/kg IV Continuous infusion: 1 mg/kg/hr IV (1–2 mg/kg)	Start infusion at same time as loading dose Slow IV push (no faster than 50 mg/min)

Anesthetic

Drug	Dose	Clinical pearls
Propofol	Initial bolus: 20–50 mg IV in emergency Continuous infusion: 10 mg/hr Rescue dose: 50% of bolus dose	Titrate infusion by 10 mg/hr every 15–20 min Non-sedative benefits

should be titrated to the dose effective at alleviating suffering and help with quality at the end of life. Finally, a palliative care specialist should generally be involved to assist with symptom management and the procedure of PS.

KEY POINTS TO REMEMBER

- Palliative sedation is a controversial, yet highly effective method for treating refractory severe pain at the end of life.
- Documentation of informed consent is paramount.
- Numerous medications can be used to achieve palliative sedation with little to no data to support the use of one medication over another medication.
- Frequent monitoring of sedation level should occur under the supervision of a skilled clinician in the practice of palliative sedation.

Further Reading

AAHPM. Statement on palliative sedation. Approved by the AAHPM Board of Directors on December 5, 2014. http://aahpm.org/positions/palliative-sedation

Cherney N. ESMO Clinical Practice Guidelines for the management of refractory symptoms at the end of life and the use of palliative sedation. *Ann Oncol.* 2014;25(3):iii143–iii152.

Cherny N, Radbruch L. European Association for Palliative Care (EAPC) recommended framework for the use of sedation in palliative care. *Palliat Med.* 2009;23(7):581–583.

Jaffe E, Knight CF. *UNIPAC 6 Ethical and Legal Dimensions of Treating Life-Limiting Illness.* 3rd ed. American Academy of Hospice and Palliative Medicine. New York: Mary Ann Lieber; 2008.

Kirk TW, Mahon MM, Palliative Sedation Task Force of the National Hospice and Palliative Care Organization Ethics Committee. National Hospice and Palliative Care Organization (NHPCO) position statement and commentary on the use of palliative sedation in imminently dying terminally ill patients. *JPSM.* 2010;39(5):914–923.

Olsen ML, Swetz KM, Mueller PS. Ethical decision making with end-of-life care: Palliative sedation and withholding or withdrawing life-sustaining treatments. *Mayo Clin Proc.* 2010;85(10):949–954. doi:10.4065/mcp.2010.020 https://www.ncbi.nlm.nih.gov/pmc/articles/PMC2947968/

Quill T, et al. Last-resort options for palliative sedation. *Ann Intern Med.* 2009. 151: 421–424.

Schildmann EK, Schildmann J, Kiesewetter I. Medication and monitoring in palliative sedation therapy: A systematic review and quality assessment of published guidelines. *J Pain Symptom Manage*. 2015;49(4):734–746.

Sinclair C, Stephenson R. Palliative sedation: Assessment, management, and ethics. *Hospital Phys*. 2006;43:33–38.

Six S, Laureys S, Poelaert J, et al. Comfort in palliative sedation (Compas): A transdisciplinary mixed method study protocol for linking objective assessments to subjective experiences. *BMC Palliat Care*. 2018;17:62.

ten Have H, Welie JV. Palliative sedation versus euthanasia: An ethical assessment. *J Pain Symptom Manage*. 2014;47(1):123–136.

30 Bone Pain in Metastatic Disease: NSAIDs and Corticosteroids

Michael A. Smith

Case Study

BJ is a 50-year-old woman diagnosed with widely metastatic clear cell sarcoma of the left foot 1 year ago. She is status post excision of the left foot mass and partial amputation. An x-ray revealed mild scattered degenerative changes with no evidence of fracture. Ten days later, a computed tomography (CT) scan revealed new pathologic compression fractures of the T2 vertebral body and lucencies within T3, T7, T8 and heterogeneous lucencies throughout the thoracolumbar spine. Two weeks later, a magnetic resonance imaging (MRI) study showed numerous patchy bone lesions throughout the lumbosacral spine concerning for metastatic disease. She was admitted with severe cancer-related pain, and she received morphine, cyclobenzaprine, and dexamethasone for pain, and pamidronate for hypercalcemia. An MRI revealed diffuse osseous metastatic disease involving the length of the spine and pelvis. Despite her multimodal analgesia regimen and high doses of opioids, her pain remains severe, with descriptors consistent with metastatic bone pain.

What Do I Do Now?

As a clinician approaching this case, it is important to understand the 10,000-foot view of metastatic bone pain and its underlying pathophysiology. Patients with solid tumors frequently suffer from metastatic disease to the bone, particularly those with breast or prostate cancer.[1] Bone metastases have been associated with shortened survival and significant morbidity related to skeletal complications, a.k.a. *skeletal-related events* (SREs) and are often present within 1 year of cancer diagnosis.[1-3] Historically, bone metastases were thought to be either osteolytic or osteoblastic; however, it is now known that there is really a spectrum of bone metastases.[4] As an example, breast cancer primarily produces osteolytic bone metastases, while prostate cancer primarily produces osteoblastic bone metastases. Each of these, however, is not solely osteolytic or osteoblastic, with features of the opposite morphology being present. In any case, what occurs is known as the "vicious cycle," where tumor cells invade the normal bone structure and release a number of growth factors from the bone. This further promotes tumor cell growth and increases the disruption of the normal bone physiology.[4] Stopping this cycle is step one. Step two is pain management.

It has been reported that more than 90% of patients with metastatic bone disease will have pain, with more than one-third reporting severe pain.[5] Therefore, understanding the pathophysiology of bone pain and how to manage it is all the more important. The pathophysiology of metastatic bone pain is not fully understood but is likely a sequela of the "vicious cycle," with osteolysis, cytokine involvement, nerve infiltration, and stimulation of ion channels being involved.[6] This cycle also leads to pathologic fractures and spinal cord compression (i.e., SREs). Thus, interrupting this cycle remains the treatment of choice. Bisphosphonates and denosumab are the primary treatments of choice for this purpose. These therapies also have been shown to decrease pain severity for sustained periods of time and improve quality of life; however, they are often inadequate as monotherapy for analgesia.[7]

Bones are highly innervated, with an abundance of nociceptors that become activated to transmit pain signals.[8] Therapies to target nociception locally are likely of benefit.

In the case of BJ, it would be a good time to review her medication list: controlled-release (CR) morphine 100 mg orally twice daily, immediate-release (IR) morphine 15 mg orally every 4 hours as needed (using 12 tablets per day), acetaminophen 1,000 mg orally three times daily, dexamethasone 4 mg orally daily, and cyclobenzaprine 10 mg orally three times daily. An odd combination of medications and doses, but one that is too often seen in patients with metastatic bone disease.

Acetaminophen 1,000 mg three times daily is adequately dosed but is not likely of benefit given the patient's progressive disease. In patients on strong opioids, acetaminophen is of little benefit and could be discontinued to decrease medication burden. Cyclobenzaprine is also not likely effective in this setting and appears to play the role of a sedative for BJ. This, too, should be discontinued. Opioids, while often utilized to treat pain associated with boney metastases, may also contribute to overall symptom burden via their potential adverse effects. This only leaves us with dexamethasone to think about.

Corticosteroids and nonsteroidal anti-inflammatory drugs (NSAIDs) are both modulators of the arachidonic acid pathway, important to the production of prostaglandins. In short, prostaglandins can activate nociceptors to begin the ascending pain pathway. Phospholipids are converted to arachidonic acid, which is then converted to prostaglandins. The first step in this pathway is mediated by phospholipases, which are inhibited by the action of corticosteroids. The second step in this pathway is mediated by cyclooxygenases, which are inhibited by the action of NSAIDs with varying degrees of selectivity. Using these drugs in patients with metastatic bone pain is targeting the pathophysiology of the pain as far upstream as possible.

To date, head-to-head data on any NSAID versus a corticosteroid are lacking. The choice of one class versus the other has to do primarily with other compelling indications or contraindications for each drug. As an example, corticosteroids may be more beneficial in patients with fatigue, nausea, or loss of appetite, while NSAIDs may be preferred in patients with diabetes mellitus or agitation. Certainly, given their mechanisms of action and risk of gastroduodenal ulcers, the combination should be avoided, but many of the common side effects of these drugs can be well managed if they are effective analgesics for the patient.[9] Consideration should also be given to the patient's prognosis and goals of care as it relates to use of these drugs concomitantly with active cancer treatment or not and the least additive effects of toxicities.

Dosing and duration specific to metastatic bone pain is also lacking; however, from understanding the disease and other literature on these drugs, the basic rules of "lowest effective dose" and only for the duration of pain are appropriate. Bone pain may abate or be present long term, so the judicious use of these drugs is important given they both have side effects related to prolonged use.

Coming back to BJ, she should likely have her dexamethasone dose doubled to 4 mg twice daily (with the second dose no later than early afternoon due to risk of insomnia). If this is inadequate, a trial of 8 mg twice daily may be warranted. If that is unsuccessful and she remains without benefit or other compelling indications, a rotation to an NSAID is reasonable should renal function and platelet counts allow, although she may not experience earth-shattering relief compared to monotherapy with a corticosteroid. At this time, it would be wise for BJ to be evaluated for other therapies for bone pain, including surgical options, radiotherapy, and osteoclast inhibitor therapy.

KEY POINTS TO REMEMBER

- Bone metastases are common and are associated with reduced survival and significant morbidity.
- Pharmacologic options for treatment to stop the vicious cycle are bisphosphonates and denosumab; these also reduce pain and improve quality of life.
- Pain management for bone pain includes the use of NSAIDs or corticosteroids which target upstream nociception.

References

1. Hernandez RK, Wade SW, Reich A, Pirolli M, Liede A, Lyman GH. Incidence of bone metastases in patients with solid tumors: Analysis of oncology electronic medical records in the United States. *BMC Cancer.* 2018;18(1):44.

2. Svensson E, Christiansen CF, Ulrichsen SP, Rorth MR, Sorensen HT. Survival after bone metastasis by primary cancer type: A Danish population-based cohort study. *BMJ Open.* 2017;7(9):e016022.

3. Poon M, Zeng L, Zhang L, et al. Skeletal morbidity rates over time in patients with bone metastases from solid tumors reported in bone modifying agents randomised trials. *J Bone Oncol.* 2012;1(3):74–80.

4. Mundy GR. Metastasis to bone: Causes, consequences, and therapeutic opportunities. *Nat Rev Cancer.* 2002;2(8):584–593.

5. Vieira C, Fragoso M, Pereira D, Medeiros R. Pain prevalence and treatment in patients with metastatic bone disease. *Oncol Lett.* 2019;17(3):3362–3370.

6. Coleman RE. Clinical features of metastatic bone disease and risk of skeletal morbidity. *Clin Cancer Res.* 2006;12(20S):6243–6249.

7. Costa L, Major PP. Effect of bisphosphonates on pain and quality of life in patients with bone metastases. *Nat Clin Prac Onc.* 2009;6(3):163–174.

8. Aielli F, Ponzetti M, Rucci N. Bone metastasis pain, from the bench to the bedside. *Int J Mol Sci.* 2018;20(2):280.

9. Jaward LR, O'Neil TA, Marks A, Smith MA. Differences in adverse effect profiles of corticosteroids in palliative care patients. *Am J Hosp Palliat Care.* 2019;36(2):158–168.

31 Bone-Directed Therapy for Metastatic Cancer

Keith A. Hecht

Case Study

A 68-year-old woman with advanced breast cancer comes to clinic for follow-up after a bone scan. Two weeks ago, she presented with pain in her upper right arm that worsened over several weeks. At that time, her pain was 10/10, with a typical score of 6/10. She was prescribed immediate-release (IR) oral oxycodone 5 mg to take as needed and a bone scan was ordered. She states the oxycodone helps blunt the pain but the pain persists with severity significant enough to impair activities of daily living. The bone scan showed multiple bone metastases, including small metastases on right-sided ribs 2, 3, and 4 and a large mass on the head of the humerus near the lesser tubercle. Her current cancer therapy is docetaxel, and she has received 1 dose, with her second dose scheduled for next week. Current lab values include hemoglobin of 9.2 g/dL, platelets of 48 k/µL, white blood cell count 3.2 k/µL, 82% neutrophils, and creatinine 0.8 mg/dL. She is wanting something in addition to oxycodone to help with her arm pain.

What Do I Do Now?

This patient is suffering from pain directly related to the metastases to the humerus. Aside from opioid analgesics, the most immediate relief of her pain can be achieved with external beam radiation therapy (EBRT) in a single-dose fraction directly to the mass growing in the humerus. Her current absolute neutrophil count is 2,624 (3,200 × 82%), indicating her marrow has sufficiently recovered from her most recent docetaxel dose and EBRT can be administered. Additionally, since the patient has multiple other bone metastases, she should be considered for bisphosphonate therapy that can stabilize her bone metastases. Radiopharmaceutical treatment would not be appropriate at this time since the patient is undergoing an active myelosuppressive chemotherapy regimen.

Pain from cancer that has spread to the bone is common in patients with advanced cancers, especially cancers of the prostate, breast, or lung. Systemically active analgesics such as opioids, nonsteroidal anti-inflammatory drugs, and corticosteroids offer significant pain relief for these patients, but they do not affect the underlying cause of disease. Bone-specific therapy can offer the opportunity to decrease pain by treating the cancer itself or limiting the effects of the cancer on the bone. Bone-specific therapies include radiation therapy, radiopharmaceuticals, and bone-modifying agents (BMAs). These bone-specific therapies are useful adjuncts in the management of pain from cancer that has spread to the bone.

RADIATION THERAPY

External Beam Radiation Therapy

Radiation therapy to treat pain from bone metastases is highly effective, with trials demonstrating pain response in 60–80% of patients. EBRT is the use of highly focused radiation from an outside source targeted to a specific location in the body, typically the location of a cancer. There are several types of EBRT that offer variations on this concept. EBRT has long been used in the treatment of various forms of cancer in the curative setting and also as part of palliative care. In patients with pain from cancer bone metastases it can help with symptom management, as well as treat consequences of cancer-weakened bones such as fractures and spinal cord compression. EBRT is most useful in the treatment of bone pain from a limited number of sites of involvement. There is no official maximum number of sites that can be radiated concurrently, although it is typically reserved in the setting of three or fewer target sites.

EBRT can be administered as multiple fractions over the course of several days or as a single fraction of therapy. Historically, for palliation of bone metastases, multiple-fraction schemes have been most utilized. However, evidence shows similar efficacy for pain relief from single-fraction radiation therapy with a smaller total dose of radiation (8 Gy from a single fraction vs. 20–30 Gy over multiple fractions). It should be noted that single-fraction radiation therapy is associated with a higher rate of need for later retreatment (20%) than is multiple-fraction (8%). When considering retreatment, total radiation exposure of the target site must be considered and should occur at least 1 month after initial treatment. Single-fraction therapy is more convenient for patients and more cost efficient, even when considering potential need for retreatment.

Because courses of EBRT for palliation of pain are more limited than radiation therapy used for curative intent, side effects are typically less intense. Side effects of EBRT will vary depending on the target site of the radiation. A universal side effect is damage to the skin. This may manifest as redness and irritation, which can be severe in some patients. In patients who are immunocompromised, skin damage could lead to infection. Other EBRT side effects will depend on what other tissue is in the treatment field. For example, radiation to the upper lumbar or lower thoracic vertebrae may reach the stomach, causing nausea and vomiting. Radiation to bone containing proliferative bone marrow (in adults, this is primarily flat bones such as the pelvis or mediastinum) may produce myelosuppression. Since single-fraction radiation is preferred, risk of myelosuppression is minimized. Patients who are neutropenic should wait for white blood cell count recovery prior to initiating EBRT. Due to risk of cumulative damage, specific safeguards are in place that limit the amount of radiation a specific area can receive. This is especially important if patients have received prior EBRT to the same location.

Radiopharmaceuticals

Another method of treating pain from malignant bone metastases with radiation is through the use of radiopharmaceuticals. A key difference for these agents in comparison to EBRT is that they treat multiple bone metastases rather than a single site. The radiopharmaceuticals could be potentially helpful for patients with multiple painful metastases, whereas EBRT is better suited to a limited number of targets. Radiopharmaceuticals are intravenously administered medications indicated for cancer that has metastasized to the bone and that has been confirmed by a bone scan. They exert their anti-cancer effect as calcium mimetics that deliver cytotoxic radiation directly to the site of bone metastases. Bone effects in multiple myeloma are not osteoblastic in nature and should not be treated with radiopharmaceuticals. There are three radiopharmaceuticals approved by the US Food and Drug Administration (FDA) for the treatment of cancer that has metastasized to the bone: strontium chloride Sr-89 (Metastron), samarium Sm-153 lexidronam (Quadramet), and radium Ra-223 (Xofigo). A comparison of these agents is given in Table 31.1.

Strontium-89 and samarium-153 lexidronam emit cytotoxic beta radiation. Strontium-89 also emits gamma radiation, which can be used in imaging of skeletal metastases. Both agents are approved for the treatment of pain from cancer bone metastases that have been confirmed by radionuclide bone scan, without regard to specific tumor type. However, most evidence for these agents is in patients with primary breast cancer, prostate cancer, or non-small cell lung cancer that has metastasized to the bone. These agents are specifically to treat patients with bone pain and are not recommended in a preventative setting.

Strontium-89 and samarium-153 have been shown in multiple clinical trials to decrease bone pain from skeletal metastases as determined by decreases in pain scores as well as a decreased need for opioid therapy. Pain score response rates ranged from 60% to 70% of patients. Benefit was seen in as early as 1 week, with effect sustained up to 16 weeks in some trials. Patients can receive a second dose of either agent after at least 90 days from initial dose.

The most significant adverse reactions occurring with these agents are a flare of bone pain and suppression of the bone marrow, especially leukopenia and thrombocytopenia. Within the first 72 hours of administration of these agents, patients may experience a temporary flare of bone pain that is self-limiting. It is recommended that these patients are supported with opioids during the pain flare. The effect on white blood cells and platelets

TABLE 31.1 **Radiopharmaceuticals used for the treatment of bone pain**

	Indication	Dosing	Mechanism of elimination
Strontium-89 (Metastron)	Radiographically confirmed painful bone metastases from any primary tumor	148 MBq (4mCi) infused intravenously over 1 to 2 minutes Dose may be repeated after at least 90 days	Renal
Samarium-153 (Quadramet)	Radiographically confirmed painful bone metastases from any primary tumor	37 MBq (1 mCi) /kg infused intravenously over 1 minute Dose may be repeated after at least 90 days	Renal
Radium-223 (Xofigo)	Castration resistant prostate cancer with symptomatic bone metastases and no visceral spread	55 KBq (1.49 µCi) /kg infused intravenously over 1 minute repeated every 4 weeks for 6 total administrations Course of therapy should not be repeated	Gastrointestinal in the stool

can be significant and prolonged. An approximate 30% decrease in counts can be expected. The nadir of myelosuppression typically occurs 4–8 weeks after administration of the drug with complete recovery taking up to 16 weeks without intervention. The effect on bone marrow is likely the reason these agents are not frequently utilized. Many patients who would be eligible for radiopharmaceutical therapy have experienced myelosuppression from past chemotherapy exposure, putting them at risk for a more severe effect from the radiopharmaceutical. Additionally, patients may be receiving ongoing myelosuppressive chemotherapy, causing concern for cumulative effects on the bone marrow from concurrent use of chemotherapy and radiopharmaceuticals.

Radium-223 is also a calcium mimetic; however, unlike strontium-89 and samarium-153, radium-223 emits alpha radiation. Alpha radiation has less penetration than beta radiation, resulting in a more localized effect of the radiation. Alpha radiation is more toxic to living cells. This may translate to enhanced toxicity against malignant and nonmalignant cells. It is specifically indicated for the treatment of prostate cancer with symptomatic spread to the bone and no visceral organ involvement. It is not approved in other cancers. An additional difference in comparison to the other radiopharmaceuticals, radium-223 is dosed every 4 weeks for 6 total administrations.

In clinical trials, radium-223 was shown to improve overall survival compared to placebo when used in the treatment of prostate cancer with bone-only metastases that has failed multiple hormonal therapies. Additional analysis showed an improvement in pain as well as other quality of life measures. Because of its demonstrated impact on overall survival, radium-223 is considered the preferred radiopharmaceutical in patients with prostate cancer.

Like strontium-89 and samarium-153, radium-223 causes myelosuppression. The effect on the marrow is more pronounced and includes anemia as well as leukopenia and thrombocytopenia. Peak marrow toxicity may occur 2–3 weeks after each radium-223 dose, however the myelosuppression timeline has varied in clinical trials. Complete marrow recovery is not expected until 6–8 weeks after the final dose. Radium-223 doses after the first should be withheld until the absolute neutrophil count is greater than 1×10^9/L and the platelet count is greater than 50×10^9/L. If blood counts do not recover within 6–8 weeks, any further doses of radium-223 should be discontinued. Other radium-223–related side effects are gastrointestinal in nature, including nausea, vomiting, and diarrhea.

Advances in hormonal therapies for the treatment of advanced prostate cancer have limited the utility of radiopharmaceuticals in this disease. Medications such as abiraterone and enzalutamide have demonstrated ability to slow the development of skeletal metastases from prostate cancer as well as significantly prolong overall survival. Early studies evaluating the use of radiopharmaceuticals combined with other prostate cancer therapies were mostly small trials that demonstrated inconsistent benefit. The

Evaluation of Radium-223 Dichloride in Combination with Abiraterone in Castration-Resistant Prostate Cancer trial (ERA 223) was a large trial (approximately 400 patients per arm) that compared standard abiraterone with a corticosteroid versus the regimen combined with radium-223. In ERA 223 patients receiving combined radium-223/abiraterone experienced more fractures (29% vs. 11%) and deaths (39% vs. 35%) than patients receiving abiraterone alone. Because of the results of ERA 223, combination radiopharmaceutical and hormonal therapies for prostate cancer should be reserved for the clinical trial setting.

BONE-MODIFYING AGENTS

BMAs, including bisphosphonate and denosumab, are considered standard therapy for patients with cancer that has metastasized to the bone. They have proved efficacy in decreasing the likelihood of skeletal-related events such as pathologic bone fractures and spinal cord compression. BMA use as analgesia in patients with active pain is not clearly established. Their primary benefit appears to be in preventing pain due to bone injury. Difficulty in recommending these agents for use in the treatment of pain comes from limitations in evidence. Large studies of BMAs assessed pain relief as a secondary outcome. The studies specifically designed to determine the impact of these agents on pain were typically small and had conflicting results.

Clinical practice guidelines do not recommend the use of one BMA over another. A key difference between denosumab and the bisphosphonates is in their use in patients with compromised renal function. Bisphosphonates should be used with caution in these patients as bisphosphonates are eliminated renally and can be nephrotoxic. Denosumab does not rely on renal clearance. In patients with compromised renal function, denosumab may be the preferred BMA. Studies comparing efficacy of denosumab to zoledronic acid suggest a modest benefit for the denosumab in the form of fewer patients progressing in the severity of pain and some quality of life measures. Table 31.2 lists the BMAs used in the treatment of patients with cancer that has metastasized to the bone.

BMAs have two primary safety concerns: hypocalcemia and osteonecrosis of the jaw (ONJ). These agents prevent bone resorption, decreasing

	Dosing[a]	Mechanism of elimination
Pamidronate (Aredia)	90 mg as a slow intravenous infusion over 2–3 hours, repeated every 3–4 weeks	Renal
Zoledronic acid (Zometa)	4 mg infused intravenously over 15 minutes, repeated every 4 weeks	Renal
Densoumab (Xgeva)	120 mg administered subcutaneously every 4 weeks	Enzymatic breakdown through reticuloendothelial system

[a]Extended interval dosing of every 12 weeks has been utilized for the prevention of skeletal-related events; however, the analgesic effect of extended dosing scheme has not been thoroughly investigated.

the ability of osteoclasts to contribute to calcium homeostasis. Routine calcium supplementation with vitamin D and regular monitoring of calcium levels is recommended for patients receiving BMAs. ONJ is a known adverse effect that can occur as a result of BMA therapy, happening in approximately 10% of patients. The exact mechanism is unknown; however, since bisphosphonates and denosumab cause ONJ at a similar frequency, it is hypothesized that ONJ is a direct result of the antiresorptive activity of the medications.

Bisphosphonates

Cancer cells that have spread to the bone have their deleterious effects through the inhibition of osteoblast and stimulation of osteoclast activity. Bisphosphonates exert their benefit by binding directly to the bone. Once bound, they are internalized by osteoclasts, where they have direct negative effects including inducing apoptosis. The bisphosphonates indicated for the treatment of patients with cancer that has spread to the bone are pamidronate and zoledronic acid, both of which are administered intravenously. Pamidronate and zoledronic acid are both administered intravenously every 3–4 weeks. Studies evaluating their use for prevention of fractures have suggested the interval may be extended as far as 12 weeks for zoledronic acid specifically. Unfortunately, the effects on pain with extended interval dosing have not been established.

Denosumab

Denosumab is a subcutaneously administered monoclonal antibody that inhibits RANK ligand. RANK ligand is a protein that promotes the maturation of osteoclasts. Additionally, RANK ligand stimulates the activity and prolongs the lifespan of osteoclasts. Denosumab prevents bone resorption through binding to RANK ligand, preventing it from binding to the receptor. Denosumab has been studied in patients with many different types of cancer. When compared to zoledronic acid, it has been shown to provide a longer period of time without bone complications. However, denosumab's use for treating patients with bone pain is limited, without consistent benefit across clinical trials.

COMBINING BONE-DIRECTED THERAPIES

Given the varied mechanisms of action involved with bone-directed therapies for pain it is reasonable to consider that combining these treatment strategies may be beneficial. EBRT is routinely used in combination with other therapies, including with bisphosphonates or radiopharmaceuticals. This can be a useful strategy for patients with pain at multiple bony sites that may need additional treatment to a metastatic site due to pathological fracture or risk of spinal cord compression. Cumulative radiation exposure from EBRT and radiopharmaceuticals should be considered, especially in patients who have received multiple treatments of either modality. Systemically active bone targeting agents can be used together without concern for additive toxicities or competing efficacy. Using a BMA in a patient who is being treated with EBRT is an appropriate strategy as well. The EBRT would be most beneficial for treating current bone pain while the BMA would delay the development of future painful bone involvement. Using a BMA along with radiopharmaceuticals has been done in clinical trials without raising additional safety concerns. The BMAs (bisphosphonates and denosumab) should not be used together, primarily due to concern for overlapping toxicities of hypocalcemia and ONJ.

KEY POINTS TO REMEMBER

- Radiation therapy to the site of painful bone metastases is the most effective bone-directed therapy. Single-fraction radiation is the preferred method of administration.
- Radiopharmaceuticals are most beneficial for patients with multiple bone metastases.
- Radium-223 should not be used in patients who are receiving abiraterone.
- BMAs are less useful for the management of acute pain but may be helpful in the prevention of painful bone fractures.

Further Reading

Anderson K, Ismaila N, Flynn PJ, et al. Role of bone-modifying agents in multiple myeloma: American Society of Clinical Oncology clinical practice guideline update. *J Clin Oncol.* 2018;36(8):812–818.

Fallon M, Giusti R, Aielli F, et al. Management of cancer pain in adult patients: ESMO clinical practice guidelines. *Ann Oncol.* 2018;29 (s4):iv166–iv191.

Lutz S, Balboni T, Jones J, et al. Palliative radiation therapy for bone metastases: Update of an ASTRO evidence-based guidelines. *Pract Radiat Oncol.* 2017;7(1):4–12.

National Comprehensive Cancer Network. NCCN Adult Cancer Pain Clinical Practice Guidelines in Oncology, v3.2019. 2019. https://www.nccn.org/professionals/physician_gls/pdf/nsclc.pdf

Nilsson S, Cislo P, Sartor O, et al. Patient-reported quality-of-life analysis of radium-223 dichloride from the phase III ALSYMPCA study. *Ann Oncol.* 2016;27(5):868–874.

Pandit-Taskar N, Batraki M, Dvigi, CR. Radiopharmaceutical therapy for palliation of bone pain from osseous metastases. *J Nucl Med.* 2004;45(8):1358–1365.

Porta-Sales J, Garzon-Rodriguez C, Llorens-Torrome S, et al. Evidence on the analgesic role of bisphosphonate and denosumab in the treatment of pain due to bone metastases: A systematic review within the European Association for Palliative Care guidelines project. *Palliat Med.* 2017;31(1):5–25.

Saylor PJ, Rumble RB, Tagawa S, et al. Bone health and bone targeted therapies for prostate cancer: ASCO endorsement of a Cancer Care Ontario guideline. *J Clin Oncol.* January 28, 2020. [Epub ahead of print].

Smith M, Parker C, Saad F, et al. Addition of radium-223 to abiraterone acetate and prednisone or prednisolone in patients with castration-resistant prostate cancer and bone metastases (ERA 223): A randomised, double-blind, placebo-controlled phase 3 trial. *Lancet Oncol.* 2019;20(3):408–419.

Van Poznak C, Somerfiled MR, Barlow WE, et al. Role of bone-modifying agents in metastatic breast cancer: An American Society of Clinical Oncology-Cancer Care Ontario focused guideline update. *J Clin Oncol.* 2017;35: 3978–3986

32 Chemotherapy-Induced Peripheral Neuropathy

Rachel Caplan and Kate Brizzi

Case Study

RB is a 53-year-old man who presents to the neurology clinic with burning pain in his hands and feet. He has a history of stage IIIB rectal cancer treated with resection, radiation, and a chemotherapy regimen including fluorouracil, leucovorin, and oxaliplatin. Two months after he completed chemotherapy, he developed painful paresthesias in both hands and feet and suffered several falls due to difficulty walking. His neurologic exam shows intact motor power throughout but reduced sensation to pinprick and cold temperature in the bilateral feet to mid-calf. Vibration and proprioception are mildly reduced in the toes bilaterally, and reflexes are absent in the ankles but intact everywhere else. His oncologist has prescribed gabapentin at increasing doses of up to 900 mg three times daily, but he recently discontinued the medication due to somnolence and lack of pain relief.

What Do I Do Now?

Our patient has survived a life-threatening cancer. Now, however, he has other serious problems as a result of his treatment, including chronic pain and disability from severe peripheral neuropathy. As a recipient of platinum-based chemotherapy, he was at high risk for this side effect. His pain has been challenging to treat with the usual suspects like gabapentin and pregabalin, and we worry that intractable symptoms might put him at risk for prolonged opioid use in the future if they aren't better controlled.

EPIDEMIOLOGY, PATHOPHYSIOLOGY, AND DIAGNOSIS

Chemotherapy-induced peripheral neuropathy (CIPN) is one of the most common and debilitating side effects of cancer chemotherapy. When it occurs during treatment, it may lead to early cessation of chemotherapy and, as a result, increased risk of cancer mortality. As a chronic illness, it can have serious effects on independence and quality of life for years after chemotherapy has ended. Around half of patients exposed to neurotoxic chemotherapy (and around one-third of all patients treated for cancer) will develop neuropathy.

Many chemotherapy agents are associated with CIPN, including platinum-based compounds (oxaliplatin and carboplatin), vinca alkaloids (vincristine, vinblastine, and others), taxanes (paclitaxel, docetaxel), and myeloma drugs including bortezomib and thalidomide. Newer chemotherapies, including immune checkpoint inhibitors, such as ipilimumab and nivolumab, can cause immune-mediated neuropathies, some of which may mimic Guillain-Barré syndrome.

RB was treated with oxaliplatin as part of a regimen that is standard of care for colorectal cancer. More than 90% of patients treated with this agent develop acute neuropathy during active chemotherapy treatment, and 69% have chronic neuropathy at a median of 4 years. Because 5-year survival from colorectal cancer is high, patients with treatable cancers like RB may continue to have symptoms well after they finish cancer treatment.

Chemotherapies are toxic to nerves through various mechanisms. Platinum-based chemotherapies, including carboplatin and oxaliplatin, directly damage sensory neurons in the dorsal root ganglia. Taxanes and vinca alkaloids target microtubule function in cancer cells, leading to disruption of axonal transport within nerves. The mechanism of nerve damage in myeloma drugs is not well understood.

CIPN develops during or shortly after chemotherapy, though onset is variable; symptoms often worsen as treatment progresses and the total dose increases. It is most prevalent in the first month after therapy (68.1%), but remains prevalent at 3 months (60%) and 6 months (30%). There are many patients, unfortunately, who will continue to have symptoms even a decade later. Patients who develop CIPN usually have prominent sensory symptoms in a distal symmetric pattern, including both sensory loss and positive symptoms such as burning, tingling, or aching pain. Symptoms most often start in the feet and fingers, but can spread proximally in response to increasing doses of drug. Loss of sensation in hands and feet can lead to clumsiness and sensory ataxia, and patients may be at risk of falling. Weakness is less common, but vinca alkaloids and bortezomib have been associated with distal weakness. Neuropathy can worsen progressively after treatment has ended, a phenomenon called "coasting," which has been seen in oxaliplatin, cisplatin, and vincristine.

Before diagnosing CIPN, a clinician must thoroughly evaluate for other causes of neuropathy, both those related to the patient's cancer and those possibly associated with other medical conditions. Toxic, nutritional, and endocrine neuropathies should be ruled out, and the clinician should schedule for labs including B_{12}, methylmalonic acid, HbA1c, and serum protein electrophoresis. Clinicians should ask about a history of heavy alcohol use, which can cause a toxic neuropathy when a patient has been drinking for a decade or more. Electrodiagnostic studies, as in nerve conduction studies and electromyography, are not very useful for diagnosing CIPN because they can only evaluate large myelinated fibers and not the small myelinated and unmyelinated nerves that are affected in peripheral neuropathy. However, they could be useful as complementary studies if trying to distinguish between polyneuropathy, radiculopathy, or plexopathy. If there is unilateral nerve pain radiating in a brachial or lumbar plexus distribution, for example, a clinician should think about neoplastic plexus invasion (radiation-induced plexopathy, on the other hand, is often painless and presents at a delay of several years). Novel techniques, such as laser Doppler imager scanning, or LDIflare, are being developed to assess small nerve fiber dysfunction and have been studied in CIPN, though it may take time before these are used in the clinic to diagnose polyneuropathy.

PREVENTION AND TREATMENT

While many therapies have been explored for the potential to prevent CIPN, none has proved effective. Studied methods have included vitamin and mineral supplements such as calcium, magnesium, acetyl-L-carnitine, alpha-lipoic acid, and vitamin E, as well as certain herbal supplements, anticonvulsants, and antidepressants (Table 32.1). Small studies have suggested that cryotherapy, or wearing frozen gloves and socks to decrease drug perfusion to the hands and feet during infusion sessions, can also decrease rates of CIPN with certain agents, though further research is needed.

For patients with CIPN, clinicians will often start with medications that are typically used in painful diabetic peripheral neuropathy (DPN), given the large amount of evidence and experience with this condition. Many clinicians will reach for gabapentin before pregabalin due to the latter's classification by the US Drug Enforcement Agency (DEA) as a controlled substance. However, pregabalin not only has fewer side effects than gabapentin, it is the only drug of any class that has Level A evidence to support its effectiveness for painful neuropathy, and it may be a good choice for patients who do not find gabapentin helpful. People using either drug will need to know about the potential for abuse as well as the risk of withdrawal seizures if they stop abruptly. Among other anticonvulsants, sodium valproate is also effective, but its side effects and drug interactions limit its usefulness; oxcarbazepine, lamotrigine, and others are sometimes tried in people with refractory symptoms, but there is no good evidence for these. Antidepressants, including the serotonin-norepinephrine reuptake inhibitor (SNRIs) venlafaxine and duloxetine, and the tricyclic amitriptyline are supported by Level B evidence and can be also be added to anticonvulsants. A randomized trial showed that adding venlafaxine to gabapentin was more effective in reducing pain than gabapentin and placebo alone. Tramadol and opioids are considered third line for those with refractory, severe pain.

Treating CIPN, however, can be challenging for clinicians in that symptoms often do not respond well to most medications that are typically prescribed for painful neuropathy. For example, RB's oncologist

TABLE 32.1 Pharmacologic treatment modalities for chemotherapy-induced peripheral neuropathy (CIPN)

Drug	Class, mechanism	Starting dose for CIPN	Side effects	Evidence (in PDN unless otherwise specified)
Pregabalin	Anticonvulsant; gabapentinoid	25–50 mg once a day	Sedation, dizziness, abuse potential	Small effect in 3 Class I studies
Gabapentin	Anticonvulsant; gabapentinoid	100–300 mg once a day	Sedation, dizziness, abuse potential	Small effect in Class I study
Sodium Valproate	Anticonvulsant; sodium channel blocker and GABAergic	250 mg BID	Fetal abnormalities, liver toxicity, low platelets	Moderate effect in 2 Class II studies
Lamotrigine	Anticonvulsant; sodium channel blocker	25 mg once a day	Stevens-Johnson syndrome	No better than placebo in 2 Class I studies
Duloxetine	SNRI	30 mg daily for 1 week, then 60 mg	Nausea, somnolence, dizziness	High level of evidence in CIPN
Venlafaxine	SNRI	37.5 or 75 mg once daily	Nausea, dry mouth, somnolence, dizziness, not recommended in pregnancy	More effective when added to gabapentin than gabapentin alone
Amitriptyline	Tricyclic antidepressant (TCA)	10–25 mg once daily	Dizziness, weight gain, anticholinergic	Large effect in 3 Class I and II studies
Tramadol	Opioid, opioid agonist, and SNRI	25–50 mg up to TID	Sedation, respiratory depression, not recommended in pregnancy	Moderate effect in class II studies

PDN, painful diabetic neuropathy; SNRI, serotonin-norepinephrine reuptake inhibitor.

Source: Bril, V, et al. "Evidence-Based Guideline: Treatment of Painful Diabetic Neuropathy: Report of the American Academy of Neurology, the American Association of Neuromuscular and Electrodiagnostic Medicine, and the American Academy of Physical Medicine and Rehabilitation." Neurology, vol. 77, no. 6, 2011, pp. 603–603. (cited within paper)

originally started gabapentin, but it made him sleepy and failed to reduce his pain. However, he finally experienced relief when duloxetine was started. Duloxetine is the only agent proved to be significantly more effective than placebo in a randomized trial in CIPN patients, and it is the one medication recommended for treatment by the American Society of Clinical Oncology. In that trial, 231 patients were treated for 5 weeks with duloxetine or placebo, with those receiving duloxetine showing a significant decrease in reported pain scores. Anticonvulsants like gabapentin and lamotrigine have been studied, but they have not been found to be more effective than placebo for CIPN. Other treatments which have been effective in some individuals with CIPN include topical agents like menthol rubs, topical gabapentin, and topical BAK (baclofen, amitriptyline, and ketamine). Neuromodulation techniques, including spinal cord stimulators, have been used to a great effect in a small number of patients with severe refractory symptoms.

Our patient was started on duloxetine, with the dose increased from 30 mg up to 60 mg nightly. His symptoms improved on this dose, and, while he continued to have tingling in his hands and feet, he found this more tolerable. Amitriptyline was later added at a dose of 25 mg nightly, and he also felt he got some benefit from this medication. He continued to be especially sensitive to extreme temperatures and was careful to wear thick gloves when he had to spend time in the cold.

Integrative medicine techniques are frequently offered to patients with cancer, and acupuncture is one of the best-studied therapies; this has been shown to be effective for CIPN in several studies, though further research is needed. Massage by massage therapists trained to work with oncology patients has shown promise whether or not it is directly targeted to the body area affected by neuropathy. Finally, cognitive-behavioral therapy (CBT) is often an integral part of treatment for chronic pain syndromes and has been applied in CIPN; a small randomized trial showed greater improvements in "worst pain" scores for CIPN patients who used a self-directed online CBT program than for those who only received usual care. For patients who have not responded well to neuropathic pain agents or who are reluctant to start prescription pain medications, nonpharmacologic therapies may be an excellent choice.

Unfortunately, RB suffered a fall resulting in a head strike shortly after he developed neuropathy. Physical therapy can help patients develop strategies to avoid injury, and occupational therapy can be helpful if neuropathy in the hands makes everyday tasks more difficult. A referral to a podiatrist may be helpful for strategies to prevent foot injuries.

RB is one of the many cancer patients who continue to have symptoms of painful peripheral neuropathy more than a year after their chemotherapy has ended. However, with the addition of duloxetine, as well as some trial and error with other agents for neuropathic pain, his quality of life has improved and his symptoms now interfere less with his day-to-day activities.

KEY POINTS TO REMEMBER

- One-third of patients treated for cancer will develop CIPN.
- Platinum-based chemotherapies, anti-microtubule agents, and multiple myeloma drugs are most strongly associated with peripheral neuropathy, though newer immune-based therapies can cause autoimmune polyneuropathy.
- Workup should include B$_{12}$, methylmalonic acid, HbA1c, and serum protein electrophoresis to rule out other causes of peripheral neuropathy. Electrodiagnostic testing is not typically helpful.
- Gabapentin and pregabalin are used frequently for painful diabetic peripheral neuropathy and may be helpful, but the antidepressant duloxetine is the single drug proved to be effective in CIPN.
- Acupuncture, massage, and CBT can be highly effective in certain patients.
- Refer patients to physical therapy and podiatry for gait training and injury prevention.

Further Reading

Bril V England J, Franklin GM, et al. Evidence-based guideline: treatment of painful diabetic neuropathy: Report of the American Academy of Neurology, the American Association of Neuromuscular and Electrodiagnostic Medicine, and the American Academy of Physical Medicine and Rehabilitation. *Neurology*. 2011;76(20):1758–1765.

Grisold W, Cavaletti G, Windebank AJ. Peripheral neuropathies from chemotherapeutics and targeted agents: Diagnosis, treatment, and prevention. *Neuro-Oncol*. 2012 September;14(Suppl 4): iv45–iv54.

Shah A, Hoffman EM, Mauermann ML, et al. Incidence and disease burden of chemotherapy-induced peripheral neuropathy in a population-based cohort. *J Neurol Neurosurg Psychiatry*. 2018 June; 89(6):636–641.

Smith EM, Pang H, Cirrincione C, et al. Effect of duloxetine on pain, function, and quality of life among patients with chemotherapy-induced painful peripheral neuropathy: A randomized clinical trial. *JAMA*. 2013;309:1359–1367.

Speck RM, Sammel MD, Farrar JT, et al. Impact of chemotherapy-induced peripheral neuropathy on treatment delivery in nonmetastatic breast cancer. *J Oncol Pract*. 2013;9(5):e234–e240. doi:10.1200/jop.2012.000863.

Staff NP, Grisold A, Grisold W, et al. Chemotherapy-induced peripheral neuropathy: A current review. *Ann Neurol*. 2017 June;81(6): 772–781.

33 Pain in Amyotrophic Lateral Sclerosis

Elyse A. Everett and Kate Brizzi

Case Study

DB is a 62-year-old man with limb-onset amyotrophic lateral sclerosis. He was diagnosed 1 year ago when he presented with weakness in the left arm and right leg. His disease has progressed, and he now requires a wheelchair when traveling more than a short distance. In addition to the limb weakness, he has also developed neck weakness, which has resulted in pain over the back of his neck. Over the past several weeks, he has been wakened from sleep due to painful cramping in the affected limbs. He describes this as a sudden-onset pain that feels like a muscle contraction. He was started on gabapentin 300 mg three times a day, which was gradually titrated to 900 mg three times a day without significant benefit in the cramping. He described fatigue on the higher doses of the gabapentin as well.

What Do I Do Now?

WHAT IS ALS?

Amyotrophic lateral sclerosis (ALS) is a neurodegenerative disease affecting the motor neurons that leads to progressive limb weakness, dysphagia, dysarthria, and respiratory failure. The disease is rare, affecting approximately 2/100,000. Most cases of ALS are sporadic, though approximately 10% have an affected family member. ALS can appear at any age, but it most commonly presents in the seventh decade. There are many forms of ALS, with some patients presenting with more upper motor neuron or lower motor neuron involvement. To date, there is no cure for the disease, and treatment is aimed at improving symptoms, quality of life, and function. Life span with the disease is typically 3–5 years from the diagnosis, but significant variability exists.

TYPES OF PAIN IN ALS

Although ALS is described as a disease of "painless weakness," more recent literature has revealed that pain is a prevalent part of the disease. Studies examining the frequency of pain in ALS have estimated that between 15% and 85% of patients have pain, with variability in how studies were performed. Clinicians do not always ask about pain, and patients may underreport these symptoms if not directly questioned. Pain impacts how patients view their quality of life, and it is significantly more common in patients who also have depression.

The types of pain in ALS falls into three main categories: nociceptive pain, neuropathic pain, and cramping/spasticity.

Nociceptive pain is largely secondary pain resulting from immobility and positioning due to weakness. Nociceptive pain is defined as pain that arises from injury or possible injury to non-neural tissue. There are a number of factors that can contribute to nociceptive pain in ALS. Decreased mobility can lead to increased pressure on the skin and back pain. Adhesive capsulitis can also occur as a result of decreased mobility at the shoulder. Patients who are not mobile require monitoring for skin breakdown and wound development. Neck pain can result from weakness of neck extensors with excessive neck flexion. Masks used for delivery of noninvasive ventilation (NIV) can cause pain due to excessive pressure with skin breakdown, especially as patients start using NIV during the day as well as the night.

Muscle cramps are estimated to affect two-thirds of patients with ALS. While muscle cramps can be seen in patients with both limb-onset ALS and bulbar-onset ALS, they are more common in limb-onset disease. Muscle cramps are typically described as a painful contraction of muscle or "charley horse" and are often more problematic at night. Cramps may reduce in frequency over time as the disease progresses.

Spasticity in ALS is seen most often in patients with upper motor neuron-predominant disease or primary lateral sclerosis. Spasticity is defined as a velocity-dependent increase in tone when the muscle is stretched or moved. Spasticity can cause pain but can also lead to decreased mobility and contractures.

NONPHARMACOLOGIC TREATMENTS

Daily stretching and range of motion exercises (active/assisted/passive) can be effective in preventing and treating nociceptive pain secondary to immobility, joint pain, spasticity, and cramping. Special mattresses, pillows, and custom wheelchairs can be used to improve pain related to positioning and immobility. Patients and caregivers should be educated that frequent position changes are needed to reduce the risk of pressure injuries. Neck braces and headrest attachments for wheelchairs can be used for pain related to neck weakness. Splints that hold wrists and ankles in neutral positions can help prevent contractures at those joints. Massage therapy, acupuncture, transcutaneous electrical nerve stimulation, and warm or cold compresses are also used for nonpharmacologic pain management. Physical therapists, occupational therapists, and wheelchair specialists can assist with recommending and implementing these various treatments. Durable medical equipment companies and noninvasive ventilation (NIV) clinics can help to prevent facial pain due to excessive pressure by providing a variety of masks for rotation as well as other techniques, including protective skin coverings on areas with high contact pressure. Many patients can use nasal masks during the day and oronasal masks at night to prevent continuous pressure applied to one area.

PHARMACOLOGIC TREATMENTS

Evidence for pharmacologic treatment of pain in ALS is scant and generally of low quality; guidelines for treatment are largely based on small, nonrandomized studies and clinical expertise.

Nociceptive pain is initially managed with nonsteroidal anti-inflammatory drugs (NSAIDs) and acetaminophen. Intra-articular steroid/lidocaine injections can be considered for painful joints in paretic limbs, especially the shoulder. In the cases of severe pain refractory to NSAIDs or contraindications to NSAIDs, low-dose opioids can be considered with special attention paid to respiratory status.

Pain due to muscle cramps can be very difficult to treat. Quinine sulfate was traditionally used but this medication now carries a boxed warning in the United States against its use for cramps due to risk of severe side effects such as cardiac arrhythmias, thrombocytopenia, and severe hypersensitivity reactions. Mexiletine, a sodium channel-block antiarrhythmic, was found in a small randomized controlled trial to reduce the frequency and severity of cramps in patients with ALS. Other commonly used medications to treat cramps include baclofen, magnesium, benzodiazepines, and antiepileptic drugs including gabapentin, levetiracetam, and carbamazepine.

Spasticity is also difficult to treat pharmacologically. Commonly used medications include baclofen, tizanidine, dantrolene, carbamazepine, and benzodiazepines. Intrathecal baclofen is rarely used in cases of intractable pain due to spasticity. Low-dose botulinum toxin injections can be considered if systemic medications cause unacceptable side effects and spasticity is limited to few muscle groups.

Neuropathic pain can be treated with a variety of antiepileptic drugs and antidepressants, including gabapentin, pregabalin, tricyclic antidepressants (TCAs), venlafaxine, and duloxetine.

Consideration of which medication to use should include what other medications the patient is on as well as what other symptoms the patient is experiencing, as many of the referenced medications can be used to treat other symptoms of ALS. For example, TCAs can be used for the treatment of sialorrhea and help with sleep. Opioids and benzodiazepines can improve dyspnea as well as sleep. It is important to warn patients that many of these medications can cause sedation, fatigue, and generalized weakness, especially at higher doses.

For DB, nonpharmacologic treatment of his pain could include meeting with a physical therapist to develop a stretching program to help with his nighttime cramping. He could also try using a soft neck brace during the day to improve his neck pain that is the result of neck extension weakness. Pharmacologic treatment could include acetaminophen 1,000 mg every 8 hours as needed or naproxen 500 mg every 12 hours as needed. Given the failure of gabapentin to treat DB's nighttime cramping with sedation at the higher dose, next-line treatment could be baclofen 10–20 mg nightly or mexiletine 150 mg twice daily.

KEY POINTS TO REMEMBER

- ALS is a quickly progressive neurodegenerative illness that causes more symptoms than just weakness.
- Pain in ALS is common, due to multiple mechanisms, and may not be reported by patients unless specifically asked about.
- Nociceptive pain due to immobility and positioning is best treated with nonpharmacologic methods (stretching, frequent repositioning, custom wheelchairs, braces), but NSAIDs and acetaminophen can be used as well.
- Pain due to muscle cramps can be treated with mexiletine, baclofen, magnesium, benzodiazepines, and antiepileptic drugs including gabapentin, levetiracetam, and carbamazepine.
- Pain due to spasticity can be treated with baclofen, tizanidine, dantrolene, carbamazepine, and benzodiazepines.
- Opioids can be used for refractory pain, but clinicians should "start low and go slow" due to ALS-related respiratory failure.

Further Reading

Atassi N, Cook A, Pineda CME, et al. Depression in amyotrophic lateral sclerosis. *Amyotroph Lateral Scler.* 2011;12:109–112.

Brettschneider J, Kurent J, Ludolph A. Drug therapy for pain in amyotrophic lateral sclerosis or motor neuron disease. *Cochrane Database Syst Rev.* 2013;(6):CD005226. doi:10.1002/14651858.CD005226.pub3.

Caress JB, Ciarlone SL, Sullivan EA, et al. Natural history of muscle cramps in amyotrophic lateral sclerosis. *Muscle Nerve*. 2016 Apr;53(4):513–7.

Chio A, Mora G, Lauria G, et al. Pain in amyotrophic lateral sclerosis. *Lancet Neurol*. 2017 Feb;16(2):144–157.

Foster LA, Salajegheh MK, et al. Motor neuron disease: Pathophysiology, diagnosis, and management. *Am J Med*. 2019 Jan;132(1):32–37.

Alsultan AA, Waller R, Heath PR, et al. The genetics of amyotrophic lateral sclerosis: Current insights. *Degener Neurol Neuromusc Dis*. 2016;6:49–64.

Marvulli R, Megna M, Citraro A, et al. Botulinum toxin type A and physiotherapy in spasticity of the lower limbs due to amyotrophic lateral sclerosis. *Toxins (Basel)*. 2019;11:381. doi:10.3390/toxins11070381.

Ng L, Khan F, Young CA, et al. Symptomatic treatments for amyotrophic lateral sclerosis/motor neuron disease. *Cochrane Database Syst Rev*. 2017;1:CD011776.

Oskarsson B, Moore D, Mozaffar T, et al. Mexiletine for muscle cramps in amyotrophic lateral sclerosis: A randomized, double-blind crossover trial. *Muscle Nerve*. 2018;58(1):42–48.

Raheja D, Stephens HE, Lehman E, et al. Patient reported problematic symptoms in an ALS treatment trial. *Amyotroph Lateral Scler Frontotemporal Degener*. 2016;17(3-4):198–205.

34 Uremic Neuropathy

Stefanie Pina-Escudero

Case Study

An 80-year-old man comes into the clinic because of a
recent fall due to progressively worsening decreased
sensation in his feet. He reports the sensation of
"walking on cushions" over the past week. Additionally,
he reports a painful burning sensation (6/10 on a visual
analog scale) and dysesthesia in both hands. He had
been diagnosed with chronic kidney disease at the age
of 65 secondary to poorly controlled hypertension.
He denies any other pertinent medical history. His
meds include amlodipine, furosemide, and calcitriol.
Physical exam is largely unremarkable other than
absent DTRs and impaired pinprick and light touch
sensations. His labs showed BUN 140 mg/dL, SCr 6.79
mg/dL, HbA1C 5.5%, hgb 8 g/dL, K 6 mEq/L, corrected
Ca 7.6 mg/dL, Mg 1.9 mg/dL and phosphate 0.6 mg/
dL. Nerve conduction studies were performed, and the
results were compatible with a severe sensorimotor
polyneuropathy. He no longer desires hemodialysis,
and at this point the palliative care team was consulted.

What Do I Do Now?

This case illustrates a patient with uremic neuropathy, which is one of the most common symptoms in patients with end-stage renal disease (ESRD) especially with a glomerular filtration rate below 12 mL/min. Uremic neuropathy develops more often in men compared to women and its incidence, depending on the series, ranges from 60% to 83% of patients with advanced chronic kidney disease (CKD). It presents as a distal symmetric sensorimotor polyneuropathy with greater lower limb than upper limb involvement. Sensory impairment manifests in patients as paresthesia or burning sensations in the distal parts of the limbs which are unpleasant, painful, and could impair their ability to sleep. In the physical examination, diminished perception of light touch, vibration, and temperature sensations in a stocking-and-glove distribution are evident. Regarding motor impairment, cramps might be the first symptom that indicates low motor neuron involvement. The physical examination of a patient with motor dysfunction can reveal muscle atrophy, weakness, and diminished or loss of deep tendon jerks. This case highlights that, particularly in older adults, sensorymotor deficits may lead to gait disturbances and falls that could potentially increase morbidity. Cases of cranial nerve uremic neuropathy, with visual or autonomic manifestations, have also been reported. The typical progression of uremic neuropathy occurs over months, as in this case, but rapid exacerbations of chronic renal insufficiency or sepsis might lead to an accelerated or even a fulminant course. In patients with other comorbidities such as diabetes or vasculitis, the diagnosis of uremic neuropathy becomes challenging.

In patients with CKD and neuropathic pain, electrophysiology studies are indicated only in symptomatic patients to corroborate the diagnosis. Motor nerve conduction velocity, which is often measured in the peroneal nerve, is characterized by prolongation of tibial F-wave minimum latencies. It is the most common parameter used to assess motor function. The sensory nerve conduction velocity of the sural nerve is even more sensitive in detecting early dysfunction but is not as widely used. Nerve conduction velocity tests usually show a reduction of motor and sensory-motor unit potential amplitudes indicating large-diameter axon neuropathy. Progressive cases are associated with demyelinating changes resulting in prolonged latencies and prolonged duration of sensory or motor unit potentials and reduction of nerve conduction velocities. Acute and chronic inflammatory demyelinating polyneuropathies have been described in patients with CKD due to membranous nephropathy or focal segmental glomerulosclerosis. In the context of patients with life-limiting serious illness, unless there is an important diagnostic doubt or a differential diagnosis that influences the therapy, measuring light touch and vibratory perception thresholds might be more suitable for diagnosis and follow-up than nerve conduction velocity measurements.

The pathologic features of uremic neuropathy are severe axonal degeneration in the most distal nerve trunks with secondary segmental demyelination. These findings support that uremic neuropathy is a dying-back neuropathy, with metabolic failure of the neuron causing distal axonal degeneration. The exact underlying mechanisms leading to the pathological changes remain unknown. One proposed pathway contemplates the accumulation of middle molecules like oxythiamine or guanidinosuccinic acid. These toxins inhibit the thiamin-dependent enzyme transketolase, pyridoxal phosphate kinase, and sodium-potassium ATPase, leading to destabilization of the axon-cylinder myelin sheaths, impaired tubulin polymerization, and blockage of neural transmission. The accumulation of parathyroid hormone and myoinositol has also been associated with alterations in the nerve conduction velocity. Another pathway could be mediated by electrolyte alterations such as hyperkalemia and hyperphosphatemia. Hyperkalemia leads to intracellular accumulation of calcium and reversal of the potassium/calcium (K/Ca) pump that results in axonal damage and depolarization.

Considering the pathologic features for the treatment of uremic neuropathy, the first question that needs to be answered is if the patient is a good candidate for dialytic therapy or not. If the answer is positive, hemodialysis or peritoneal dialysis becomes the first line of treatment. These therapies normalize nerve excitability parameters by removing middle molecules and reversing electrolyte abnormalities. Dialytic therapy was offered to this patient. After multidisciplinary consultations with nephrology, geriatrics, and palliative care, the patient made a fully informed choice not to start dialysis. He was then offered multidisciplinary palliative care. In patients who are not good candidates for dialytic therapy or who, as in this case, refuse it, other alternatives must be considered to treat uremic neuropathy. Relief of all symptoms is generally not possible in patients who are not going to be dialyzed, and it is important to establish realistic management expectations with the patient. The goals of the treatment need to focus on relieving symptoms to a tolerable level that allows optimal function and quality of life.

Conservative or nondialytic management of kidney disease is a high priority because fluid balance alterations, anemia, acidosis, and hyperkalemia contribute to the appearance and worsening of symptoms in uremic neuropathy. Edema may worsen neuropathic pain, and the prescription or adjustment of loop diuretics (oral furosemide 80–240 mg/day) with or without thiazide-like (metolazone, chlorthalidone, indapamide) or thiazide-type (hydrochlorothiazide) diuretics is a powerful tool to manage edema in patients with residual diuresis, as in this case. In those patients who do not have residual diuresis, fluid restriction, and comfort measures for dry mouth and metallic taste need to be implemented. However, imprudent use of diuretics or excessive fluid restriction could lead to hypovolemia and electrolyte alterations. In this case, the patient presents with anemia that can be addressed using erythropoiesis-stimulating agents and iron supplements to target ferritin levels above 200 ng/mL and hemoglobin levels between 11 and 12 g/dL. Erythropoietin has been shown to improve motor nerve conduction velocity and limb weakness but has no effect on sensory indices. It is important to monitor secondary hyperparathyroidism of ESRD because, if uncontrolled, it can lead to erythropoietin resistance. This patient has hypocalcemia and an elevated phosphate, which raises a suspicion of uncontrolled secondary hyperparathyroidism that needs to be addressed. This patient is also lacking arterial gases determination. If acidosis is present, it can be managed with oral bicarbonate (500–1,000 mg, 3–4 times a day) to keep the goal of serum bicarbonate levels above 22 mEq/L to improve symptoms attributed to uremia. Higher doses may contribute to the appearance or worsening of edema and the onset of abdominal colic and diarrhea. Potassium is also out of range in this patient. This electrolyte can be maintained within as normal ranges as possible with dietary potassium restriction, loop diuretics, and potassium-removing agents such as sodium polystyrene sulfonate. Normalizing potassium levels has shown uremic neuropathy improvement in earlier stages of CKD. In the very advanced stages of the disease, a comprehensive evaluation that considers life expectancy, nutritional status, quality of life, and severity of symptoms will help to individualize dietary recommendations. Avoiding the use of drugs such as angiotensin-converting-enzyme inhibitors or angiotensin II receptor blockers is also recommended to avoid hyperkalemia. Dietary supplements like biotin (10 mg/day), high-dose thiamine (30–45 mg/day equivalent), and pyridoxine (60 mg/day) have also been shown to improve uremic neuropathy symptoms in patients with ESRD in hemodialysis but there is no evidence in conservative management. For this patient, diuretic management was adjusted and edema was well controlled. This diuretic adjustment and mild dietary restriction helped control potassium levels. Sevelamer was added to control phosphate levels. Arterial gases were requested and due to an HCO_3 of 13 mmol/L, oral bicarbonate was prescribed. Monthly intravenous iron and weekly subcutaneous epoetin were prescribed to maintain hemoglobin target.

Once the management of the underlying pathology is instituted, uremic neuropathy symptoms must be directly addressed. Physical therapy may prevent the loss of muscle power and prevent or improve functional loss caused by uremic neuropathy. When significant weakness is present, devices such as ankle/foot orthosis, canes, walkers, or wheelchairs may help with mobility. This patient started with an at-home physical therapy program 5 days a week, focused on maintaining balance and strength. Also, a cane was prescribed to avoid further falls. He received fall prevention and fall safety protocol education. Passive mobility and postural changes are also important toward the end of life because patients with neuropathy are at an increased risk of developing foot ulcers. Proper foot and nail care are encouraged to prevent additional complications.

Regarding pain and dysesthesias, there is a paucity of literature on anticonvulsants such as gabapentin and pregabalin for uremic neuropathy. Based on studies of polyneuropathy in patients in hemodialysis, these medications need to be used judiciously since even low doses have been associated with adverse events such as altered mental status and falls. The elimination half-lives of gabapentin and pregabalin are 132 and 48.7 hours, respectively, in patients with creatinine clearance (CrCl) of less than 15 mL/min, which leads to accumulation and potential dose-dependent toxicity. Therefore, doses as low as 100 mg of gabapentin or 25 mg of pregabalin are recommended when initiating these therapies. Oral solutions may be used to administer even lower doses. Increases in dosing intervals may also be required when compounded lower doses are unavailable (e.g., three times per week). For this patient, pregabalin 25 mg three times a week was initiated and titrated to 75 mg three times per week. After the new metabolic control and anticonvulsant recommendations were followed, the patient experienced an improvement in pain to 3/10 and a reduction of paresthesias.

Another group of drugs that has been used in polyneuropathy to address pain and dysesthesias are antidepressants; however, they tend to be poorly tolerated—although not contraindicated in patients with ESRD—and could potentially exacerbate electrolyte disturbances and lower the seizure threshold. It is also important to keep in mind that the pharmacological effect starts after 4–6 weeks when considering antidepressants for a patient at the end of life.

If pain is severe and anticonvulsants are not well tolerated in higher doses, opioids may be considered. They also become the first choice of treatment toward the end of life when these patients might present with other etiologies of pain or dyspnea. Fentanyl is a potent and highly lipid-soluble synthetic opioid. It is metabolized in the liver into inactive and nontoxic metabolites with less than 10% excreted unchanged in the urine. These characteristics support fentanyl as the preferred opioid in patients with ESRD. Fentanyl's main disadvantage is primarily a limited selection of commercially available dosage forms (transmucosal, transdermal, and parenteral). Additionally, transdermal and parenteral doses may accumulate with sustained administration, requiring a dose reduction of 50% if CrCL is less than 10 mL per minute. Doses of 150–250 μg per 24 hours in a continuous subcutaneous infusion are often sufficient to control pain. Careful monitoring for toxicity is needed. Equivalent transdermal doses can be delivered through a patch once the pain is controlled, although some data suggest reduced efficacy of transdermal fentanyl in cachectic patients.

Another synthetic opioid that represents an option for patients with ESRD is methadone. Its metabolites are mostly excreted in the feces, but renal excretion of the unchanged drug is important, and it can accumulate in tissues on repeated administration. There is weak evidence that plasma concentrations are no higher than in those with normal renal function, suggesting that fecal excretion might compensate in those with renal impairment. Because of this and the limited possibilities for use of other opioids, methadone has been used particularly for neuropathic pain in patients with ESRD. Strict monitoring for adverse events and toxicity is paramount. A dose reduction of 50–75% is recommended in patients with ESRD following any previous equianalgesic calculations when converting from another mu opioid agonist. While the incidence is unclear in this patient population, methadone-associated QTc prolongation should be considered, especially given the propensity for electrolyte abnormalities.

Buprenorphine may represent an attractive opioid analgesic in those with ESRD and uremic neuropathy owing to its biliary excretion. However, it cannot be unequivocally recommended owing to its active metabolites that may undergo renal excretion, with associated accumulation in patients with ESRD. Norbuprenorphine is 40 times less potent than buprenorphine and exhibits pure mu agonist activity, while buprenorphine-3-glucuronide (B3G) has only a small antinociceptive effect. One study in rats has demonstrated B3G is a more potent respiratory depressant than buprenorphine despite its limited analgesic efficacy. Given the limited evidence, it should be used with caution, considering dose reduction, increased dose interval, and careful monitoring until more evidence is available.

Because drug treatment is associated with numerous side effects, nonpharmacologic strategies such as electroanalgesia are potential adjuvants. High-tone external muscle stimulation showed efficacy in a pilot study with 25 participants for the discomfort and pain associated with diabetic and uremic neuropathy.

It is important to consider that constipation is frequent with opioids, and, in patients with peritoneal dialysis, it may interfere with the therapy and could even worsen uremic symptoms due to microbiota production of uremic toxins. Appropriate laxatives are important in all patients receiving opioids but even more so in the context of patients receiving dialytic therapy.

A final consideration toward the end of life of these patients is that they can develop uremic encephalopathy or delirium for different reasons and these might be interpreted as an adverse effect of medication. These conditions need to be exhaustively ruled out before modifying the treatment because poor control of pain might worsen delirium and increase suffering.

After 4 months, despite all the measures, fluid retention and peripheral edema increased progressively in our case study patient. The pain progressively increased to 8/10 despite increasing the dose of pregabalin, and he started complaining about shortness of breath. At this point, he began to receive hospice care at home, and fentanyl was incorporated into the management with good control of dyspnea and pain improvement (4/10). His mental status began to deteriorate due to uremic encephalopathy, and he was unable to get out of bed. Passive mobilization helped prevent pressure ulcers. The patient died 10 days after the last consultation.

KEY POINTS TO REMEMBER

- Distal symmetric sensorimotor polyneuropathy is the most common presentation of uremic neuropathy.
- In patients who are not in dialytic therapy, conservative management of kidney disease might have a positive impact on uremic neuropathy.
- Physical therapy may prevent the loss of muscle power and improve functionality.
- Fentanyl is the first-line opioid in patients with poor pain control with anticonvulsants or with concomitant dyspnea.
- In patients prescribed opioids, management of constipation is particularly important to maintain electrolyte equilibrium and prevent drug or metabolite toxic accumulation.

Further Reading

Arnold R, Pianta TJ, Pussell BA, et al. Randomized, controlled trial of the effect of dietary potassium restriction on nerve function in CKD. *Clin J Am Soc Nephrol.* 2017 October 6;12(10):1569–1577.

Brown SM, Holtzman M, Kim T, Kharasch ED. Buprenorphine metabolites, buprenorphine-3-glucuronide and norbuprenorphine-3-glucuronide are biologically active. *Anesthesiology.* 2011;115(6):1251–1260.

Camargo CRS, Schoueri JHM, Alves BCA, Veiga GRL, Fonseca FLA, Bacci MR. Uremic neuropathy: An overview of the current literature. *Revista da Associação Médica Brasileira.* 2019;65(3):469–474.

Ishida JH, McCulloch CE, Steinman MA, Grimes BA, Johansen KL. Gabapentin and pregabalin use and association with adverse outcomes among hemodialysis patients. *J Am Soc Nephrol.* 2018;29(7):1970–1978.

Klassen A, Di Iorio B, Guastaferro P, Bahner U, Heidland A, De Santo N. High-tone external muscle stimulation in end-stage renal disease: Effects on symptomatic diabetic and uremic peripheral neuropathy. *J Renal Nutr.* 2008;18(1):46–51.

Krishnan AV, Kiernan MC. Uremic neuropathy: Clinical features and new pathophysiological insights. *Muscle Nerve.* 2007;35(3):273–290.

Murtagh FE, Chai MO, Donohoe P, Edmonds PM, Higginson IJ. The use of opioid analgesia in end-stage renal disease patients managed without dialysis: Recommendations for practice. J Pain Palliat Care Pharmacother. 2007;21(2):5–16.

Pham PC, Khaing K, Sievers TM, et al. 2017 update on pain management in patients with chronic kidney disease. *Clin Kidney J.* 2017;10(5):688–697.

Raouf M, Atkinson TJ, Crumb MW, Fudin J. Rational dosing of gabapentin and pregabalin in chronic kidney disease. *J Pain Res.* 2017;10:275–278.

Said G, Krarup C, eds. Uremic neuropathy. *Handbook of Clinical Neurology.* Elsevier. 2015;115:607–612.

Sherifa AH. Neurologic conditions and disorders of uremic syndrome of chronic kidney disease: Presentations, causes, and treatment strategies. *Exp Rev Clin Pharmacol.* 2019;12(1):61–90.

35 Cancer Pain Syndromes

Daniel Paget

Case Study

CN is a 69-year-old female with stage 4 ovarian cancer following multiple rounds of chemotherapy and known metastatic disease to the liver. She presented with several days of escalating right upper quadrant pain which she described as "deep aching pain" that referred to her right shoulder and mid-back. This pain was worsened by movement and deep breaths. The pain was constant at 8/10, and "flared" 4–5 times daily for 30 minutes with no clear precipitant. Her medication list included acetaminophen 650 mg every 6 hours as needed, immediate release morphine 15 mg every 4 hours as needed (4 doses over the past 24 hours with minimal relief), and controlled-release (CR) morphine 30 mg every 12 hours. Exam was notable for marked hepatomegaly, with tenderness to palpation diffusely at the right upper quadrant, without rebound or guarding. The shoulder exam showed no erythema or swelling on visualization, but was notable for hyperalgesia on the anterior aspect of the shoulder. Labs were notable for an albumin of 2.5, and otherwise normal liver function tests, INR, and complete blood count. A computed tomography (CT) scan of the abdomen and pelvis showed significant progression of hepatic metastatic disease but no signs of biliary obstruction. An x-ray of the right shoulder showed no bony metastatic disease. Prior to a palliative care consult, the patient was continued on CR morphine 30 mg twice a day and was started on intravenous (IV) morphine 5 mg every 2 hours as needed. She has used 30 mg of IV morphine for a total of 150 oral morphine equivalents (OME; 60 mg oral morphine + 30 mg IV morphine × 3 = 150 mg OME) over the past 24 hours. She still notes 8/10 pain with 3–4 spikes to 10/10 over the past 24 hours, which seem to return to her baseline 8/10 pain over 30 minutes with morphine dosed as needed.

What Do I Do Now?

Cancer is a highly heterogeneous disease process that presents significant burdens to patients and their families. Acute and chronic pain are common among patients with active cancer and contribute significantly to this burden. A recent meta-analysis found the prevalence rates of cancer pain to be 39.3% after curative treatment, 55% during treatment, and 66.4% in advanced disease. While many treatment guidelines have been published over the past 15 years, one review suggested that as many as 43% of cancer patients received inappropriate pain management. In many cases, the constellation of pain symptoms experienced by cancer patients can suggest specific well-characterized cancer pain syndromes. The recognition of these syndromes is an essential skill for palliative care clinicians given their important prognostic and therapeutic implications.

A palliative care approach to pain should always begin with a methodical assessment of both the phenomenology and pathogenesis of the pain. Pain is inherently subjective, and patient self-report is the gold standard for assessment. Pain should be described specifically based on temporal features (onset, pattern, and course), location and radiation, severity (typically defined by a rating scale, either mild/moderate/severe or numeric 1–10 rating), quality, and exacerbating or alleviating factors. If a patient is nonverbal, several pain rating scales are available to aid the examiner in systematic pain assessment, including the PAINAD and Doloplus-2 scales. It is important to elicit caregiver input, including observations about nonverbal pain cues or any recent behavioral changes that might suggest worsening pain.

CN has given a highly specific account of her pain, and the clinician's next step is to identify potential mechanisms behind it. Pain may be described as nociceptive, neuropathic, or a combination. The term "nociceptive" describes pain resulting from sustained tissue injury and is further classified as *somatic* when related to primary afferent nerve activation or *visceral* when visceral afferents are activated. Visceral pain tends to be poorly localized and described as vague, gnawing, or crampy. The reason for this mechanistically is that visceral nerves have much lower innervation density than somatic nerves, as well as afferent projections to a much larger number of levels in the spinal cord: one visceral sensory nerve may innervate multiple visceral organs. In addition, the phenomenon of referred pain occurs because visceral and somatic afferent fibers can converge on the same part of the spinal cord. As a result, nociceptive signals from a visceral site may be processed by higher brain centers and associated with seemingly unrelated areas of the body. The referral sites are quite specific based on the location of the primary tumor: esophageal distention refers to the chest and back, and cervical distention refers to the lower abdomen and back. Hepatic distention leads to pain in the region of the ipsilateral scapula, and hyperalgesia and allodynia can also occur at the site of referral. Neuropathic pain results from damage to the nervous system itself and has varied subtypes including deafferentation pains (central pain, phantom pain, and postherpetic neuralgia), mono/polyneuropathies, and complex regional pain syndromes. Neuropathic pain syndromes are often less responsive to opioid drugs; therefore, determination of pathophysiology is essential in guiding appropriate therapy. CN's description of her abdominal pain suggests that it is visceral in nature, given its nonspecific aching quality, location, and reference to the right shoulder.

Another helpful step in the diagnosis process is to determine if a patient's presentation falls under the rubric of a pain syndrome. The majority of pain syndromes in cancer patients are chronic syndromes and as many as three-quarters of these result from direct effect of the neoplasm on surrounding tissues. Of these chronic syndromes, somatic pains (71%) are more common than neuropathic (39%) and visceral pains (34%). Bony metastases are the most common cause of chronic pain in patients with cancer, accounting for 30–35% of all cancer pain among patients with advanced disease. The vertebrae are the most common site of metastasis, and up to 85% of patients with vertebral metastases may experience multi-level disease. Bony pain typically presents with a triad of background pain, spontaneous pain, and movement-related pain, and, because it is due to local inflammation, it is often responsive to nonsteroidal anti-inflammatory drugs (NSAIDs), steroids, and, to a lesser extent, bisphosphonates. Other common pain syndromes include neuropathic pain syndromes, a heterogeneous group of pain conditions which are typically sequelae of either cancer treatments or direct cancer invasion into nerve structures (e.g., plexopathies). These tend to have both nociceptive and neuropathic components. Acute cancer pain syndromes are less common and typically associated with diagnostic or therapeutic interventions, such as such as surgery or cancer-directed treatments.

Hepatic distention due to increasing tumor burden can cause a common pain syndrome. Pain-sensitive structures in the region of the liver include the liver capsule, blood vessels, and biliary tract. These are variably innervated by the celiac plexus, the phrenic nerve, and the lower right intercostal nerves. This syndrome classically causes visceral pain in the right upper quadrant with a pleuritic component and referral to the ipsilateral supraclavicular, neck, and scapular regions. CN's symptomatology is most consistent with this syndrome, and a recognition of this can help guide further workup and therapeutic decision-making.

The approach to treatment should be multimodal, with careful consideration of the individual's goals of care. CN made clear through multiple conversations with providers that her priority was comfort and being close to her family. A holistic plan for CN should include psychosocial support, disease-modifying treatments, interventional modalities, and a broad-based pharmacological approach using opioid and non-opioid analgesics and appropriate adjuvants. As such, the medical oncology and radiation oncology teams were consulted for consideration of interventions to target her hepatic tumor burden. Because her disease had been previously unresponsive to multiple rounds of chemotherapy, it was agreed that further systemic therapy was unlikely to give her symptomatic benefit, and, similarly, the burden of multiple fractions of radiation therapy was also felt to outweigh its potential benefit. Consideration was given to celiac plexus block; however, given the multiple innervations of the liver capsule and marked hepatomegaly, it was felt that the risk of the procedure outweighed the potential for symptomatic benefit.

Pharmacological pain treatment should always occur in a stepwise manner. Patients with mild pain should start with non-opiate and adjuvant analgesics with titration to affect. Both acetaminophen and NSAIDs produce dose-dependent analgesic effects. Acetaminophen is safer when given at therapeutic and non-hepatotoxic doses (less than 3–4 g daily) but does not have substantial anti-inflammatory effects and may be less effective when used for bony pain or in perioperative settings. The chronic use of NSAIDs may be limited by renal and gastrointestinal side effects as well as by potential situations of thrombocytopenia. Corticosteroids may also be considered for their anti-inflammatory effects and have shown particular efficacy in bony metastatic pain and pain due to hepatic distention.

Topical lidocaine applied to the site of referred pain has also been shown to improve pain. CN was started on oral acetaminophen 650 mg every 6 hours, dexamethasone 4 mg daily, and a lidocaine patch was applied to her right shoulder.

Opioid analgesics are the mainstay of pain treatment in cancer patients, and, given their effectiveness and overall safety profile when appropriately prescribed, should be administered routinely to patients with moderate to severe pain. The oral route is the preferred route for chronic opioid therapy, though transdermal and IV routes may have benefit in select patients. When initiating therapy, dosing should be based on severity of pain and previous opioid exposure. Thereafter, dosing should be titrated to achieve a favorable balance between analgesic effect and side effects. Most common side effects include gastrointestinal (constipation, nausea, vomiting) and neuropsychological (somnolence and impaired cognition). Tolerance, a physiological adaptation to chronic drug exposure resulting in decreased effectiveness, should be expected with long-term opioid use and can be managed with appropriate titration and consideration of opioid rotation with adjustment for incomplete cross-tolerance. Given CN's continued severe pain, the decision was made to transition her to morphine patient-controlled analgesia (PCA). When making decisions about basal dose, rate is typically set to match 50–100% of prior 24-hour usage depending on the level of pain control. She had used a total of 150 oral morphine equivalents (OMEs) over the prior 24 hours with continued poor control, so the decision was made to initiate morphine PCA at a basal rate of 2 mg/hr to match 100% of her previous 24 hour use (2 mg/hr × 24 hours × 3 mg oral morphine/ 1 mg IV morphine = 144 OME). Bolus dosing for breakthrough pain on a PCA is recommended to be 50–100% of the hourly rate every 10–15 minutes, so she was also given morphine 1 mg every 10 minutes as needed. Over the next 24 hours she used a total of 250 OME and noted significant improvement of her pain (down to a level of 3/10). She was transitioned to 50 μg transdermal fentanyl (targeted at 50% of the previous 24-hour use and adjusted for incomplete cross tolerance; 250 OME × 1/2 previous 24-hour use × 0.75 for cross-tolerance × 1 μg fentanyl/2 OME = 47 μg fentanyl) with a cross titration of basal PCA dose over the course of 24 hours by halving the basal morphine rate 12 hours after placement of transdermal fentanyl and then discontinuing basal morphine 24 hours after placement.

Her breakthrough pain medication was transitioned to oral morphine 25 mg every 2 hours as needed (10% of prior 24-hour use). On initiation of PCA, she was also started on a bowel regimen with sennosides, 2 pills every 12 hours, and polyethylene glycol as needed.

There is a distinct interplay between pain and emotional state, and psychosocial and spiritual support can be important adjuncts to the previously mentioned interventions and pharmacotherapy. Among the most useful approaches for pain management include mind-body approaches, relaxation training, and guided imagery. For CN, a multidisciplinary approach was employed through pain psychology, social work, and spiritual care involvement.

KEY POINTS TO REMEMBER

- Pain management for patients with cancer should include psychosocial support, consideration of disease-modifying treatments, interventional modalities, and a broad-based pharmacological approach.
- The recognition of pain syndromes and the ability to distinguish between them is an essential skill for palliative care clinicians, given their important prognostic and therapeutic implications.
- Opioids are the mainstay of symptomatic treatment for cancer pain. Effective dosing depends on appropriate selection of a drug and route and should be titrated to achieve a favorable balance between analgesic effect and side effects.
- The addition of an NSAID to opioid treatment can provide benefit, but careful attention should be paid to side-effect profiles.
- Adjuvant analgesic drugs (glucocorticoids, antidepressants, and anticonvulsants) can provide supplementary benefit to an opiate regimen.
- Many nonpharmacological treatments can be used to improve pain control, including mind-body approaches, relaxation training, and guided imagery.

Further Reading

Caraceni A, Portenoy RK. An international survey of cancer pain characteristics and syndromes: IASP Task Force on Cancer Pain. International Association for the Study of Pain. *Pain.* 1999;82:263–274.

Chang V, Janjan N, Jain S, Chau C. Regional cancer pain syndromes. *J Palliat Med.* 2006;9(6):1435–1453.

Cherny NI. Cancer pain: Principles of assessment and syndromes. In Berger AM, Portenoy RK, Weissman D (eds.). *Principles and Practice of Palliative Care and Supportive Oncology.* 2nd ed. Philadelphia: Lippincott Williams and Wilkins; 2003: 3–52.

Deandrea S, Montanari M, Moja L, Apolone G. Prevalence of undertreatment in cancer pain: A review of published literature. *Ann Oncol.* 2008;19:1985–1991.

Grond S, Zech D, Diefenbach C, Radbruch L, Lehmann KA. Assessment of cancer pain: A prospective evaluation in 2266 cancer patients referred to a pain service. *Pain.* 1996;64:107–114.

Keefe FJ, Ahles TA, Porter LS, et al. The self-efficacy of family caregivers for helping cancer patients manage pain at end-of-life. *Pain.* 2003 May;103(1–2):157–162.

Kwekkeboom KL, Cherwin CH, Lee JW, Wanta B. Mind-body treatments for the pain-fatigue-sleep disturbance symptom cluster in persons with cancer. *J Pain Symptom Manage.* 2010;39:126–138.

Stockler M, Vardy J, Pillai A, et al. Acetaminophen (paracetamol) improves pain and well-being in people with advanced cancer already receiving a strong opioid regimen: A randomized, double-blind, placebo-controlled cross-over trial. *J Clin Oncol.* 2004;22(16):3389–3394.

van den Beuken-van Everdingen MH, Hochstenbach LM, Joosten EA, Tjan-Heijnen VC, Janssen DJ. Update on prevalence of pain in patients with cancer: Systematic review and meta-analysis. *J Pain Symptom Manage.* 2016;51(6):1070–1090.

36 Breakthrough Pain

Nathan Boehr and Zachary Macchi

Case Study

A 55-year-old man with advanced colorectal cancer presents to clinic for follow-up of chronic abdominal pain. He recently started chemotherapy and imaging shows his disease is stable. He currently takes oxycodone 10 mg every 4 hours as needed and a transdermal fentanyl patch 25 µg/hr changed every 72 hours. He reports using 2–3 doses of oxycodone per day within the first 2 days of changing his patch, and 4–6 doses on day 3. He reports daily bowel movements. His pain is a deep ache and poorly localized, currently rated 2/10. He takes oxycodone when the pain reaches 6 or 7/10, and reports improvement to a tolerable level of 3/10. He denies any inciting factors of these pain episodes and says they occur gradually. He has good support through his family and synagogue, denies anxiety or depression, and feels "at peace" with his diagnosis. Exam is unremarkable, and you note the patient is wearing his fentanyl patch on his chest and the area is free of excess hair.

What Do I Do Now?

reakthrough pain is defined as a transient worsening of pain in a patient whose underlying pain is otherwise adequately managed at baseline. Formulating a clinical plan to address breakthrough pain begins with a comprehensive pain assessment. Be aware that pain can be due to physical, emotional, spiritual, or social stressors. Use a unidimensional or multidimensional numeric pain scale to assess the patient's pain level. Patients who are unable to communicate pain should be assessed using a validated pain rating scale for the cognitively impaired. Asking about the quality or characteristics of pain typically helps differentiate neuropathic pain from nociceptive pain, although mixed presentations are not uncommon. Neuropathic pain is caused by injured or dysfunctional nerve fibers and is typically described as a burning, shooting, tingling, or numb sensation. Nociceptive pain, on the other hand, is caused by injury at peripheral pain receptors. It can be further classified as somatic (sharp, well-localized) or visceral (cramping, poorly localized). The physical exam is a key element in assessing pain etiology and is therefore instrumental in formulating a clinical plan.

END-OF-DOSE FAILURE BREAKTHROUGH PAIN

End-of-dose failure breakthrough pain occurs when medication levels in the bloodstream fall below the analgesic threshold prior to the next scheduled dose. Pain tends to return in a predictable manner at the end of a dosing interval. It often has a gradual onset. Treatment strategy includes giving doses of a scheduled long-acting opioid at more frequent intervals versus increasing the dose. Rescue doses of a short-acting opioid should be used to control pain while the long-acting regimen is being titrated.

INCIDENT BREAKTHROUGH PAIN

Incident breakthrough pain has an identifiable cause. It is related to activity and generally has a fast onset. Examples include pain from a pathologic fracture, metastatic disease/tumors, or wounds. Premedicating before activity is advised. Consider treating predictable causes of incident pain with a nonopioid medication when possible. Examples include using an adequate bowel regimen to prevent colorectal spasm secondary to constipation, or using an antitussive to treat a cough that is causing incident breakthrough pain.

IDIOPATHIC BREAKTHROUGH PAIN

Idiopathic breakthrough pain occurs spontaneously without a predicable cause. It is recommended that the patient's long-acting opioid regimen be optimized with rescue doses available. Consider adding a scheduled adjuvant or nonopioid analgesic to the patient's regimen.

OPIOIDS FOR BREAKTHROUGH PAIN

Opioids are the cornerstone of pharmacologic management of breakthrough pain in palliative care, although it is advisable to maximize nonopioid adjuvants prior to initiation of opioid therapy if possible. Both long- and short-acting opioid formulations are available. Administration of a short-acting opioid is often referred to as a "breakthrough" or "rescue" dose. Commonly available oral short-acting opioids include morphine, oxycodone, hydrocodone, and hydromorphone. Note that hydrocodone is only available in a combination with acetaminophen in the United States. Limits on daily acetaminophen intake place a ceiling on dose titration of any opioid-acetaminophen combination product.

In an inpatient setting, intravenous opioids can be used to treat breakthrough pain. This is often used for pain that does not respond to oral medications or when the oral route is lost. Common intravenous opioids include morphine, hydromorphone, and fentanyl. Note that oxycodone and hydrocodone are not available as an intravenous formulation in the United States.

A reasonable starting dose for a short-acting opioid would include morphine 5 mg, or oxycodone 5 mg, or hydromorphone 1 mg. In general, dosing intervals of oral short-acting opioids should not exceed 4 hours in patients with normal renal function who are able to tolerate the opioid without signs of sedation. Longer dosing intervals may lead to gaps in adequate analgesia. Opioid-acetaminophen combination products may be limited to dosing intervals of every 6 hours. If more frequent dosing is needed, consider switching to an opioid-only formulation or reassess the long-acting opioid regimen.

Having an adequate long-acting opioid regimen is vital for controlling breakthrough pain. If the long-acting regimen is ineffective, patients may require an excessive number of breakthrough doses. If a patient consistently requires more than 4 or 5 breakthrough doses per day, or consistently wakes from sleep to take a breakthrough dose, consider adding a long-acting opioid. When initiating a long-acting opioid, conservative starting doses are often used. When titration is needed, a common method used by clinicians is to calculate 50% of the daily short-acting opioid requirement and add this to the long-acting regimen. The dose of the short-acting opioid should equal approximately 10% of the total 24-hour opioid requirement. Commonly used regimens include long-acting formulations of morphine or oxycodone. The total daily dose of oral long-acting opioids is often divided into two scheduled doses (i.e., every 12 hours). If end-of-dose failure breakthrough pain occurs, providers can consider dividing the total daily dose into three scheduled doses (i.e., every 8 hours). Please note that the manufacturer of controlled-release oxycodone does not recommend dosing intervals more often than every 12 hours, so prudent clinical judgment should be used.[4] As discussed earlier, transdermal fentanyl is another option for long-acting opioid therapy. It has an advantage over oral medications in that the patch only needs to be replaced every 72 hours (every 48 hours for certain patients). The transdermal route of administration ensures the medication will be delivered even if patients are unable to tolerate oral intake, thus reducing the risk of withdrawal in those scenarios. Transdermal fentanyl is generally not recommended in opioid-naïve patients. Noteworthy data suggest that transdermal fentanyl may become less efficacious in patients with cachexia.

The use of methadone for analgesia is beyond the scope of this chapter, and it should only be used by providers who are experienced with it.

NONOPIOID ADJUVANTS

Although opioids are commonly used to treat breakthrough pain in palliative care, their use can be limited by adverse effects. Constipation, urinary retention, nausea, sedation, hyperalgesia, and the risk of respiratory depression all must be considered when initiating and titrating an opioid regimen. Due to the risk of opioid-induced constipation, a proper bowel regimen should be in place for all patients taking opioids and should include a stimulant laxative. Nonopioid adjuvants and disease-directed treatment and procedures should all be considered when developing a comprehensive plan to treat breakthrough pain.

Nonopioid adjuvants should be considered early and often. This can potentially benefit the patient by reducing the 24-hour opioid requirement, therefore decreasing the risk of adverse effects from opioids as well as opioid tolerance. Both nonsteroidal anti-inflammatory drugs (NSAIDs) and acetaminophen are commonly used adjuvants. Their analgesic effects may be additive to opioids, thereby providing an opioid-sparing effect. The use of NSAIDs is contraindicated in patients taking corticosteroids due to the increased risk of gastrointestinal toxicity.

Corticosteroids can be useful for bony pain (i.e., bone metastasis). Dexamethasone has a longer half-life than prednisone and therefore can be dosed daily. Starting doses between 1 mg and 4 mg daily are generally used. Dosing in the morning is recommended to avoid insomnia. Short-term adverse effects (i.e., insomnia, psychosis) and long-term adverse effects (i.e., moon facies, osteoporosis) must be considered when initiating and continuing a corticosteroid regimen. Bone pain due to osteolytic lesions can also be treated with intravenous bisphosphates such as zoledronic acid or pamidronic acid. Analgesic effects can take a week or longer, and this medication can be given every 4 weeks.

Muscle relaxants can be considered as adjuvants for the treatment of incident breakthrough pain due to muscle spasms. This class includes medications such as cyclobenzaprine, baclofen, and tizanidine. Caution should be used with elderly patients or those taking opioids or other sedating medications.

Several classes of adjuvants, such as anticonvulsants, serotonin-norepinephrine reuptake inhibitors (SNRIs), and tricyclic antidepressants (TCAs), can be useful for the treatment of neuropathic pain. Neuropathic pain is caused by injured or dysfunctional nerve fibers and is typically described as a burning, shooting, tingling, or numb sensation. Anticonvulsants such as gabapentin or pregabalin can be useful, but caution should be used as both can cause drowsiness. Clinicians should also be mindful that dose reduction is needed for patients with renal impairment. SNRIs (i.e., duloxetine, venlafaxine) can be considered as well, but analgesic benefits may not be observed for a week or longer. TCAs such as nortriptyline can also be used to treat neuropathic pain. Clinicians should be mindful of the risk of anticholinergic effects, sedation, and cardiac arrhythmias.

The use of ketamine has become more common to treat pain that is refractory to opioids. A thorough discussion of this topic is beyond the scope of this chapter. Please refer to the "Further Reading" section at the end of this chapter for more information.

DISEASE-DIRECTED TREATMENT AND PROCEDURES

When possible, consider disease-directed treatments that may help minimize the patient's breakthrough pain burden. For example, breakthrough pain secondary to malignancy may benefit from chemotherapy or immunotherapy. Other examples include vertebroplasty for pathologic compression fractures, surgical debulking of solid tumors, or nerve blocks (i.e., celiac plexus block for pain secondary to pancreatic cancer). Radiation therapy can be considered for palliation of pain secondary to bone lesions. Patients with pain that is refractory to oral analgesics and who have chronic pain below the neck that is in a focal location may benefit from a pain anesthesia consult to evaluate them for an intrathecal pain pump.

The patient in our case is likely experiencing breakthrough pain due to end-of-dose failure. It is unlikely that emotional, spiritual, or social stressors are contributing to his physical pain. A reasonable approach would include having the patient change the fentanyl transdermal patch every 48 hours, given that his need for more frequent breakthrough doses only occurs between 48 and 72 hours after patch change. Prior to making this change, it is advisable that the clinician verifies the patient is applying the patch to non-irradiated skin on a flat surface of the torso or upper arms. Hair at the application site should be clipped but not shaved.

The patient reports good relief with his current dose of oxycodone, therefore this should not be changed. Although an increase in the dose of his fentanyl patch can be considered as an alternative to replacing the patch more frequently, his daily opioid requirement does not justify that at this time.

SUMMARY

Breakthrough pain can be classified as end-of-dose failure, incident, or idio-pathic. When formulating a clinical plan to treat breakthrough pain, a comprehensive pain assessment should be performed. Clinicians must consider physical, emotional, spiritual, and social causes of pain. In the palliative care setting, opioids are commonly used to treat breakthrough pain. An opioid regimen should be custom-tailored for each patient and both short- and long-acting opioids should be considered when appropriate. Adverse effects of opioids may limit their use and should always be considered when initiating or titrating an opioid regimen. Nonopioid analgesics and disease-directed therapy and procedures should all be considered when forming a plan to address breakthrough pain.

KEY POINTS TO REMEMBER

- Breakthrough pain is classified as end-of-dose failure, incident, or idiopathic.
- Always start with a comprehensive pain assessment and consider physical, emotional, spiritual, and social causes of pain.
- If a patient consistently requires more than 4 or 5 breakthrough doses per day, or consistently wakes from sleep to take a breakthrough dose, consider adding a long-acting opioid.
- The use of nonopioid adjuvants should be considered early and often.
- Disease-directed treatment and procedural interventions to treat pain should be considered when appropriate.

References

1. Closs SJ, Barr B, Briggs M, et al. A comparison of five pain assessment scales for nursing home residents with varying degrees of cognitive impairment. *J Pain Symptom Manage*. 2004;27(3):196–205.

2. Driver LC. Case studies in breakthrough pain. *Pain Med*. 2007 January;8(Suppl 1):S14–S18.

3. Quill T, Periyokoil V, Denney-Koelsch E, et al. *Primer of Palliative Care*. 7th ed. Chicago, AAHPM; 2019.

4. Rudowska J. Management of breakthrough pain due to cancer. *Contemp Oncol (Pozn)*. 2012;16(6):498–501.

Further Reading

Bolash R, Mekhail N. Intrathecal pain pumps: indications, patient selection, techniques, and outcomes. *Neurosurg Clin N Am*. 2014;25(4):735–742.

Medicines. Summary of product characteristics Durogesic Fentanyl DTrans. DataPharm. https://www.medicines.org.uk/emc/product/6939/smpc#gref. Accesed November 13, 2021

See S, Ginzburg R. Choosing a skeletal muscle relaxant. *Am Fam Physician*. 2008 Aug 1;78(3):365–370.

Vadivelu N. Role of ketamine for analgesia in adults and children. J *Anaesthesiol Clin Phmarmacol*. 2016 July-Sep;32(3):298–306.

37 Abdominal Pain in Palliative Care

Dharma Naidu and John Hausdorff

Case Study

A 62-year-old woman presents to the emergency room with increasing abdominal bloating, pain, and vomiting, with a history of advanced, metastatic mucinous adenocarcinoma of the appendix. At the time of diagnosis 6 months earlier, she had undergone appendectomy, tumor debulking, and total abdominal hysterectomy with bilateral salpingo-oophorectomy. Following surgery, she was treated with fluorouracil, leucovorin, and oxaliplatin (FOLFOX). She was then admitted to the hospital a month ago for gastric outlet obstruction requiring esophago-gastro-duodenoscopy (EGD) with placement of a pyloric stent. Now, in the emergency room, physical examination shows obvious distention and hyperactive bowel sounds, and plain films and computed tomography show obstruction again, this time involving the small bowel.

What Do I Do Now?

Malignant bowel obstruction is an all-too-common complication of advanced cancer and brings with it particular issues: the need to weigh the benefits and risks of surgical intervention, which requires special attention to the individual patient's prognosis and goals of care, and major challenges in providing good symptom management.

While there is a high likelihood that obstruction in a patient with cancer is due to advancing disease, patients may also have benign conditions such as adhesions. Malignant bowel obstruction is commonly seen in gynecological malignancies and may also develop in patients with gastric, pancreatic, appendiceal, biliary duct, and colorectal cancers, and occasionally in others such as breast and lung cancers, when the pattern of spread includes peritoneal carcinomatosis. After a thorough workup, if the diagnosis of malignant bowel obstruction is made, the most definitive therapeutic interventions may be surgery, particularly if the presentation is early in the course of the disease. This decision is based in large part on the patient's functional status and life expectancy. Unfortunately, the presence of malignant ascites may greatly complicate wound healing subsequently. Also critical is the distinction between small bowel and large bowel obstruction because in patients who are poor surgical candidates one nonsurgical palliative intervention for *large* bowel obstruction is the placement of a self-expandable metallic stent. Abbott and colleagues reported on 146 patients, almost all of whom had colorectal cancer as the cause of large bowel obstruction; they had a 97% success rate in stent placement and a perforation rate of less than 5%, with a 30-day mortality rate of 2.7%. In this study, 30% of patients required at least one further intervention for their bowel obstruction.

Typically, regardless of the ultimate interventions, a nasogastric tube is used for initial decompression and management of symptoms. For some patients, the conservative approach of decompression, bowel rest, and intravenous (IV) hydration will prove effective. If obstruction persists and definitive surgery is not felt to be a good option, a percutaneous surgically or endoscopically placed venting gastrostomy tube can be considered. Nasogastric tubes tend to be quite uncomfortable, especially long term, while a venting gastrostomy provides relief of pain, nausea, and vomiting, as well as allowing patients to continue to eat and drink—whatever they take in is then drained out through the gastrostomy tube, so intake must be of thin consistency.

For patients in whom none of the above interventions is appropriate or acceptable, we then look at pharmacological modalities. These include opioids for pain, octreotide for decreasing bowel function and intraluminal secretions, dexamethasone for edema and nausea, and aggressive use of antiemetics.

Octreotide can be used in doses that start with 100 µg subcutaneous (SC) injections every 12 hours and are dose-titrated as needed to control nausea and vomiting. More aggressive, and generally more effective, would be an octreotide IV infusion, starting at 25 µg/hour with flexible titration up to 100 µg/hour. When planning discharge from the hospital, octreotide infusions can be continued indefinitely, or use of intramuscular (IM) octreotide in a long-acting release (LAR) preparation can be tried, and lasts a month. Unfortunately, many reimbursement models do not support expensive interventions like octreotide.

Hospice organizations will frequently utilize dexamethasone at doses of 6–16 mg/day. Dexamethasone has a relatively low incidence of adverse effects (insomnia, agitation, hunger, fluid retention), does not impact survival, and is significantly less expensive than octreotide.

In patients with incomplete bowel obstruction, metoclopramide at starting doses of 10 mg IV every 6 hours and increased up to 20 mg IV every 4 hours can provide relief. Haloperidol and olanzapine have also been used for refractory nausea and vomiting management in patients with malignant bowel syndrome. In a retrospective study of patients with incomplete bowel obstruction, olanzapine at a starting dose of 5 mg/day proved effective, with minimal side effects. One added advantage of olanzapine over haloperidol is the availability of an orally dissolving formulation that is well-tolerated by patients and can be placed on the tongue.

Given what is often a short life expectancy (days to months) of patients with advanced cancer who present with inoperable malignant bowel obstruction, aggressive symptom management of pain, nausea, and vomiting, as well as balancing patient and family expectations with realistic goals of care, is of the utmost importance.

DIFFERENTIAL DIAGNOSIS OF ABDOMINAL PAIN

Abdominal pain is a complex and challenging complaint that is frequently of benign cause but is often secondary to extremely serious and potentially life-threatening conditions. The differential is extremely broad, including

- the "surgical" abdomen (e.g., bowel perforation or infarction, diverticular or other abscess, advanced cholecystitis, appendicitis, aortic or other aneurysmal rupture);
- peritonitis from infectious, inflammatory, or other nonsurgical causes,
- vascular occlusion (e.g., splenic infarction) or mesenteric ischemia;
- stretching or irritation of Glisson's capsule (secondary to expanding peripheral liver metastases, hepatitis, hemorrhage, or surface tumor implants);
- bowel obstruction, volvulus, ileus, diverticulitis, colitis, constipation, gastritis/ulcer disease, and irritable bowel syndrome;
- renal or ureteral infection or obstruction;
- malignancy from any number of primary or metastatic sources;
- pancreatitis or related conditions;
- referred pain (e.g., from lung, pleura, heart, or pericardium);
- medical conditions, both common (e.g., diabetic ketoacidosis or migraine) and uncommon (e.g., acute intermittent porphyria);
- gynecologic conditions, including pelvic inflammatory disease, ectopic pregnancy, ovarian torsion or ruptured cyst, endometritis, endometriosis, uterine fibroids, and pregnancy;
- psychiatric conditions including anxiety, depression, somatization, and psychosis; and
- side effects of various medications or ingested toxins.

Critical to the approach is to start with a thoughtful and skillfully taken history (which very often provides the probable diagnosis), supplemented with a careful physical examination. These two time-honored fundamentals of clinical medicine should then lead to directed and appropriate laboratory and radiographic testing.

Pain perception is usually from mechanical and/or chemical stimuli that activate the receptors in the viscera. Stretching, pressure, or distention also can add to the pain stimulus. A good medical history starts with the description of the pain: dull, achy, cramping, sharp, or intermittent. We want to know what precipitates and what relieves the pain, the location of the pain (generalized, upper, lower, left or right), if it radiates and to where, how it has changed over time, and particular timing: when did the pain start, and is it intermittent or constant? In patients presenting with chronic abdominal pain, a detailed psychosocial history is important to investigate if abdominal symptoms correlate with life stressors or psychological trauma.

Given that a thorough discussion of the evaluation of abdominal pain and its extensive differential diagnosis is beyond the scope of this chapter, we instead highlight three less well known and underappreciated causes of abdominal pain: chronic abdominal wall pain (CAWP), centrally mediated pain syndrome (CAPS), and narcotic bowel syndrome (NBS). While opioids are an important tool for the immediate relief of many serious abdominal pain syndromes, opioids are *not* the agents of choice in any of these three conditions.

CHRONIC ABDOMINAL WALL PAIN

CAWP, also referred to as anterior cutaneous nerve entrapment syndrome (ACNES), is a common cause of chronic abdominal pain that is often underrecognized and mistaken for visceral abdominal pain. This condition is estimated to occur in 1 of 1,800 individuals in the general population. CAWP was seen in 2% of all patients presenting to a Dutch emergency department with abdominal pain and may comprise as many as 10% of all patients with chronic abdominal pain. This chronic condition is four times more prevalent in women than men and commonly presents in patients in their fifties and sixties. Patients with CAWP also tend to have comorbid conditions such as obesity, gastroesophageal reflux disease, irritable bowel syndrome, and fibromyalgia. Patients with abdominal wall pain are usually able to point to a single area where the pain is located, as opposed to diffuse, generalized abdominal pain. Practitioners can assess for Carnett's sign, which entails palpation of the area of maximal tenderness with the patient in a resting position. Then the patient is to tense the abdominal muscles, either by raising the legs or lifting the head and shoulders off the table. Carnett's sign is considered positive if pain on palpation during tension of the muscles is more than it was in a resting position. A trigger point injection using steroids and local anesthetic serves to both confirm the diagnosis and is also the treatment of choice. Trigger point injections can provide immediate relief, which can last up to a month. Patients may need repeat trigger point injections; in the event the pain proves refractory and other diagnoses have been ruled out, patients may need chemical neurolysis or, in severe cases, surgical neurectomy.

CENTRALLY MEDIATED ABDOMINAL PAIN SYNDROME

CAPS was formerly referred to as *functional abdominal pain syndrome*. As a functional gastrointestinal disorder, CAPS is less well known than irritable bowel syndrome. The prevalence is reported to be from 0.5% to 2%, and it peaks in the fourth decade of life. It is seen slightly more commonly in women than men (60/40 ratio). Given the high healthcare utilization by these patients, CAPS can cause a significant economic burden.

The distinguishing features of CAPS (vs. other functional gastrointestinal disorders) are the presence of continuous or nearly continuous abdominal pain; pain not related to eating, defecation, or menses; and some loss of daily functioning. Patients also tend to have certain symptom-related behaviors, including expressing high levels of pain, an increase in pain when discussing psychologically distressing issues, and a decrease in severity when the patient is distracted. Patients tend to deny psychosocial factors as contributing causes and often have unrealistic expectations regarding appropriate treatment. Many may request exploratory surgeries and continue to aggressively seek diagnostic workup despite repeatedly negative findings. Patients may often request opioids, despite non-opioid or nonpharmacological interventions being implemented.

There is emerging evidence that functional gastrointestinal disorders such as this are due to dysregulation in the complex communication between the central nervous system and the enteric nervous system, which manifests as gastrointestinal symptoms that are influenced by anxiety and stress. This has led to the development of neurogastroenterology as a subspecialty, and treatment plans for this condition include antidepressants, cognitive-behavioral therapy, relaxation techniques, and biofeedback.

Kilgallon and colleagues described their 7-year experience with 103 consecutive patients referred to their neurogastroenterology clinic. The mean age of patients was 40, and 85% were female. Two-thirds had undergone surgery previously, and two-thirds of this group had a surgical procedure in an attempt to explain their pain. Eighty-one percent of the patients described allodynia (where a nonpainful stimulus evokes pain), which was strongly associated with opioid use. As treatment at the clinic, almost all patients received centrally acting neuromodulators, including tricyclic antidepressants (TCAs), gabapentin, pregabalin, or duloxetine. Of the 51 patients who continued follow-up at the clinic, 67% exhibited a positive response, 19% showed no response, and 14% were unable to tolerate the chosen pharmacotherapy. TCAs had the lowest response rates, with 7/32 (22%) responding to amitriptyline and 5/21 (24%) responding to nortriptyline. Out of 40 patients, 15 (38%) responded to gabapentin and 10/26 (38%) responded to pregabalin. Duloxetine was the only neuromodulator significantly better at achieving a response than amitriptyline, with 12/16 (75%) responding, and it was the only drug tolerated by all patients in whom it was tried.

NARCOTIC BOWEL SYNDROME

NBS has an estimated prevalence of 4.2–6.4% in those who chronically take opioids. Diagnosis of NBS is difficult as the symptoms are easily mistaken for constipation, ileus, and pseudo-obstruction. It may be also difficult to diagnose in patients with a comorbid condition that requires continued opioid therapy, particularly when the provider is not familiar with the hyperalgesic effects of chronic opioid use. While frequently considered similar, NBS is quite distinct from opioid-induced constipation (OIC). With OIC, there is a reduction in abdominal pain after the use of appropriate interventions aimed at alleviated the underlying constipation. In NBS, patients have chronic or recurring abdominal pain which continues to worsen as opioid doses are increased. This is thought to be associated with a hyperalgesia phenomenon, so treatment focus should be opioid *de-escalation*. Opioid doses should be reduced slowly and symptoms of acute withdrawal managed effectively. Early recognition is key to ensure that patients are able to understand the negative effects of opioids in this condition, and referral to appropriate therapists for implementation of nonpharmacologic interventions is timely.

On presentation to ER, our case study patient had a nasogastric tube placed. She had immediate relief of her nausea, but clearly she did not want to have to live with a nasogastric tube. She was started on some fluids, and a surgical referral to consider her for venting gastrostomy. She was placed on octreotide 100 mg SQ every 8 hours and IV dexamethasone 4 mg every 12 hours while her surgery could be scheduled. Her nausea was significantly improved. Her surgeon was able to do a venting gastrostomy, and, post procedure, she was discharged with hospice care, given that her goals were not to pursue further treatments and return to the hospital. She was given a diet for pleasure and sublingual olanzapine, along with tapering doses of dexamethasone for nausea.

KEY POINTS TO REMEMBER

- Abdominal pain and distension must be aggressively managed in malignant bowel obstruction. Surgical interventions can be considered in patients with adequate disease control and good performance status. Stents and venting gastrostomies may be helpful for some palliative patients. Nasogastric tubes provide immediate relief but may not be tolerated by patients for prolonged periods. Pharmacological interventions include octreotide, steroids, opioids, and antiemetics. Presence of malignant bowel obstruction in the inoperable patient requires frank discussions with patient and family regarding goals of care based on patient preferences and a realistic assessment of prognosis.
- In patients with CAWP and a positive Carnett's sign, consider trigger point injections.
- CAPS is a complex diagnosis of exclusion, with biopsychosocial treatment modalities including antidepressants, psychotherapy, cognitive-behavioral therapy, biofeedback, and relaxation techniques.

- NBS is easily overlooked and ideally should be recognized early. Treatment goals should include compassionate opioid taper. Having protocols in place for managing opioid withdrawal symptoms and managing any comorbid pain disorders with non-opioid interventions is paramount.

Further Reading

Abbott S, Ellington TW, Ma Y, et al. Predictors of outcome in palliative colonic stent placement for malignant obstruction. *Br J Surg*. 2014 January;101(2):121–126.

Clouse RE, Mayer EA, Aziz Q, et al. Functional abdominal pain syndrome. *Gastroenterology*. 2006;130:1492–1497.

Kilgallon E, Vasant DH, Green D, et al. Chronic continuous abdominal pain: Evaluation of diagnostic features, iatrogenesis and drug treatments in a cohort of 103 patients. *Aliment Pharmacol Ther*. 2019 May;49(10):1282–1292.

Farmer AD, Gallagher J, Bruckner-Holt C, et al. Narcotic bowel syndrome. *Lancet Gastroenterology Hepatol*. 2017 2(5):361–368.

Franke AJ, Iqbal A, Starr JS, et al. Management of malignant bowel obstruction associated with GI cancers. *J Oncol Pract*. 2017 July;13(7):426–434.

Mayer EA, Tillisch K. The brain-gut axis in abdominal pain syndromes. *Annu Rev Med*. 2011;62:381–396.

Srinivasan R, Greenbaum D. Chronic abdominal wall pain: A frequently overlooked problem: Practical approach to diagnosis and management. *Am J Gastroenterol*. 2002; 97: 824–830.

Tuca A, Guell E, Martinez-Losada E, Codorniu N. Malignant bowel obstruction in advanced cancer patients: Epidemiology, management, and factors influencing spontaneous resolution. *Cancer Manag Res*. 2012;4:159–169.

38 Pain Management in Calciphylaxis

Jennifer Ku

Case Study

SN is a 43-year-old White woman with diabetes, hypertension, hyperlipidemia, obesity, and end-stage renal disease (ESRD) on hemodialysis. She was admitted with newly diagnosed calciphylaxis. Eight months ago, she developed skin discoloration and subsequent formation of plaques after starting warfarin for deep vein thrombosis (DVT). On admission, she had painful palpable subcutaneous nodules with a reticulate pattern of erythema on her thighs. Three weeks later, the lesions have ulcerated and progressed to her abdomen, buttocks, and proximal lower extremities. She reports 10 out of 10 pain that worsens during wound care and dialysis. She describes her pain as a burning sensation in her wounds and endorses both hyperalgesia and allodynia. Previous attempts to manage her pain with hydromorphone and gabapentin resulted in excessive sedation and concerns for myoclonus with minimal pain relief. Now, she refuses to receive dialysis until her pain is better controlled.

What Do I Do Now?

One of the most challenging aspects of symptom management in calciphylaxis is the complex etiology of pain. Experts hypothesize that pain in calciphylaxis is caused by progressive vascular calcification and microvascular thrombosis, resulting in ischemia-induced tissue and nerve damage. Due to ongoing tissue injury, pain typically presents with somatic, neuropathic, and inflammatory components that may be poorly responsive to traditional analgesics, as seen in SN's case. Therefore, a clinician should aim to limit further ischemic damage by utilizing interventions to inhibit vascular calcification, minimize thrombosis, and promote wound healing to manage SN's pain. As there are currently no approved treatments or clinical practice guidelines for managing these issues in calciphylaxis, a clinician may find it helpful to collaborate with colleagues from dermatology, nephrology, plastic surgery, and wound care in building SN's treatment plan.

INHIBITING VASCULAR CALCIFICATION

Mineral bone metabolism abnormalities are common in calciphylaxis and contribute to vascular calcification and wound progression. Thus, the clinician should consider interventions focused on correcting abnormal calcium-phosphate-parathyroid hormone (PTH) metabolism. The clinician should minimize exogenous sources of vitamin D and calcium by discontinuing vitamin D analogs, calcium supplements, and calcium-containing phosphate binders. Switching from peritoneal dialysis to hemodialysis may also help a clinician gain better control of bone mineral metabolism, with some experts recommending dialysis sessions up to 5–6 times weekly. However, intensifying dialysis may not be possible for patients like SN who struggle to adhere to dialysis treatment at baseline.

Pharmacological options for minimizing vascular calcification include a variety of off-label treatments. Oral calcimimetics like cinacalcet have been shown to lower the rate of lesion progression but not the rate of mortality. For patients who are unresponsive to calcimimetics, parathyroidectomy is an option to restore normal calcium-phosphate-PTH metabolism. Surgical patients should be selected carefully due to high risk of postoperative complications. A meta-analysis showed that patients who underwent parathyroidectomy had improved wound healing but were also younger and had higher serum albumin than nonsurgical patients.

Furthermore, calciphylaxis has been reported to recur or occur de novo after a parathyroidectomy. Sodium thiosulfate (STS) is a common intervention in calciphylaxis that forms highly soluble complexes with calcium and decreases calcium-phosphate precipitation in the vascular wall. It is often administered intravenously (IV) at 25 g three times a week after dialysis to help minimize vascular calcification with an anticipated onset of benefit within months for wound healing and decreased calcification. However, not all patients may respond to STS; a meta-analysis with a pooled cohort of 151 patients showed no benefit with STS on wound healing and mortality despite most individual studies suggesting otherwise. STS also has antioxidant and vasodilatory effects that may decrease tissue ischemia and provide pain relief within a few weeks of treatment initiation. IV bisphosphonates have been used in some patients with calciphylaxis to reduce extraosseous mineralization and decrease systemic inflammation contributing to pain. Safety and efficacy of bisphosphonates in calciphylaxis has been demonstrated in cohort studies, while a meta-analysis using a pooled cohort of 37 patients showed a decreased rate of amputation with bisphosphonates. Yet the clinician should be cautious about using bisphosphonates given the limited evidence available in regards its optimal dosing and safe use in calciphylaxis patients, especially in individuals with impaired renal function. Phytonadione is a relatively new intervention for calciphylaxis treatment. Vitamin K-dependent matrix Gla protein is a potent inhibitor of arterial calcification and may be impaired in patients with vitamin K deficiency or exposed to vitamin K antagonists like warfarin. In addition to discontinuing warfarin, a clinician may consider supplementing a patient with oral or parenteral phytonadione 10 mg three times a week, with dialysis to minimize vascular calcification. Of note, hepatic thrombosis is an uncommon side effect of vitamin K supplementation, so the risks and benefits of using phytonadione should be carefully considered in patients like SN who have active or are at high risk of thrombosis.

MINIMIZING MICROVASCULAR THROMBOSIS

Direct anticoagulants are preferred in calciphylaxis and preferred over heparin products when possible due to the concern of recurrent skin trauma from subcutaneous (SQ) injections promoting progression of skin lesions.

In cases where SQ injections cannot be avoided, rotating injection sites and decreasing dosing frequency is preferred. Apixaban is now approved for use in end-stage renal disease (ESRD) and has been shown to be safe and effective in calciphylaxis patients on hemodialysis. Several case reports also discuss use of pentoxifylline as an adjunct in combination with STS to help reduce blood viscosity to minimize risk of thrombus formation, but its independent efficacy in calciphylaxis is still unclear and onset of benefit may take weeks. Although there are reports of other treatments to minimize microvascular thrombosis, two interventions are not recommended: tissue plasminogen activator due to its significant bleed risk and limb revascularization due to poor outcomes status-post intervention in patients with calciphylaxis.

PROMOTING WOUND HEALING

Many medications may delay wound healing and should be discontinued if possible, depending on the patient's goals of care. Examples include cytotoxic antineoplastic agents, immunosuppressants, corticosteroids, and nonsteroidal anti-inflammatory drugs (NSAIDs). Surgical debridement is frequently used in calciphylaxis to remove necrotic tissue to improve wound healing and has been shown to improve survival in retrospective studies in combination with comprehensive wound care. Benefit may be limited, though, if skin lesions are widespread across multiple body parts. Outside of adequate wound care, hyperbaric oxygen treatment (HBOT) is often used as salvage therapy for patients unresponsive to conventional treatments to improve wound healing in calciphylaxis. HBOT is believed to promote wound healing via increased oxygen delivery to hypoxic tissues, promotion of angiogenesis, and enhanced oxygen-dependent neutrophil activity. However, there are several limitations to this therapy. HBOT requires patients to be in a sealed treatment chamber for at least an hour per session for an average of 20–30 sessions, so may be inappropriate for those who suffer from claustrophobia. Cost and availability of this treatment are also major barriers to consider. Furthermore, efficacy is unclear; individual cohort studies show benefit in wound healing but no benefit in rate of amputation, progression of skin lesions, and mortality when examined as part of a meta-analysis of pooled cohort studies.

SAFE AND EFFECTIVE ANALGESIC REGIMEN

A common challenge a clinician faces when selecting analgesics is choosing agents that are both effective for calciphylaxis pain and safe in the setting of renal impairment. Fentanyl and its analogs are the opioids most commonly used in calciphylaxis due to their lack of renal metabolites; other preferred opioids in patients with poor renal function include buprenorphine and methadone. Alternative opioids may be used depending on the degree of renal impairment but carry an increased risk of opioid toxicity due systemic accumulation, and they may be dialyzed out, resulting in worsening pain during or after dialysis sessions. Regardless of opioid selection, a clinician may expect to rapidly titrate opioids to high doses in order to achieve adequate analgesia given the progressive nature of this disease. Setting patient expectations is paramount as pain may not fully respond to opioids given the underlying ischemic nerve damage in calciphylaxis. In these cases, starting a neuropathic pain agent is essential. Case reports support the use of IV ketamine for neuropathic pain in calciphylaxis, and methadone may also be helpful given its similar N-methyl-D-aspartate (NMDA) receptor antagonism. Experts also recommend use of other neuropathic pain agents such as gabapentinoids, tricyclic antidepressants, and serotonin-norepinephrine reuptake inhibitors. However, a clinician should trial these other agents with caution and close monitoring for benefit since there is a paucity of evidence regarding the efficacy of these therapeutic drug classes for calciphylaxis pain. There is a case series that mentions use of parenteral ketorolac to treat pain secondary to nerve inflammation in calciphylaxis although NSAIDs should be used with extreme caution given their negative impact on wound healing and associated nephrotoxicity. In refractory cases, consulting an interventional pain specialist may also be helpful, given that lumbar sympathetic blocks have shown to provide pain relief in calciphylaxis.

PROGRESSIVE NATURE OF CALCIPHYLAXIS AND NEED FOR ADVANCE CARE PLANNING

Calciphylaxis is a progressive disease with a 1-year mortality rate of 45–80% in patients with ESRD and 24–45% in patients without ESRD. Moreover, patients with calciphylaxis also experience high rates of hospitalization, immobility, and poor quality of life. Advance care planning conversations should occur early on and throughout the disease trajectory.

An important decision point for patients with calciphylaxis is whether to withdraw dialysis, especially for those who wish to pursue hospice options where continued dialysis is not possible. Discussions regarding dialysis should also include decisions regarding other treatments that are frequently administered with dialysis, such as STS and phytonadione. A desire to continue these interventions may affect a patient's decision to stop dialysis or even to pursue hospice.

Another important topic to discuss is whether a patient who is a transplant candidate should delist from the transplantation wait list. Continued pursuit of transplantation is a controversial topic as calciphylaxis is not an absolute contraindication to kidney transplant. However, it is important to consider that patients with calciphylaxis may not survive the time to transplant given potentially long wait times. Furthermore, despite case reports of calciphylaxis resolution after kidney transplant, calciphylaxis has also been reported to occur de novo after kidney, liver, and simultaneous liver-kidney (SLK) transplants. Predictive factors for development of and/or resolution for calciphylaxis in transplant patients is still unknown.

Last, it is essential that the clinician elicit the patient's wishes for end-of-life care. Palliative care is often underutilized in this patient population, especially during a patient's terminal hospital admission. Only half of patients with calciphylaxis who died in the hospital received inpatient palliative care consults, with most consults occurring a few days prior to patient death and at the request of patient and family. With advance planning and understanding of the patient's perception of "a good death," the clinician will be able to help the patient achieve their desired end-of-life experience in a setting of their choice.

CREATING A COMPREHENSIVE PAIN MANAGEMENT PLAN

In summary, a comprehensive plan to manage SN's calciphylaxis pain should include treatments that address underlying vascular calcification, microvascular thrombosis, and poor wound healing while taking into account her goals of care and sensitivity to renally cleared medications. First steps in SN's case include discontinuing offending agents such as vitamin D analogs, calcium supplements, calcium-containing phosphate binders, medications known to inhibit wound healing, and warfarin. Instead of warfarin, SN can be started on apixaban if anticoagulation is needed. To inhibit vascular calcification, initial treatment with cinacalcet 30 mg once daily is recommended given its low cost and low risk. If SN is interested in continuing dialysis, STS 25 mg IV three times a week with dialysis can also be started if it is available and covered by insurance. Phytonadione may be unsafe given SN's risk for clots, but can be considered at 10 mg three times a week, IV or orally, with dialysis if she has vitamin K deficiency and is therapeutically anticoagulated. Parathyroidectomy and bisphosphonates are not recommended given SN's comorbidities. To encourage healing of SN's skin lesions, she should be started on comprehensive wound care and, if consistent with goals, surgical debridement of necrotic tissue. HBOT may be considered if wound healing remains poor but only if cost, access, and claustrophobia are not barriers to treatment. For her neuropathic pain, we recommend discontinuing gabapentin and trialing an agent with NMDA receptor antagonism, such as low-dose ketamine or methadone. Venlafaxine is a second-line neuropathic pain agent that could also be considered. Other non-opioid analgesics for neuropathic pain are not recommended given her renal function. Given SN's intolerance of renally cleared opioids and severe pain, she would benefit most from switching her hydromorphone to patient-controlled analgesia (PCA) with IV fentanyl. Her PCA will likely require rapid dose titration and subsequent addition of a basal rate as her condition progresses. When her pain is better controlled, her fentanyl PCA may be transitioned to a fentanyl patch or to methadone with oral oxycodone for breakthrough pain. Transition to methadone as her primary long-acting opioid is especially recommended if her pain is responsive to NMDA receptor antagonists.

KEY POINTS TO REMEMBER

- Pain in calciphylaxis is contributed to by ischemia-induced tissue and nerve damage secondary to vascular calcification and ongoing thrombosis.

- Efficacy of various interventions to manage vascular calcification, thrombosis, and poor wound healing in calciphylaxis is still unclear. Patients may respond to some interventions and not others.
- Management of calciphylaxis pain may require aggressive titration up to high opioid doses and the addition of neuropathic pain agents.
- Patients with calciphylaxis often have renal impairment. Minimize use of medications that have renal metabolites and renally dose adjust as appropriate.
- Early and ongoing discussions on goals of care are important given rapid progression and high symptom burden of calciphylaxis.

Further Reading

Nigwekar SU, Kroshinsky D, Nazarian RM, et al. Calciphylaxis: risk factors, diagnosis, and treatment. *Am J Kidney Dis.* 2015;66(1):133–146.

Nigwekar SU, Thadhani R, Brandenburg VM. Calciphylaxis. *N Engl J Med.* 2018;378(18):1704–1714.

Roza K, George JC, Bermudez M, Mehta Z. Uremic calciphylaxis #325. *J Palliat Med.* 2017;20(4):424–425.

Seethapathy H, Nigwekar SU. Revisiting therapeutic options for calciphylaxis. *Curr Opin Nephrol Hypertens.* 2019;28(5):448–454.

Udomkarnjananun S, Kongnatthasate K, Praditpornsilpa K, Eiam-Ong S, Jaber BL, Susantitaphong P. Treatment of calciphylaxis in CKD: A systematic review and meta-analysis. *Kidney Int Rep.* 2019;4(2):231–244.

39 Pain Management in Palliative Care for Infants

Alexis Dallara-Marsh and Sarah Ermer

Case Study

A 35-year-old G2P0010 woman gave birth to a 37-week baby boy with macrocephaly. The baby was born via caesarean section and was vigorous at birth with Apgars 9 and 9 at 1 and 5 minutes. Birth weight was 3.9 kg (90th percentile) and head circumference was 49 cm (>97th percentile). Vital signs were normal. Physical exam was significant for large, full anterior and posterior fontanelles and widely spread sutures. The neurological exam was otherwise normal. Neurosurgery was consulted for hydrocephalus, and a ventriculoperitoneal shunt was placed. Repeat imaging subsequently revealed a compressed cerebral aqueduct secondary to a collection of fluid and blood products within and above the cerebellar hemispheres. The patient's head circumference decreased to 40 cm after the procedure. The patient re-presented at 3 months of age after having 12 hours of difficulty breathing. On exam, the patient was hypothermic (35°C), tachypneic (respiration rate = 50), and dyspneic with occasional apnea. The head circumference was now at 45 cm. Physical exam displayed flat fontanelles, wide sutures, left cranial nerve VI and VII palsies, hypotonia, and 2+ reflexes throughout. The patient had a magnetic resonance imaging (MRI) study which was consistent with a high-grade posterior fossa tumor. MR spectroscopy showed a large choline-to-creatine ratio, further supportive of neoplasm. The patient underwent craniotomy and brain biopsy for definitive diagnosis. Pathology was suggestive of medulloblastoma with high-grade features.

What Do I Do Now?

Pediatric palliative care is provided to children with a wide variety of primary care conditions. In 1900, children 5 years of age or younger accounted for 30% of all deaths in the United States; in 1999, that number dropped to 1.4%. Today, more deaths occur in the first year of life than all other years of childhood combined, with two-thirds of these deaths occurring in the first month of life. The leading cause of infant mortality in the United States is "congenital anomalies," with genetic disorders involving 22% of infant deaths and neuromuscular diseases involving 15%. The etiology of most of these birth defects remains unknown and thus hampers our ability to manage and prevent such diseases. Compared with adult patients, pediatric patients who receive hospital-based palliative care services tend to have a greater diversity of medical conditions as well as longer duration of survival, which in turn may require a longer duration of services. The Association for Children's Palliative Care describes palliative care for neonates with life-threatening conditions as "an active and total approach to care from the point of diagnosis or recognition, throughout the child's life, death and beyond. It embraces physical, emotional, social and spiritual elements and focuses on the enhancement of quality of life for the baby and support for the family. It includes the management of distressing symptoms, provision of short breaks, and care through death and bereavement." In one study, the most frequent clinical signs and symptoms at time of entry into a pediatric palliative care included neurologic symptoms such as cognitive impairment (46.8%), speech difficulties (45.8%), problems with enteral intake (25.6%), seizures (24.5%), and fatigue (23.3%), with other concerns including paralysis, edema, sepsis, sweating, and dry mouth. As previously suggested, many of these symptoms will necessitate neurologic consultation.

There remain multiple barriers to use of palliative care in pediatrics. Palliative care for newborns was introduced in the 1980s. Not until 1987 did the American Academy of Pediatrics state that it is no longer ethical to perform surgery on babies without anesthetic. Fast forward 30 years and barriers to pediatric pain management and palliative care continue to be problematic. These include lack of experience on the part of healthcare professionals, lack of time and reimbursement, and uncertainty with disease prognostication. Other factors include families not being ready to accept that a condition may be incurable. At times there may be multiple ethical issues surrounding the care of infants and children. Professional societies such as the American Academy of Pediatrics and the American Academy of Neurology have written and approved statements about end-of-life decision-making. Intensive care is generally not recommended when early death is very likely and when survival would be accompanied by a high risk of unacceptably severe morbidity. Key reasons that lead to decision to discontinue support include predicted suffering, high risk of severe physical and mental disability, and incapacity for verbal and nonverbal communication. Limited data to guide prognostication with each patient's specific clinical scenario often make these discussions increasingly difficult to perform.

Comfort care protocols are abundant in the adult world and fairly standardized across institutions. However, this is not the case in neonatal palliative care. One survey addressing neonatal comfort care protocols was sent to neonatal practitioners in the United States and Canada. Nearly half reported their institution did not have protocols in place, and, of those reporting comfort care guidelines, 19.1% did not address pain symptom management. This is problematic as pain is the leading cause of physical and psycholo gical distress in neonates receiving palliative care. One barrier to providing adequate pain control in infants is correctly identifying and evaluating pain. Assessing pain in newborns can be challenging and time-consuming. Because of this, utilizing validated pain scales to regularly assess pain is essential. Various tools, such as Faces, Legs, Activity, Cry, Consolability (FLACC) and Neonatal Infant Pain Score (NIPS) can be used for evaluation of *acute* procedural or postoperative pain in infants. Three validated scales for neonatal *prolonged or chronic* pain include the Échelle de Douleur et d'Infconfort du Nouveanu-né (EDIN), Neonatal Pain, Agitation, and Sedation Scale (N-PASS), and COMFORTneo. Like other pain scales for pediatric patients, the signs and symptoms assessed are not necessarily specific indicators of pain. Hunger, agitation, or desire for human interaction can all cause distress in infants. A partnership of healthcare providers and parents in managing pain may improve communication and encourage parents to take an active role in pain management. Infants with uncontrolled pain should be evaluated at least every 15 minutes until pain is controlled, including after pharmacologic and nonpharmacologic interventions.

During a single neonatal intensive care unit (NICU) stay, critically ill infants may experience greater than 480 painful procedures. Because of the rapidly developing nervous system in neonates, these painful experiences may permanently modify pain processing. Around 22-weeks' gestation, pain transmission and modulation in infants rapidly grow. By 2 months of age, these processes are matured and fully functioning. Preterm neonates in particular experience much greater pain than term neonates. The single best way to avoid pain is to avoid painful procedures. Consider discontinuing unnecessary interventions and grouping disruptive interventions, such as diaper changes and heel sticks, to increase time without pain and external stimuli. Nonpharmacologic options should always be employed and include breastfeeding, swaddling, skin-to-skin contact, and non-nutritive sucking. Oral sucrose has been shown to reduce acute procedural pain and should be considered in combination with other nonpharmacologic and pharmacologic interventions.

Opioids are the drug of choice for moderate to severe pain in infants. The preferred medication is morphine, which can be administered in a variety of preparations including oral, rectal, intravenous, and subcutaneous. Rectal administration can be considered if no other access is available, however absorption is erratic in infants. When administering opioids, the need for titration due to high metabolic variability in this population and occurrence of tolerance should be anticipated. Changes in renal function, maturation of hepatic enzymes, and protein binding are all factors that play a role in analgesic efficacy and variability. In preterm neonates, fentanyl is frequently used for pain due to a more rapid onset of action, less histamine release than morphine, and no reliance on hepatic enzyme maturity for activation and metabolism. Boluses need to be administered slowly to prevent chest wall rigidity. Although effective for acute pain, tolerance to fentanyl develops after 5–9 days of *continuous* infusion, requiring escalation of doses and even causing precipitation of withdrawal. Consider administration of benzodiazepines if prolonged sedation is needed in neonates. Off-label, fentanyl can be administered intranasally via a mucosal atomization device for rapid pain relief. Opioid-related side effects to monitor in infants under palliative care include constipation and urinary retention. Use of other analgesics in neonates, such as nonsteroidal anti-inflammatory drugs (NSAIDs), ketamine, and acetaminophen, are often administered based on experience, but these lack sufficient evidence of safety and efficacy in this population. In general, it is crucial to combine nonpharmacologic interventions with medications to optimize pain management.

Palliative care practices in infants remains a challenge as practices vary significantly among institutions. More research needs to be done regarding best practices for palliative care in many of the pediatric subspecialties, such as child neurology. Many of the articles in the palliative care literature in this area are of patients with neurodegenerative diseases. On the other hand, pediatric brain tumors, which comprise 25–30% of all childhood cancers and are the leading cause of death by cancer in children under 15, have had minimal research guiding palliative care practices. Research in oncology, in addition to neonatal neurology, is greatly needed as neonates often have a very uncertain long-term prognosis, leading to difficult decisions occurring on a fairly common basis. Similar to adults, these children are commonly living longer, with the advancements of neuroimaging techniques, new antiepileptic treatments, and whole-body cooling. The highest proportion of seizures in children occur in infancy; the highest proportion of stroke in children is also in newborns. The families of patients with hypoxic ischemic encephalopathy, or intraventricular hemorrhage and periventricular leukomalacia, often have many questions and concerns that may go unanswered. The preceding case highlights how less common neurologic disorders, such as brain tumors, can also present in the newborn period.

It should be our obligation to help patients and families with the difficult decisions that arise regarding life planning along with evaluating and optimizing pain control. In the words of Mattie Stepanek, a 9-year-old boy who died from a neurologic disorder, "Palliative care no longer means helping children die well, it means helping children and their families to live well and then, when the time is certain, to help them die gently."

Pain management following craniotomy is challenging due to the lack of studies evaluating analgesia in this population and potential for serious postoperative complications. Undertreated pain may lead to an increase in intracranial pressure which could cause bleeding. Excessive sedation with opioids may cause respiratory depression and/or mask new neurologic deficits, making postoperative monitoring difficult. This delicate balance has been a source of controversy for determining the optimal safe and effective analgesic regimen post-craniotomy.

For the baby boy in our case study, the FLACC score should be used to evaluate his postoperative pain. Multimodal pain management should be utilized, and, in this case, acetaminophen should be given around the clock. NSAIDs are typically avoided immediately after craniotomy due to risk of postoperative hemorrhage. However, this depends on the neurosurgeon's preference and extent of tumor resection. Following surgery, the baby boy scored a 5 on the FLACC scale, indicating moderate pain. Enteral morphine every 3 hours as needed and intravenous morphine as needed for severe pain (FLACC >6) should be available. Patients experiencing persistent moderate to severe pain postoperatively may require nurse-controlled analgesia for adequate pain management. Uncontrolled pain should be reassessed at least every 15 minutes to prevent severe complications and psychological distress.

KEY POINTS TO REMEMBER

- Utilization of validated pediatric pain assessment tools is necessary for appropriate pain management.
- Never underestimate the importance of nonpharmacologic interventions!
- Challenges of optimizing pharmacologic interventions for pain in infants include maturity of hepatic enzymes, protein binding, and renal function.
- Opioids are the key medications for pain relief in infants; however, other pharmacologic options are utilized based on expert-experience in pediatric palliative care.

Further Reading

Chambers L. *A Guide to the Development of Children's Palliative Care Services*. In Goldman A, eds. Together for short lives, 4th ed. Bristol, 2018.

Dallara A, Meret A, Saroyan J. Mapping the literature: Palliative care within adult and child neurology. *J Child Neurol*. 2014;29(12):1728–1738.

Davies B, Sehring SA, Partridge JC, et al. Barriers to palliative care for children: perceptions of pediatric health care providers. *Pediatrics*. 2008;121(2):282–288.

Feudtner C, Kang TI, Hexem KR, et al. Pediatric palliative care patients: A prospective multicenter cohort study. *Pediatrics*. 2011;127(6):1094–1101.

Garten L, Bührer C. Pain and distress management in palliative neonatal care. *Semin Fetal Neonat Med*. 2019;24:101008. doi: 10.1016/j.siny.2019.04.008.

Hain R, Goldman A, Rapoport A, Meiring M, eds. *Oxford Textbook of Palliative Care for Children,* 3rd ed. New York: Oxford University Press; 2021.

Haug S, Farooqi S, Wilson CG, et al. Survey on neonatal end-of-life comfort care guidelines across America. *J Pain Symptom Manage*. 2018;55(3):979–984.

40 Pediatric Pain

Erinn Louttit and Jessica L. Spruit

Case Study

BN is a 2-year-old boy with dystrophic epidermolysis bullosa, a condition characterized by fragile skin that causes abnormal blistering or eroding of the skin from minor injury or friction.[1] BN's normal skin care routine involves a bath every 3 days with part bleach solution and sterile lancing of any new blisters, followed by extensive topical wound care and dressing. Recently, BN has been screaming, crying, hitting, and kicking in attempts to get away from his parents as they prepare the needle for lancing. He is causing more skin damage during these episodes. He currently is taking oral morphine solution 6 mg (0.4 mg/kg) via his gastrostomy (G) tube about 20 minutes prior to his bath. He has had two 15% increases in his opioid dose in the past 2 months. Prior to those increases, his doses were increased about every 4 months. The family uses his iPad for distraction during baths but this has recently proved futile. Mom worries his pain is not controlled.

What Do You Do Now?

Pediatric pain is a serious complaint that can have significant impact on a child and family's quality of life. For children living with serious illness, pain control often becomes an important consideration in their total care. Treatment should start with the identification of the pain source, as well as the type of pain that the child is experiencing: nociceptive, inflammatory, and/or neuropathic. This is often a challenging task in younger children who have not yet developed verbal skills or children with developmental delays, but success can be promoted by caregiver input and interpretation, direct provider observations, and the use of standardized pain scales. With this information collected, the provider can begin to formulate an appropriate plan for treatment. In BN's case, we know that his regular medical care involves painful processes to address his wound health and that he has a baseline wound burden. The pain associated with wounds is both nociceptive and dependent on stimulus as well as non-stimulus dependent, neuropathic pain. Nociceptive pain is defined by the International Association for the Study of Pain (IASP) as "An unpleasant sensory and emotional experience associated with, or resembling that associated with, actual or potential tissue damage." I n BN's case, the pain he experiences with lancing is likely an acute spike in nociceptive pain in the cutaneous areas. Opioids are known to work well for nociceptive pain by blocking the transmission of input into mu, kappa, and delta opioid receptors, supporting the decision to utilize this as an appropriate medication to assist with pain control during episodes of recurrent pain.

Inflammatory pain is associated with tissue damage and the subsequent inflammatory process, which has the benefit of eliciting physiologic responses that result in healing. Neuropathic pain is the result of nerve damage in either the peripheral or central nervous system and results from the sensitization of neurons. Ongoing nociceptive pain can actually produce neuropathic pain in the neurons involved due to damage, dysfunction and, exacerbation by the nociceptive pain. BN also likely has peripheral sensitization, meaning that peripheral nociceptors become hyperexcited due to inflammation, normal healing mechanisms, and surrounding tissues reacting to the injury, and this results in amplified pain signals in the associated central neurons, causing central sensitization.

The World Health Organization (WHO) created a pain ladder in response to an overuse of opioids in treating pain. Though specifically created for adult patients with chronic cancer pain, the principles of the ladder offer a starting point in considering how to approach pain in all patients presenting for treatment. Modifications of the original ladder have been created to assist with systematic management of acute and assorted types of chronic pain and remain a useful visualization for the clinician to reference. The ladder is divided into "steps," advising the clinician on specific pain medications to consider at each point. The WHO pain ladder refers to general classes of medications rather than specific medications. Of note, the modified ladder does not mention the use of adjuvants, which are present on the WHO pain ladder, so it may be beneficial to use both resources together.

While incredibly effective for nociceptive pain, opioids also have a broad spectrum of centrally and peripherally mediated effects including respiratory depression, feelings of euphoria or dysphoria, itching, decreased gastrointestinal motility, sedation, and nausea. As a patient is consistently exposed to an opioid medication, they can develop a seemingly rapid tolerance or loss of analgesic effect while continuing to experience the untoward side effects, to which tolerance develops more slowly. Ideally, the approach to pain control in patients should be performed systematically, working to achieve adequate control while minimizing side effects. In treating pediatric patients, these ladders offer evidence-based guidance directing the clinician to start with medications such as nonsteroidal anti-inflammatory drugs (NSAIDs) and acetaminophen, which have a relatively low side-effect profile at proper doses in younger patients.

If NSAIDs and acetaminophen have not been trialed before, the first recommendation could be to attempt using both agents as a combination without opioid use for the acute pain episode. It may be presumed that over-the-counter medications are not as strong or beneficial for pain as those available by prescription. However, more recent evidence has shown that non-opioid approaches to pain management can be as effective as opioid medications and have the added benefit of negating serious risks associated with opioid use including respiratory depression, tolerance, and addiction.[3] In cases where this is not a reasonable initial approach to pain control, there is evidence supporting concomitant use of NSAIDs, acetaminophen, and opioids for an opioid-sparing effect.[3] As BN will likely be using opioids for recurrent acute pain episodes throughout his life, putting him at risk for increasing tolerance to opioid medications, it is important to implement approaches that attempt to control this phenomenon early in the course of his medical care.

Looking specifically at BN's pain management, the clinician should consider and discuss the timing of the morphine that is given prior to the start of his bath time. It is optimal for the morphine peak effect to occur at the most painful part of his care process, which his mother has identified as lancing new blisters with a needle. Morphine generally has an onset of action of around 30 minutes, with peak effect around 1 hour and duration of effect around 3–5 hours. While this is variable among individual patients due to patient metabolism, it is important to educate his mother about the administration time of the morphine in relation to activities during his bathing process. One strategy may include creating a timeline of the bathing process, identifying the points during the process when his pain appears to be the worst. Visualization of this timeline can help the provider and the caregiver determine the best time to administer the medication based on the pharmacokinetics. A family may trial different administration times to understand when their son experiences the peak effect of the morphine, as pharmacogenetics influence an individual patient's response to a medication.

What happens if, in your conversation with his mother, you find that they are already using NSAIDs, acetaminophen, and appropriate timing for the morphine to have peak effect? What would be your next step in working toward better pain management?

An important note in this case is that the morphine dose has been titrated with increasing frequency in the past month compared to months prior. Though there are many reasons to consider an opioid rotation, this alone should prompt the provider to consider a planned switch of opioids, as BN's tolerance of morphine appears to be increasing at a higher rate. Rotation is done by using an estimate of relative potency between the chosen opioids. Morphine, hydromorphone, hydromorphone, and oxycodone are common short-acting opioids used in pediatric patients for acute pain. Codeine, another short-acting opioid, should be avoided in pediatric patients due to genetic variability in metabolism that results in some patients having high sensitivity and risk for serious adverse effects, including respiratory depression and death. The selection of an opioid depends on the patient's prior experience with opioids or provider preference. There are combination opioid analgesics, such as hydrocodone-acetaminophen; however, many providers choose to avoid these in pediatric patients due to the increased the risk of acetaminophen toxicity. In the setting of guarded or impaired kidney function, hydromorphone is generally considered the safest short-acting opioid to use based on metabolism. When prescribing pharmacologic interventions for children, the provider must consider available formulations and concentrations of the solutions. Young children may not be able to swallow tablets, and small doses may be difficult to draw up into syringes depending on the solution concentrations. Additional considerations include

- Insurance coverage or financial considerations
- Prior opioids trialed or taken
- Drug-drug interactions
- Local availability

Once an opioid has been selected, standard variables are used to convert dosing based on the potency of each medication. In addition, it is recommended to reduce the new opioid medication dose by 25–50% to account for incomplete cross-tolerance, or the belief that, although the medications are of the same class and act on the same receptors, their unique profiles are different enough to not be exclusively interchangeable with the same level of tolerance. In BN's case, we might recommend a rotation to hydromorphone.

As identified earlier, BN's pain is both nociceptive and neuropathic in origin. While NSAIDs, analgesics, and opioids are effective for nociceptive pain, an additional agent may need to be considered for the neuropathic pain. Gabapentin, a gamma-aminobutyric acid (GABA) analogue, is an anticonvulsant used in the treatment of epilepsy and for postherpetic neuralgia in adults. Off label, it had been used for chronic headaches, fibromyalgia pain, and anxiety. It has been used in pediatrics for many different conditions, but most notable to this case are neuropathic pain and pruritus. BN could benefit from reduced neuropathic pain in addition to gabapentin's potential effects on itching and, as demonstrated in adult patients, decreasing anxiety. Polypharmacy is an important consideration in pediatric pain treatment, and the use of a medication that may have dual benefits is encouraged. Patients with epidermolysis bullosa often experience poorly controlled pruritus that impacts their quality of life. This pruritus is not completely understood, but likely multifactorial and related to persistent inflammation, hyperthermia secondary to dressings, local sensitizers, and systemic opioid therapy. Though gabapentin's action is not entirely clear, there is some modulation of mu receptor, which has an effect on central perception of itching. Additionally, gabapentin is known to inhibit the release of a peptide known to mediate itching in the spinal cord. The pharmacokinetics of the medication makes drug interaction unlikely, and it does not affect liver enzymes. Due to its relatively short half-life, gabapentin works best when dosed two to three times per day. The severity of the neuropathic pain or itching and the child's age may guide the clinician in determining the dose. A starting dose of 5 mg/kg up to 300 mg at bedtime would be appropriate in this case, although data are limited. Dosing at bedtime is recommended when starting since a common side effect is drowsiness. The dose of gabapentin may be increased to twice daily on the second day of therapy and three times daily on the third day of therapy. Once the three times a day dosing is achieved, additional dose increases, administered at the same frequency, may be prescribed, continuing until the desired effect or burdensome side effects are noted. The drowsiness experienced during titrations should abate within 1 week; if it persists, it would be appropriate to decrease back to the prior dose and remain there. The maximum daily dose is 3,600 mg/day. As discussed previously, it may be beneficial to consider when the gabapentin is being given in relation to the bath, as the goal remains for peak effect to occur at the time that induces the most pain.

Acute anxiety may also contribute to the distressing experiences of bath time and wound care for BN and his family. Used carefully, with consideration for the potential for oversedation in combination with opioids, benzodiazepines may be helpful for anxiolysis. Another agent that could be considered as an adjuvant to his opioid regimen would be clonidine. An alpha-2 agonist, clonidine influences norepinephrine, which affects blood pressure, heart rate, anxiety, attention, and arousal. Approved for use in hypertension in adults, off-label uses in pediatrics include attention deficit hyperactivity disorder (ADHD), sleep disorders, and anxiety due to its sedative and analgesic properties. It should be used cautiously due to its vasoactive effects, but it can have great benefit in inducing a sense of calm in patients faced with a stressful encounter such as a procedure. Conservative dosing strategies should be applied, especially in a child this young, with careful monitoring of his blood pressure. Again, the medication should be given to time the peak effect with the most distressing part of his bath time.

In addition to medication management of BN's pain, it would be important to consider nonpharmacological strategies to support his bathing process. Encouraging the family to normalize bath time by including favorite toys or letting BN assist with aspects of his bath may aid in distraction. Though his bath time is medicalized, it does not have to be treated as a procedure. Prepping all the necessary tools and supplies prior to the bath helps to decrease time between important steps, particularly when approaching the lancing stage. Creative interventions, such as the application of ice on his blisters prior to them being lanced, may also assist with his tolerance. Though BN is likely to have many specialists involved in his care, a referral to play therapy may be extremely beneficial for him and his family. With a focus on understanding BN's routines and necessary medical care, the play therapist can recommend developmentally appropriate ways for the family to encourage and react to BN throughout his bath time. Additionally, they can help BN explore his medical norms and cope with his experiences as a child living with a chronic, complex medical condition.

KEY POINTS TO REMEMBER

- It is critical that the clinician considers the timing of painful care interventions and guides administration of interventions according to that timeline. For this consideration, a visual timeline may be helpful.
- All sources and types of pain experienced should be considered, with attention to each as a pain management regimen is created.
- Complicated pain, such as chronic wound pain in various states of healing, requires a multifaceted approach that balances pharmacological treatment and nonpharmacological approaches for a safe and successful plan.

- In addition to knowledge of the type of pain that pharmacological treatment targets, it is especially important to consider formulations and concentrations in pediatrics. For example, some children cannot swallow tablets, and some liquid preparations may be very difficult to draw in to a syringe.
- Multiple variables contribute to the experience of pain or discomfort, including anxiety and pruritus. To adequately address each factor contributing to this experience, it is valuable for the clinician to consider all possible variables.
- The care plan of a child with chronic pain will continually evolve as the child grows and develops. Establishing a trusting relationship with the family in addition to careful observation, engagement of the pediatric patient (if possible), listening to the family, and provider patience are all important factors in successful modifications to the plan. It is unlikely that one change will result in complete resolution or control of the pain.

References

1. National Institutes of Health (NIH). Epidermolysis bullosa. 2018. https://rarediseases.info.nih.gov/diseases/6359/epidermolysis-bullosa
2. International Association for the Study of Pain (IASP). IASP terminology: Nociceptive stimulus. 2017. https://www.iasp-pain.org/Education/Content.aspx?ItemNumber=1698#Nociceptivestimulus. Accessed November 13, 2021.
3. Sullivan D, Lyons M, Quinlan-Colwell A. Exploring opioid-sparing multimodal analgesia options in trauma: A nursing perspective. *J Trauma Nurs.* 2016;23(6):361–375.

Further Reading

Dumas EO, Pollack GM. Opioid tolerance development: A pharmacokinetic/pharmacodynamic perspective. *AAPS J.* 2008;10(4):537–551.

Fine PG, Portenoy RK, Ad Hoc Expert Panel on Evidence Review and Guidelines for Opioid Rotation. Establishing "best practices" for opioid rotation: Conclusions of an expert panel. *J Pain Symptom Manage.* 2009;38(3):418–425.

Goldschneider KR, Good J, Harrop E, et al. Pain care for patients with epidermolysis bullosa: Best care practice guidelines. *BMC Med.* 2014;12:178. doi:10.1186/s12916-014-0178-2

Martin K, Geurent S, Asche JK, et al. Psychosocial recommendations for the care of children and adults with epidermolysis bullosa and their family: Evidence based guidelines. *Orphanet J Rare Dis.* 2019;14(1):133.

Mendham JE. Gabapentin for the treatment of itching produced by burns and wound healing in children: A pilot study. *Burns.* 2004;30(8):851–853.

Pope E, Lara-Corrales I, Mellerio J, et al. A consensus approach to wound care in epidermolysis bullosa. *J Am Acad Dermatol.* 2012;67(5):904–917.

Yesudian PD, Wilson JE. Efficacy of gabapentin in the management of pruritus of unknown origin. *Arch Dermatol.* 2005;141:1507–1509.

41 Pain Management in Liver Disease

Michelle Krichbaum and Maura Miller

Case Study

RM is a 63-year-old White woman with known history of type 2 diabetes, solitary kidney, and cryptogenic cirrhosis (CC). She presented to the ED with abdominal pain and hematemesis. Endoscopy showed esophageal varices, and she received 2 units of packed red blood cells and underwent endoscopic variceal ligation. She subsequently was given platelets and fresh frozen plasma, intubated to protect her airway, and admitted with diagnoses of hepatic encephalopathy and acute respiratory failure secondary to this. Octreotide was initiated. She improved, was extubated, and was transferred to the general floor. She then developed recurrent gastrointestinal bleeds with intensification of abdominal pain and distension, reporting a pain score of 8/10, characterized as a diffuse, dull ache with tightness. RM then suffered acute respiratory failure, with her SCr increasing to 3.0 mg/dL from 1.6 mg/dL. Her International Normalized Ratio (INR) is 1.4, ammonia 126 µmoles/L. Surgery was consulted to evaluate the abdominal distension, but determined she was not a surgical candidate.

What Do I Do Now?

TRANSITIONS TO END-STAGE LIVER DISEASE

Chronic liver disease accounts for approximately 1 million deaths annually, with an additional 1 million deaths from liver cancer and acute hepatitis. Accurate estimates of mortality are important in determining timing of care interventions, including pain control. The two most common indices to predict long-term outcomes are the Child-Pugh score and the Model for End Stage Liver Disease (MELD). Child-Pugh and MELD are limited because they do not align with patients' subjective reports of well-being. Diagnostic paracentesis should be completed if possible. Nursing assessment of patient's functional status and ability to manage daily activities are especially important measures in assessing and discussing desired patient-centered outcomes and should be considered in addition to Child-Pugh and MELD scores, especially if prognosis is terminal.

End-stage liver disease (ESLD), or decompensated cirrhosis, can result from a wide range of disorders, including viral hepatitis, nonalcoholic fatty liver, chronic alcohol use, and vascular injury. The most significant complicating feature of decompensated cirrhosis is portal hypertension, which is responsible for the development of symptoms of gastroesophageal variceal hemorrhage, splenomegaly, ascites, hepatic encephalopathy (HE), spontaneous bacterial peritonitis (SBP), and hepatorenal syndrome (HRS). These complications can come with severe and distressing symptoms, and pain control can be complex.

GASTROESOPHAGEAL VARICEAL HEMORRHAGE

Gastroesophageal varices are an immediate, life-threatening problem with a 20–30% mortality rate associated with each episode of bleeding. Signs and symptoms include vomiting blood; black, tarry, or bloody stools; dizziness; and fatigue. If abdominal pain is present, aspirin and nonsteroidal anti-inflammatory drugs (NSAIDs) should be avoided as they significantly increase the risk of further gastroesophageal bleeding.

ASCITES

As cirrhosis progresses, decreased protein synthesis by the liver results in loss of oncotic pressure. With the loss of pressure, fluid leaks into the peritoneal cavity causing ascites. Ascitic symptoms include dyspnea, abdominal pain and distention, and peripheral edema. The treatment of ascites secondary to portal hypertension includes abstinence from alcohol, sodium restriction, and diuretics. While abstinence from alcohol is preferred for patients with ascites, consider dietary sodium restriction of less than 2,000 mg/day only if the patient is not terminally ill. The decrease in protein synthesis is a concern when picking analgesic options that may be highly protein bound, including tricyclic antidepressants (TCAs) and increasingly, cannabidiol (CBD) and tetrahydrocannabinol (THC). Analgesic modalities that may contribute to worsening edema (e.g., gabapentinoids) should be use judiciously. Additionally, with the likely use of diuretics, medications known to contribute to hyponatremia should be avoided (e.g., oxcarbazepine, carbamazepine).

HEPATIC ENCEPHALOPATHY

Ammonia is a neurotoxin produced in the intestinal tract and metabolized by the liver. As cirrhosis progresses, there is loss of brain function when ammonia is not removed, causing the symptoms of HE. These include forgetfulness, confusion, and breath with a sweet musty odor, progressing to tremor, disorientation, lethargy, delirium, and coma. These symptoms can decrease the ability to accurately assess pain, therefore a reliable scale such as the Pain Assessment in Advanced Dementia (PAINAD) or Pain Assessment Checklist for Seniors with Limited Ability to Communicate (PACSLAC-II) should be used for verbal and nonverbal patients experiencing cognitive impairment.[1] As in the case of RM, HE-related confusion caused impaired medical decision-making capacity. Identification of a healthcare surrogate to assume medical decision-making responsibilities was needed to guide further treatment.

The mainstay of treatment for encephalopathy is lactulose, an osmotic laxative, to eliminate ammonia. Lactulose is initiated at 20–30 g (30–45 mL) 2–4 timer per day with a goal of 2–3 soft stools per day. If minimal or no improvement on lactulose, the oral antibiotic rifaximin can be added to lactulose. Rifaximin kills gut bacteria that produce nitrogenous compounds that can cause HE and has been found to be safe and well-tolerated in long-term treatment.

When ESLD patients are in the terminal stages, treatment goals may shift to comfort and palliation of symptoms. For symptoms of terminal delirium and agitation, the use of antipsychotics is preferred over benzodiazepines. Benzodiazepines have been shown to predispose patients to HE and are highly protein bound and metabolized through the liver. Even a low dose of the short-acting benzodiazepine midazolam can become toxic in cirrhotic patients as half-life greatly increases and protein binding is reduced from 97% to 5%, resulting in more free drug. The antipsychotics haloperidol, ziprasidone, and olanzapine have oral and short-acting parenteral dosage forms and can be used at lower initial doses for delirium and agitation in ESLD. Routine use of analgesics versus as-needed dosing should be considered. Drugs requiring biotransformation for analgesic activity may be negatively impacted by ESLD (e.g., tramadol and codeine). Hepatic dosing for most opioids is required, with the exception of fentanyl.

HEPATORENAL SYNDROME

Approximately 20% of patients with advanced cirrhosis or acute liver failure will develop HRS. Goal of therapy is to reverse the acute kidney injury if improvement in liver function is not possible. Management includes discontinuing diuretics and initiating vasoconstrictors, often with intravenous (IV) albumin. NSAIDs should be avoided due to their increased risk for HRS.

Vasoconstricting agents such as norepinephrine or vasopressin can increase ICU survival time, but they have serious side effects including myocardial ischemia and cardiac arrhythmias. Their use should be carefully evaluated in the palliative setting to ensure patient's end-of-life preferences are being met.

HYPONATREMIA

Hyponatremia is common in cirrhotic patients and is associated with increased mortality. Symptoms include fatigue, confusion, dizziness, and muscle cramps. Correction of hyponatremia has no current data to suggest improvement in morbidity or mortality, however it can improve symptoms. Management includes discontinuing antihypertensives and diuretics, correcting hypokalemia if present, and, if hyponatremia is severe and symptomatic, considering the use of albumin infusion or hypertonic saline. If muscle cramps and spasms are unremitting, the skeletal muscle relaxants baclofen and low-dose methocarbamol have been used successfully in cirrhotic patients. Baclofen is renally dose-adjusted, and methocarbamol is initiated at a lower dose due to its prolonged half-life in cirrhotic patients.

PAIN AND SYMPTOM MANAGEMENT

Patients with liver disease often complain of a mixed nociceptive and neuropathic pain in their abdomen that can be worsened by skin stretching and tightness secondary to ascites. Drug choice for palliative symptoms can be a confusing problem as many drugs are metabolized in the liver. Increased accumulation of highly protein bound drugs is also a concern as the increasingly cirrhotic liver decreases protein synthesis. Renal dose adjustment may also play a role as the liver becomes increasingly cirrhotic.

Acetaminophen can be used at less than 2 g/day, but NSAIDs should be avoided due to their increased risk for gastroesophageal bleeding and HRS. Systemic inflammation or pain secondary to metastases can be managed using a steroid such as prednisone or dexamethasone.

As RM's condition deteriorated, her symptom burden increased with worsening ascites, dyspnea, and pain. Advance care planning meetings were held with the healthcare team and surrogate; the terminal nature of disease process, poor response to treatment, and treatment options were discussed. The decision was made to consult palliative care, which provided additional education and support. RM was admitted to hospice. Palliative treatment of RM's symptoms of severe pain and dyspnea required use of opioids. If her oral route was available, hydrocodone or oxycodone initiated at dose reductions of 30–50% could be used.[2] Morphine or hydromorphone may also be used at lower initial doses, but both have toxic metabolites in renal failure. Low-dose fentanyl was used. Fentanyl is highly protein bound and metabolized by CYP 3A4, but it does not produce toxic metabolites and is preferred in renal impairment. Methadone is another option because it has oral and parenteral routes and is a multimodal analgesic that reduces both nociceptive pain via mu opioid agonism and neuropathic pain by N-methyl-D-aspartate (NMDA) receptor antagonism and serotonin and norepinephrine reuptake inhibitor (SNRI) action. It is highly protein bound and metabolized in the liver by the cytochrome system but does not have toxic metabolites and can also be used if patient has renal insufficiency.

For neuropathic pain, gabapentin or pregabalin may be useful as neither are metabolized in the liver nor highly protein bound. However, both drugs need to be renally dose-adjusted for a creatine clearance (CrCl) of less than 60 mL/min. Tricyclic antidepressants (TCAs), such as amitriptyline and nortriptyline, have also been used for neuropathic pain, despite their high protein binding and metabolism by the cytochrome P450 system. If TCAs are to be trialed, nortriptyline, which is the active metabolite of amitriptyline, is recommended at low doses due to its lower anticholinergic side-effect profile. Hospice treatment goals should focus on palliation of symptoms with the goal of comfort at the end of life. Use of nonpharmacological nursing comfort interventions, aromatherapy, repositioning, skin care, massage, music therapy, spiritual care, social support, and ongoing family education were offered in addition to pharmacotherapy. RM's symptoms were palliated to comfort and she died peacefully in hospice care.

In the case of RM, IV fentanyl 25 μg every hour as needed for pain was initiated with the palliative team regularly evaluating efficacy and recurrence of use. As RM's symptoms progressed, a continuous IV infusion of fentanyl 25 μg/hour was needed to manage her pain and dyspnea. Spironolactone and furosemide for abdominal stretching and distension were discontinued due to her renal failure. The palliative care team also ordered olanzapine oral disintegrating tablets 2.5 mg every 4 hours as needed for delirium or agitation, though this order went unused as RM's agitation declined once pain was appropriately managed.

KEY POINTS TO REMEMBER

- ESLD, marked by hepatic insufficiency and cirrhosis, can arise from a variety of specific diagnoses.
- Clinical indicators for poor prognosis include refractory ascites, high systolic blood pressure, hepatorenal syndrome, recurrent hepatic encephalopathy, recurrent variceal bleeding, and unrelieved suffering.
- Assess pain using the right tool for mentation status, including a PAINAD or PACSLACII for patients with cognitive impairment.

- Diuretics, paracentesis, and TIPS can help manage abdominal pain, stretching, and tightness secondary to ascites.
- Muscle cramps can be managed with baclofen or low-dose methocarbamol in patients without electrolyte imbalance or if electrolytes are unable to be corrected.
- When choosing analgesic options, considerations for patients with ESLD must include protein binding, renal dose adjustments, and active and/or toxic metabolites.

References

1. Hadjistavropoulos T, Herr K, Prkachin KM, et al. Pain assessment in elderly adults with dementia. *Lancet Neurol.* 2014;13(12):1216–1227.
2. Soleimanpour H, Safari S, Nia KS, et al. Opioid drugs in patients with liver disease: a systematic review. *Hepatitis Mon.* 2016;16(4):e32636. doi:10.5812/hepatmon.32636.

Further Reading

Abd-Elsalam S, Arafa M, Elkadeem M, et al. Randomized-controlled trial of methocarbamol as a novel treatment for muscle cramps in cirrhotic patients. *Eur J Gastroenterol Hepatol.* 2019;31(4):499–502.

Chandok N, Watt K. Pain management in the cirrhotic patient: The clinical challenge. *Mayo Clin Proc.* 2010;85:451–458.

Dinis-Oliveira RJ. Metabolomics of Δ9-tetrahydrocannabinol: implications in toxicity. *Drug Metabol Rev.* 2016;48(1):80–87.

Dwyer JP, Jayasekera C, Nicoll A. Analgesia for the cirrhotic patient: A literature review and recommendations. *J Gastroenterol Hepatol.* 2014;29(7):1356–1360.

EASL. EASL Clinical Practice Guidelines for the management of patients with decompensated cirrhosis. *J Hepatol.* 2018;69(2):406–460.

Elfert AA, Ali LA, Soliman S, et al. Randomized placebo-controlled study of baclofen in the treatment of muscle cramps in patients with liver cirrhosis. *Eur J Gastroenterol Hepatol.* 2016;28(11):1280–1284.

Garcia-Tsao G, Abraldes JG, Berzigotti A, et al. Portal hypertensive bleeding in cirrhosis: Risk stratification, diagnosis, and management: 2016 practice guidance by the American Association for the study of liver diseases. *Hepatology.* 2017;65(1):310–335.

Oliverio C, Malone N, Rosielle DA, Drew A. Opoid use in liver failure. *J Palliat Med.* 2012;15(12):1389–1391.

Runyon BA. Management of adult patients with ascites due to cirrhosis: Update 2012. *Hepatology.* 2013;57(4):1651–1653.

42 Pain Management in Chronic Kidney Disease

Scot Born, Ashley Unger, and
Christopher M. Herndon

Case Study

Our patient is a 72-year-old woman with a long-standing history of poorly controlled type 2 diabetes mellitus (DM). She has had numerous complications related to DM, including retinopathy and painful peripheral neuropathy, coronary artery disease (CAD) with catheterization and stent placement × 1 4 years ago, and stage V chronic kidney disease (CKD) with an estimated glomerular filtration rate (GFR) of 14 mL/min. She has been followed closely over the past several years and is presently on an angiotensin receptor blockers (ARB), statin, beta-blocker, aspirin, and insulin. She has been having difficulty with progressive peripheral neuropathy pain in her feet and was started on gabapentin 6 months ago at a dose of 300 mg before bed, which provided some relief of her neuropathy pain initially but is no longer controlling her symptoms. She has recently fallen and suffered a fragility fracture of her wrist. Approaching symptomatic uremia, she has determined that she is not interested in renal replacement therapy.

What Do You Do?

GENERAL APPROACH TO PAIN MANAGEMENT IN THE PALLIATIVE CARE PATIENT WITH CHRONIC KIDNEY DISEASE

The approach to pain management in patients with chronic kidney disease (CKD) will follow the core principles of good pain management in the general population. Additional considerations in this patient population should include knowledge of the altered pharmacokinetics/pharmacodynamics and potentially altered toxicity and efficacy. Generally, patients with advanced CKD will also have multiple other medical comorbidities that need to be considered, often attended by a complex medical regimen that needs to interface with any new therapeutic additions.

Approaching the management of this specific patient, one should first characterize the specific character and chronicity of her pain, recognizing that patients often will have multiple concurrent syndromes. These considerations include characterizing pain as either chronic or acute, which will require different approaches to management. Specific pain subtypes to consider would include nociceptive, neuropathic, or combined. Thoughtful consideration must also be given to the extensive array of adjunctive and complementary pharmacologic and nonpharmacologic therapies available to these patients.

ACUTE PAIN MANAGEMENT IN THE CKD PATIENT

Modification of the general approach to acute pain management in the CKD patient is necessary because use of nonsteroidal anti-inflammatory drugs (NSAIDs) should be restricted in patients with stage III CKD, avoided in patients with stage IV CKD, and strictly contraindicated in patients with stage V CKD who are not yet on dialysis. It well known that NSAIDs have several potential negative effects on renal function, most notably impairing production of vasodilatory prostaglandins regulating afferent renal artery tone and thereby substantially reducing renal plasma flow and hence glomerular filtration rate (GFR). The renal hemodynamic sensitivity to these agents is also amplified by other agents commonly used in these patients, including angiotensin converting enzyme (ACE) inhibitors, angiotensin II receptor blockers (ARBs), and diuretics. This could likely precipitate a potentially fatal drop in GFR, especially in this patient in whom dialysis is not being pursued. As with most severe CKD patients, our patient is medically quiet frail and at high risk of other NSAID adverse effects including an increased risk of gastrointestinal ulceration, hypertension, volume retention, and myocardial infarction. Even those on dialysis should avoid NSAIDs except in rare circumstances because these agents can adversely impact residual renal function, which is strongly correlated with survival on dialysis. This is often a poorly appreciated toxicity of these and other nephrotoxic medications that providers feel they can prescribe with impunity once a patient is on dialysis. With an enhanced emphasis on alleviation of pain and acceptance of increased risk to achieve that endpoint in the palliative care patient, there may be rare instances where these medications can be used with close monitoring, but in general they should be avoided. Topical NSAID formulations can be considered in this setting and would be preferable where NSAIDs are believed to be needed. They are generally considered be safe but are inadequately studied to make any definitive conclusions. When NSAIDs are clinically required, they should be used for the shortest possible time and in the minimum effective dose.

For patients with pain not adequately controlled by acetaminophen, consideration should next turn to opioid management options. A review of opioid prescribing habits in patients on dialysis revealed that more than 60% of these patients received a prescription for opioids during the study period. The most commonly prescribed agents in order of use were hydrocodone, oxycodone, and tramadol, which collectively accounted for 86% of opioid prescriptions written for chronic pain in this patient population.

Patients who continue to experience moderate to severe pain will require consideration for more potent therapies. These agents would typically include hydrocodone, codeine, oxycodone. Of these, hydrocodone is the most widely prescribed in both the CKD and general population, but it is associated with unpredictable pharmacokinetics in patients with significantly impaired renal function. Oxycodone has been shown in limited studies to accumulate in CKD patients, with the area under the curve (AUC) and maximum concentration (C_{max}) doubling in patients with severe CKD. Use of these agents, in addition to codeine, are also prone to wide intraindividual variations in efficacy/toxicity depending on their metabolic status. Oxycodone, hydrocodone, and codeine are all metabolized to active metabolites via CYP 2D6 and inactive metabolites via CYP

3A4. Pharmacogenomic polymorphisms may predispose these patients to either supratherapeutic opioid effects or, more importantly in this context, accumulation of renally cleared neurotoxic metabolites. The potential for significant adverse drug interactions resulting from concomitant use of multiple other medications commonly used in these medically fragile patients is also a serious consideration. Together with the general lack of proven safety in this population, use of these agents, including tramadol, should generally be avoided. Additionally, meperidine should be strictly avoided in patients with renal impairment due to accumulation of the metabolite normeperidine, which is associated with significant neurotoxicity, including seizures.

Moving up the potency ladder of opioid medications we come to a group of agents with a more favorable risk profile in CKD. Hydrocodone, fentanyl, methadone, and buprenorphine all appear to have negligent half-life changes in severe CKD. None of these agents is burdened with significant accumulation of active or toxic metabolites and all are considered preferable agents for use in the CKD population. It has been advocated that use of these agents in doses appropriate to the level of pain is as safe as use of agents considered less potent and does not confer increased addiction potential (which is of lesser concern in our palliative care population).

Our patient would be better served by either renally dosing gabapentin or pregabalin and the addition of low-dose hydromorphone for short-term use for management of her wrist pain. While considered safe for short periods in this patient population, accumulation of the renally cleared hydromorphone-3-glucuronide may contribute to neuroexcitatory symptoms. If she requires continuous dosing beyond several days, one could consider starting her on a fentanyl transdermal patch with hydromorphone as needed for breakthrough pain.

CHRONIC PAIN MANAGEMENT IN THE CKD PATIENT

Recall that our patient suffers from diabetic peripheral neuropathy. Diabetes in the leading cause of ESRD in this country, and management of diabetes-associated comorbidities in these patients is very common. The approach to patients with chronic pain is much different from acute pain: the use of opioids has a much more restricted role in management, with complementary and adjunctive therapies assuming a more central role.

Pharmacologic management of chronic neuropathic pain is generally initiated with an adjunctive agent such as a gabapentinoid, anticonvulsant, or tricyclic antidepressant (TCA). Commonly used agents include gabapentin, pregabalin, carbamazepine, and amitriptyline. The former two agents are generally considered to be first-line agents due to more widespread experience in this population. Both are excreted almost exclusively through the kidneys, and therefore the half-life of these agents increases proportionately with progressive impairment of the eGFR. This will require very significant dose reductions in patients with stage IV–V CKD and ESRD. Gabapentin has been used most extensively in this population, and with an eGFR the maximal daily dosage should not exceed 300 mg (Table 42.1). In our experience gabapentin has been associated with more overt neurotoxicity (confusion, somnolence, gait disturbance) than any other agent used for chronic pain, and maximal dosage guidelines should be strictly adhered to. Pregabalin similarly needs to have appropriate dosage reduction with progressive impairment of kidney function.

Carbamazepine has shown efficacy for management of chronic neuropathic pain in the non-CKD population and has been long used for conditions such as peripheral neuropathy and postherpetic neuralgia. Its pharmacokinetics are unchanged in patients with renal impairment and should not alter dosing. However, as with all such agents, it should be initiated cautiously and titrated to the minimum effective dose. Some clinicians may wish to monitor serum drug levels of 10,11-carbamazepine epoxide in lieu of traditional carbamazepine levels as this active metabolite is renally cleared and may be disconcordantly elevated in the renally compromised patient. TCAs, such as amitriptyline and nortriptyline, may be used as third-line agents, but should be used at low dosages due to significant anticholinergic and sedative side effects and should largely be avoided in this patient given her advanced age and significant cardiovascular history.

If pain management is inadequate with maximal titration of these agents, one would next consider addition of a non-opioid analgesic such as acetaminophen or a topical agent such as lidocaine, capsaicin, or diclofenac gel. Failing to achieve acceptable control of symptoms, one would next turn to the introduction of an opioid agent. Appropriate agents for consideration

TABLE 42.1 Select analgesics, excretion, hemodialysis, peritoneal dialysis

Medication	Metabolism	Excretion	Renal dose adjustment	Dialyzable?
Pure opioid agonists				
Morphine	Hepatic conjugation	Mostly urine Feces (~7%)	CrCl ≥60: No dose adjustment CrCl 30 to <60: Administer 50–75% of initial dose CrCl 15 to <30: Administer 25–50% of initial dose CrCl <15: Avoid use HD/PD/CRRT: Avoid use	Yes
Codeine	Hepatic CYP2D6 CYP3A4	Urine (90%) Feces	GFR >50: No dose adjustment GFR 10 to 50: Administer 75% of initial dose GFR <10: Administer 50% of dose CRRT: Administer 75% of dose	No
Fentanyl	Hepatic CPY3A4	Urine (75%) Feces (~9%)	Transdermal Patch: • CrCl 10–50: Administer 75% of initial dose • CrCl <10: Administer 50% of initial dose • HD: Administer 50% of initial dose IV: • CrCl <50: Decrease dose to avoid accumulation	No data
Hydrocodone	Hepatic CYP2D6 CYP3A4	Urine	Mild impairment: No dose adjustment Moderate to severe impairment: Administer 50% of initial dose ESRD: administer 50% of initial dose	No data
Hydromorphone	Hepatic glucuronidation	Mostly urine Feces (1%)	Injectable: • Administer 25–50% of initial dose Oral: • CrCl >60: No dose adjustment • CrCl 40–60: Administer 50% of initial dose • CrCl <30: Administer 25% of initial dose	No data

Drug	Metabolism	Elimination	Renal dose adjustment	Hepatic
Levorphanol	Hepatic	Urine	No dose adjustments per manufacturer's labeling. Use with caution.	No data
Methadone	Hepatic CYP3A4 CYP2B6 CYP2C19 CYP2C9 CYP2D6	Urine	CrCl ≥10: No dose adjustment CrCl <10: Administer 50–75% of initial dose	No
Meperidine	Hepatic CYP3A4 CYP2D6	Urine	Avoid use in renal impairment	No
Oxycodone	Hepatic CYP3A4 CYP2D6	Urine	CrCl ≥60: No dose adjustment CrCl <60: Administer 33–50% of initial dose	No data
Oxymorphone	Hepatic glucuronidation	Urine, feces	CrCl ≥50: No dose adjustment CrC; <50: Use with caution	No data
Partial opioid agonist				
Buprenorphine	Hepatic CYP3A4	Feces (~70%) Urine (~30%)	No dose adjustments per manufacturer's labeling. Use with caution.	No data
Central opioid agonists				
Tapentadol	Hepatic glucuronidation	Urine (99%)	CrCl ≥30: No dose adjustment CrCl <30: Avoid use	No data

Continued

TABLE 42.1 **Continued**

Medication	Metabolism	Excretion	Renal dose adjustment	Dialyzable?
Tramadol	Hepatic CYP3A4 CYP2D6	Urine	IR: • CrCl ≥30: No dose adjustment • CrCl <30: Increase dosing interval to q12h (max 200 mg/day) • Dialysis: Increase dosing interval to q12h (max 200 mg/day) ER: • CrCl ≥30: No dose adjustment • CrCl <30: Avoid use	Yes (IR)
SNRIs				
Duloxetine	Hepatic CYP1A2 CYP2D6	Urine (~70%) Feces (~20%)	CrCl ≥30: No dose adjustment CrCl <30: Avoid use HD/PD/CRRT: Avoid use	No
Milnacipran	Hepatic	Urine	Mild impairment: No dose adjustment Moderate impairment: Use with caution Severe impairment (CrCl ≤29): Reduce dose to 25 mg BID ESRD: Avoid use	No data
Venlafaxine	Hepatic CYP2D6	Urine (~87%)	CrCl ≥30: No dose adjustment CrCl <30: Initial 37.5 mg/day, do not exceed 50% of max dose HD/PD/CRRT: Initial 37.5 mg/day, do not exceed 50% of max dose	No
TCAs				
Amitriptyline	Hepatic	Mostly urine, also feces	No dose adjustments per manufacturer's labeling. Use with caution.	No

Drug	Metabolism	Elimination	Dose adjustment	
Desipramine	Hepatic	Urine (~70%)	No dose adjustments per manufacturer's labeling. Use with caution.	No
Nortriptyline	Hepatic	Urine	No dose adjustments per manufacturer's labeling. Use with caution.	No
Skeletal muscle relaxants				
Carisoprodol	Hepatic CYP2C19	Urine	No dose adjustments per manufacturer's labeling. Use with caution.	Yes
Cyclobenzaprine	Hepatic CYP3A4 CYP1A2 CYP2D6	Mostly urine, also feces	No dose adjustments per manufacturer's labeling.	No data
Metaxalone	Hepatic CYP1A2 CYP2D6 CYP2E1 CYP3A4	Urine	No dose adjustments per manufacturer's labeling. Use with caution. Contraindicated with significant renal function.	No data
Methocarbamol	Hepatic	Urine	No dose adjustments per manufacturer's labeling.	No data
Orphenadrine	Hepatic	Urine	No dose adjustments per manufacturer's labeling.	No data
Tizanidine	Hepatic CYP1A2	Urine (60%) Feces (20%)	CrCl ≥25: No dose adjustment CrCl <25: Use with caution	No data

Continued

TABLE 42.1 **Continued**

Medication	Metabolism	Excretion	Renal dose adjustment	Dialyzable?
Baclofen	Hepatic	Mostly urine, also feces	CrCl >80: No dose adjustment CrCl 50-80: Initial dose 5 mg q12h CrCl 30-59: Initial dose 2.5 mg q8h CrCl <30: Initial dose 2.5 mg q12h HD: Avoid use	Yes
Anticonvulsants				
Carbamazepine	Hepatic cytochrome p450 CYP3A4	Urine (72%) Feces (28%)	Mild to severe impairment requires no initial dose adjustment. Subsequent dose adjustments should be based on serum concentrations.	No
Oxcarbazepine	Hepatic	Urine (94%) Feces (<4%)	Mild to moderate impairment: No dose adjustment Severe impairment (CrCl <30): Initiate at 50% of initial dose (300 mg/day) ESRD: Use IR formulations over ER	No data
Topiramate	Hepatic	Urine	CrCl ≥70: No dose adjustment CrCl <70: Reduce dose by 50% HD: 50 to 100 mg twice daily	Yes
Zonisamide	Hepatic CYP3A4	Urine (62%) Feces (3%)	GFR ≥50: No dose adjustment GFR <50: Avoid use	No data

Gabapentin	N/A	Urine	IR:	Yes

IR:
- CrCl >79: Max 3,600 mg/day in 3 doses
- CrCl 50–79: Max 1,800 mg/day in 3 doses
- CrCl 30–49: Max 900 mg/day in 2–3 doses
- CrCl 15–29: Max 600 mg/day in 1–2 doses
- CrCl <15: Max 300 mg/day in 1 dose
- HD: 100 mg 3 times per week
- PD: 100 mg every other day
- CRRT: 100 mg twice daily

ER:
- CrCl ≥60: No dose adjustment
- CrCl 31–59: 600–1,800 mg once daily
- CrCl <30: Avoid use
- HD/PD: Avoid use

Pregabalin	N/A	Urine			Yes

CrCl	Total daily dose		Doses per day
≥ 60	150	300	450	600	2–3
30–60	75	150	225	300	2–3
15–30	25–50	75	100–150	150	1–2
<15	25	25–50	50–75	75	1
HD	25–50	50–75	75–100	100–150	1

Continued

TABLE 42.1 Continued

Medication	Metabolism	Excretion	Renal dose adjustment	Dialyzable?
Levetiracetam	N/A	Urine	IR: • CrCl 80–130: 500–1,500 mg q12h • CrCl 50–79: 500–1,000 mg q12h • CrCl 30–49: 250–750 mg q12h • CrCl 15–29: 250–500 mg q12h • CrCl <15: 250–500 mg q24h • HD: 500–1,000 mg q24h • PD: 250–500 mg q24h • CRRT: 750–1,000 mg q12h ER: • CrCl >80: 1–3 g q24h • CrCl 50–80: 1–2 g q24h • CrCl 30–49: 500–1,500 mg q24h • CrCl <30: 500–1,000 mg q24h • HD/PD: Avoid use	Yes
Miscellaneous				
Acetaminophen	Hepatic CYP2E1	Urine	Mild to severe impairment: No dose adjustment	Yes
Lidocaine patch	Hepatic	Urine	No dose adjustments per manufacturer's labeling.	No

CrCl, creatinine clearance; CRRT, continuous renal replacement therapy; GFR, glomerular filtration rate; HD, hemodialysis; PD, peritoneal dialysis.

would again include methadone, hydromorphone, or a fentanyl patch. As discussed previously these agents provide the safest and most reliably effective activity in this class and should be used preferentially. Both methadone and transdermal fentanyl also offer the advantage of a prolonged duration of action, which is also generally desirable in these patients.

Our patient is currently being managed with a combination of gabapentin and now hydromorphone. Failing to achieve adequate pain control with this, and the addition of acetaminophen as a second agent, we would next consider the addition of fentanyl or methadone. Consider that fentanyl transdermal patch efficacy may be attenuated in cases of cachexia. Methadone may provide an extended duration of analgesia, and, due to additional N-methyl-D-aspartate (NDMA) receptor antagonism, provide superior relief for patients with combined nociceptive and neuropathic pain. Careful consideration of methadone use in those patients with preexisting cardiac disease is necessary given the possible electrocardiographic changes associated with methadone use.

UREMIC NEUROPATHY

Uremic neuropathy is a complex and incompletely understood neurologic injury characterized by both axonal degeneration and demyelination that can present with both motor and sensory deficits. Multiple metabolic derangements, inflammation, and poor clearance of uremic toxins all likely play a pathologic role. Prevalence is high and progressive with worsening renal function, such that findings can be demonstrated in most patients with clinical uremic syndrome and ESRD. The severity of symptoms is variable but increasingly manifest with higher degrees of renal impairment. Typical sensory symptoms can include paresthesia, pin-prick needle sensations, and deep burning pain. Unfortunately, isolating the etiology of symptoms to renal failure can be difficult because neuropathy is a frequent concomitant of other common etiologies that can affect renal function, such as diabetes (leading cause of ESRD), amyloidosis, myeloma, vasculitis, etc. Thus, this important condition is all too often overlooked in clinic practice.

Definitive treatment is renal transplantation, which is most able to effectively reverse the multiple metabolic derangements of uremic syndrome. Hemodialysis can significantly improve symptoms in those patients with severe renal failure who have yet to initiate renal replacement therapy and would represent the next best option. For those patients on dialysis, an intensification of their treatment regimen to help promote enhanced removal of causative uremic toxins may improve symptoms significantly. There are also currently studies evaluating the efficacy of renal replacement techniques that allow for enhanced middle molecule removal (larger uremic toxins poorly cleared by conventional dialyzers that are felt to contribute to a number of uremic manifestations), such as hemodiafiltration, but results are currently pending.

Medical therapy generally involves use of typical agents used in the management of peripheral neuropathy including gabapentin, pregabalin, and TCADs. Dosages need to be strictly adjusted for impairment in renal function due to both the accumulation of poorly cleared drugs and metabolites as well as enhanced penetration of the blood–brain barrier in patients with uremia.

KEY POINTS TO REMEMBER

- The approach to pain management in the end-stage CKD patient should follow the basic framework appropriate for patients with normal renal function, including consideration of all adjunctive and complementary modalities.
- Medication selection must consider significant alterations in drug pharmacokinetics that may have important effects on drug safety, efficacy, and dosage requirements.
- Opioids are commonly used in this population, with recent reports showing almost 50% of class IV–V CKD patients receive at least one opioid prescription annually.
- Review of use by specific agent has revealed that up to 90% of opioids prescribed for chronic pain in this patient subset are for agents that are considered inappropriate, with hydrocodone, oxycodone, and tramadol collectively accounting for 81% of these prescriptions.

- Inappropriate dosing, particularly with gabapentin and pregabalin, further complicates management and contributes to excessive patient morbidity.
- Careful consideration of renal clearance for analgesics and their metabolites is paramount for patients with CKD in pain.

Further Reading

Li T, Wilcox CS, Lipkowitz MS, Gordon-Cappitelli, Dragoi SD. Rationale and strategies for preserving residual kidney function in dialysis patients. *Am J Nephrol.* 2019;50:411–421.

Kimmel PL, Fwu C, Abbott KC, Eggers AW, Kline PP, Eggers PW. Opioid prescription, morbidity, and mortality United States dialysis patients. *J Am Soc Nephrol.* 2017;28:3658–3670.

Davison SN. Clinical pharmacology considerations in pain management in patients with advanced kidney failure. *Clin J Am Soc Nephrol.* 2019;14:917–931.

Novick TK, Suprapaneni A, Shin J, et al. Prevalence of opioid, gabapentinoid, and NSAID use in patients with CKD. *Clin J Am Soc Nephrol.* 2018;13:1886–1888.

43 Pain Management in Mechanically Ventilated Patients

Kourtney Engele

Case Study

RS is a 71-year-old man who presented to the ED with shortness of breath for approximately 6 hours prior to arrival. The patient has a past medical history of coronary artery disease (CAD), status post coronary artery bypass graft, congestive heart failure (CHF), hypertension, and morbid obesity (weight 210 kg, BMI 89). RS's medication profile includes aspirin, furosemide, and metoprolol. Upon further evaluation, his troponin was elevated to 15.8 ng/mL but electrocardiogram showed no acute infarction. The patient decompensated overnight and experienced a cardiac arrest with monomorphic ventricular tachycardia (VT) and ultimately became unresponsive. A stat electroencephalogram (EEG) was performed, and no seizure activity was seen. At this time, family was notified, and the patient's code status was changed to do not resuscitate (DNR). His pain and sedation regimen includes fentanyl at 200 µg/hr and propofol at 5 µg/kg/min. The Critical Care Pain Observation Tool (CPOT) score has been 0 for the past 4 hours.

What Do I Do Now?

Several factors could be contributing to this patient's unresponsiveness, and a differential diagnosis for neurological compromise should be performed. An assessment to rule out four major etiologies of unresponsiveness should be considered including neurological, metabolic, psychiatric, and medication-induced. A neurological workup should be completed including a head computed tomography (CT) scan to rule out intracranial bleeding, especially in the setting of RS's coagulopathies. Metabolic and psychiatric abnormalities are unlikely contributing factors due to the rapidly improving blood gas, minimal metabolic derangements on repeat laboratory evaluation, and lack of psychiatric conditions in the past medical history. Hypoxia during the cardiac arrest could be adding to his decreased mental status, but this is less likely as he was neurologically intact immediately after the arrest. RS does, however, have potential for medication-induced encephalopathy.

Mechanically ventilated patients require medications to keep them calm and comfortable while life-saving interventions are performed. Unfortunately, several of these medications can accidently cause unwanted encephalopathy. Appropriate pain management is therefore vital to facilitate high-quality care for our ICU patients. As one can see from our patient case, inappropriate pain management can not only cause clinical issues such as oversedation but can also lead to wasted hospital resources and unnecessary diagnostic tests.

PAIN ASSESSMENT IN THE MECHANICALLY VENTILATED PATIENT

The first step a clinician should take when addressing a pain management regimen is to see whether the patient is indeed in pain. The 2018 Clinical Practice Guidelines for the Prevention and Management of Pain, Agitation/Sedation, Delirium, Immobility and Sleep Disruption in Adult Patients in the ICU (PADIS) recommend using the Behavioral Pain Scale (BPS) or the Critical Care Pain Observation Tool (CPOT) to assess pain in the mechanically ventilated patient.[1] A patient is "in pain" if the CPOT is greater than 2 or the BPS is greater than 3. In the case of RS, the nursing staff had charted his CPOT score as 0 for the past 4 hours but proceeded to increase his fentanyl drip to 200 μg/hr. While RS is likely experiencing some degree of pain following cardiopulmonary resuscitation (CPR), a consistent CPOT score of 0 without dose adjustment is inappropriate. Opiates are commonly misconstrued as medications used to facilitate sedation in the ICU even though they have been shown to increase time to mechanical ventilation liberation in comparison to sedatives. While the 2018 PADIS guidelines recommend using opiates to treat pain in critically ill patients, they should be used and titrated via the preceding assessment tools and should not be ordered or titrated for sedation.

FACTORS THAT AFFECT DRUG SELECTION

A clinician should then review the pain regimen for the correct drug, dose, route, and frequency. Pharmacokinetics (PK), pharmacodynamics (PD), and adverse effects should be considered for each drug and patient. PK/PD parameters in critically ill patients are drastically different from those in other hospitalized patients. Absorption of drugs given by mouth (PO) may be decreased due to limited blood flow to the gastrointestinal tract during shock states. Some PO drugs can bind to enteral feedings or the tubes used to administer enteral feedings. Volume of distribution may be altered, particularly if large fluid volumes are administered. Medication delivery can be decreased because of vasoconstriction caused by vasopressors. Drug metabolism may be significantly altered due to reduced perfusion to the liver, and drug elimination is often decreased because of poor urine output during hemodynamic compromise. A quick onset of action is preferred in critically ill patients since urgent management of conditions is often required. A short duration of action is usually favorable, especially for opioid medications, as neurological status needs to be constantly monitored and assessed.

Adverse effects of medications should be carefully evaluated and monitored in all patients. Many critically ill patients have multisystem organ failure, which cause adverse effects to be exacerbated. Like RS, several patients have some degree of coagulopathy, acute kidney injury, coronary artery disease, or hypotension which could be worsened by pain management regimens. Overall, the pain management regimen for mechanically ventilated patients should be tailored to each patient by evaluating their PK/PD profile, adverse effects, and other pertinent clinical characteristics.

ADJUVANT MEDICATIONS FOR PAIN CONTROL

Several adjuvant medications for pain management in the ICU are recommended in both the 2013 and 2018 PADIS guidelines. Acetaminophen is a relatively low-risk intervention in most critically ill patients without hepatic dysfunction. It has been shown to improve pain scores and decrease need for opiates in mechanically ventilated patients. While most of the data surrounding acetaminophen use in critically ill patients are in the surgical population, it can often be used in other critically ill patients due to its reasonable tolerability. Acetaminophen can be either scheduled or used as needed for uncontrolled CPOT scores. Intravenous (IV), PO, and rectal preparations are available in the United States although many hospitals do not carry the IV formulation because of high cost and risk for hypotension during infusion. IV and PO acetaminophen have similar effectiveness on pain control, but IV may be preferred in patients who have decreased perfusion to their GI tract, such as in those in shock states or receiving high-dose vasopressors.

Nonsteroidal anti-inflammatory drugs (NSAIDs) are an attractive option to treat pain due to their analgesic and anti-inflammatory properties; however, the PADIS 2018 guidelines recommend against the use of cyclo-oxygenase (COX-1)-selective NSAIDs in critically ill patients. Two small studies evaluated COX-1-selective NSAID use, and, although a significant reduction in morphine equivalents were seen, NSAIDs were not associated with an improvement in pain control at 24 hours. No studies to date are available to assess the use of COX-2 selective agents in critically ill patients and thus PADIS 2018 did not recommend for or against their use. In addition to lack of positive data for efficacy, concerns also exist regarding the risk of adverse effects from NSAIDs. NSAID use has been associated with an increased risk for acute kidney injury (AKI) and major bleeding events. Since many ICU patients exhibit significant renal dysfunction or a high risk for bleeding, the guidelines recommend extreme caution with their use from this aspect as well. NSAIDs are not preferred for RS due to his thrombocytopenia and AKI. Certain low-risk patient populations, such as relatively uncomplicated postsurgical patients, may benefit from NSAID use, but risk versus benefit should be evaluated.

Medications such as gabapentin, carbamazepine, and pregabalin may be used to treat neuropathic pain in critically ill patients. Neuropathic pain is extremely hard to identify in mechanically ventilated patients as no validated pain scale is available for this patient population. Most of the positive data supporting the use of neuropathic patient medications in the ICU are in postsurgical patients or in patients with Guillain-Barré syndrome, and they have been shown to decrease pain intensity and opioid consumption within 24 hours of therapy. Although these drugs are recommended as first-line agents for the treatment of neuropathic pain, they are not commonly used in mechanically ventilated patients due to the inability to reliably assess this type of pain.

Ketamine, another adjuvant agent recommended by the PADIS guidelines, is used for a wide array of indications. As an N-methyl-D-aspartate (NMDA) receptor antagonist, it is an option for sedation, status epilepticus, and alcohol withdrawal. Its ability to mitigate the risk of opioid-induced hyperalgesia makes it an appealing option as an adjuvant pain medication in critically ill patients. Most of the data available to support ketamine's use in the ICU reside in the surgical population. Ketamine can cause an increase in mean arterial pressure which, while not recommended for patients with coronary artery disease, may be preferred in a patient who is on multiple vasopressors for septic shock. Ketamine is not a preferred agent in patients with a history of psychosis due to the risk of hallucinations and emergence reactions.

OPIOID ANALGESICS FOR MECHANICALLY VENTILATED PATIENTS

Opioids are commonly chosen to manage pain in mechanically ventilated patients due to the lack of other more suitable options. Each opioid regimen has its own advantages and disadvantages. Fentanyl, as was used in the case of RS, is often preferred in the ICU due to its low risk for histamine release, quick onset, and short duration of action. As a synthetic compound, it exhibits a lower risk of allergic reactions and hemodynamic instability. Because of its large volume of distribution and lipophilicity, fentanyl is easily distributed into the central nervous system, which leads to a quick onset of action. While its lipophilicity may be a useful property, it also results in an increased duration of action with prolonged use, especially in obese patients like RS.

Morphine, a natural compound, is one of the most well-studied opiates used in modern practice. It is metabolized by the liver into three metabolites: morphine-3-glucuronide, morphine-6-glucuronide, and normorphine. Both the parent compound and the active metabolites are renally cleared and have a substantial risk of accumulation in renal failure. In addition, morphine-3-glucuronide has been shown to cause hyperalgesia instead of analgesia. While morphine does not have a favorable pharmacokinetic profile in critically ill patients, some physicians insist on its use in patients presenting with acute myocardial infarction. New data suggest that utilizing morphine in this setting could decrease the effectiveness of antiplatelet agents and increase adverse cardiac outcomes and in-hospital mortality, and it is therefore no longer recommended as a first-line agent for this indication.

Hydromorphone, a semi-synthetic compound, is significantly more potent than morphine and must be used cautiously in opioid-naïve patients. Unlike morphine, hydromorphone is metabolized to inactive compounds. The parent drug will, however, still accumulate in renal failure, prolonging its already increased half-life. Hydromorphone may be used as an alternative to fentanyl if a longer duration of pain control is needed.

Remifentanil, a newer synthetic opioid, is an attractive option for mechanically ventilated patients. It is metabolized by esterases into relatively inactive compounds and would theoretically not be affected by organ dysfunction. Remifentanil is, however, an ultra-short-acting opioid and caution should be taken when discontinuing the medication. Withdrawal could happen quickly, and pain may be difficult to control without appropriate taper and reintroduction of longer-acting opiates.

DOSE EVALUATION

After assessing for the correct drug in the pain management regimen, the dose should also be evaluated for appropriateness. The dose of fentanyl that RS is receiving is more than 1,000 mg of oral morphine equivalents per day, which is a significantly higher starting dose than recommended for an opioid-naïve patient. RS is not a baseline opioid user and does not have any history of illicit drug use. He will theoretically be more sensitive to the effects of opioids than a patient with opioid use history. Although preventing respiratory depression is not necessarily our priority in someone who is already mechanically ventilated, high-dose opioids can prolong time to extubation and cause oversedation, as seen in our patient. Although fentanyl was likely an appropriate initial choice for pain management in RS, the dose should have been limited to the minimum dose needed to achieve a controlled CPOT score.

Overall, a pain management regimen for mechanically ventilated patients should be chosen based on both patient- and drug-specific clinical characteristics using the preceding general principles for therapy choice.

KEY POINTS TO REMEMBER

- The presence of pain in mechanically ventilated patients should be evaluated by using either the CPOT or BPS.
- Pharmacokinetics, pharmacodynamics, and adverse effects of each drug should be carefully considered to choose an effective and safe pain management regimen.
- Appropriate drug, dose, route, and frequency should be evaluated for each regimen.
- Adjuvant pain medications should be considered in all patients to reduce opioid consumption.
- Fentanyl is one of the most preferred opioid medications in critically ill patients due to its low risk of histamine release, quick onset of action, and short duration of action.

Reference

1. Devlin JW, Skrobik Y, Gelinas C, et al. Clinical practice guidelines for the prevention and management of pain, agitation/sedation, delirium, immobility, and sleep disruption in adult patients in the ICU. *Crit Care Med.* 2018;46(9):e825–e873.

Further Reading

Barr J, Fraser GL, Puntillo K, et al. Clinical practice guidelines for the management of pain, agitation, and delirium in adult patients in the intensive care unit. *Crit Care Med.* 2013;41(1):263–306.

Cooksley T, Rose S, Holland M. A systemic approach to the unconscious patient. *Clin Med (Lond)*. 2018;18(1):88–92.

Duarte GS, Nunes-Ferreira A, Rodrigues FB, et al. Morphine in acute coronary syndrome: systematic review and meta analysis. *BMJ Open*. 2019;9(3):e025232.

Jibril F, Sharaby S, Mohamed A, Willby KJ. Intravenous versus oral acetaminophen for pain: Systemic review of current evidence to support clinical decision-making. *Can J Hosp Pharm*. 2015;68(3):238.

Patel SB, Kress JP. Sedation and analgesia in the mechanically ventilated patient. *Am J Respir Crit Care Med*. 2012;185(5):486–497.

Smith BS, Yogaratnam D, Levasseur-Franklin KE, Forni A, Fong J. Introduction to drug pharmacokinetics in the critically ill patient. *Chest*. 2012;141(5):1327–1336.

44 Pain Management in Opioid-Tolerant Patients

Stephanie Abel

Case Study

AB is a 42-year-old woman with metastatic breast cancer and a complex pain history. She was started on opioids more than a decade ago for chronic pain related to a traumatic car accident. Her opioid doses increased slowly over the years prior to her cancer diagnosis but remained stable overall. Recently, however, she has been admitted for acute uncontrolled pain monthly for the past 4 months, and her home opioid regimen has been aggressively up-titrated. Her cancer is now widely metastatic to bone and lung and she has developed a fungating breast wound. She has documented bone metastases in her thoracic spine (no spinal cord compression) and her ribs. She also has concomitant diabetes mellitus type 2, posttraumatic stress disorder from her car accident, anxiety, and depression. AB has diabetic nephropathy (chronic kidney disease stage 3), hepatic function tests are within normal limits, blood glucose is 200 mg/dL. Upon evaluation, you determine that AB's pain is complex and a mix of somatic, visceral, and neuropathic components. She is writhing in pain and her heart rate, blood pressure, and respiratory rate are elevated from baseline. The team has done an infectious workup which has come back negative, she is not febrile, nor is she showing any signs of high-acuity illness.

What Do I Do Now?

As a clinician approaching this complex case, we must triage the acuity of symptomatic treatment needs. The priority should be getting the severe and intractable pain to a tolerable level. The rationale is several-fold: it is causing significant suffering, affecting her vital signs, and she will be unable to engage in conversation to address a more comprehensive and targeted approach to her pain, symptoms, and goals. As we think through optimal management of acute pain in this opioid tolerant patient (OTP), there are a few particularly challenging aspects of this case that will be addressed throughout. The first is that this patient has a long history of opioid use and tolerance for chronic pain. Furthermore, her opioid regimen has been up-titrated without an observable proportionate response in analgesia. The second is that she has multiple etiologies of pain with a mixed pain syndrome. Third, she has concomitant psychiatric conditions which may be contributing to her experience of pain. Fourth, she has various comorbidities of which we need to be mindful when considering our therapeutic treatment options. Last, AB's metastatic cancer is progressing and causing significant suffering. It is unknown at this point how it is impacting her physically, psychologically, socially, and spiritually. This information will be crucial to understanding her "total pain" and to form a comprehensive treatment plan. Please see Figure 44.1 for a treatment algorithm for acute pain in an OTP; this chapter provides further discussion and insight into these concepts and how they may be applied.

Patients with opioid tolerance and chronic pain experience physiologic changes from chronic opioid exposure that make it more difficult to treat acute pain. Opioid receptors may become desensitized, signaling pathways become altered, and N-methyl-D-aspartate (NMDA) receptors show increased sensitivity, all of which contribute to hyperalgesia. Furthermore, the opioids themselves may induce hyperalgesia, a phenomena often called *opioid-induced hyperalgesia* (OIH). Due to the current climate surrounding opioid dosing and prescribing as a result of the opioid crisis, OTPs may receive significantly reduced equianalgesic doses in the acute care setting. Clinician fears and unfamiliarity with equianalgesic dosing and conversions, as well as misconceptions of acute pain management in OTPs may all contribute. AB has known opioid tolerance and should be evaluated for OIH because her opioid doses have increased without a proportionate analgesic response. One of the first steps for the palliative clinician in assessment of

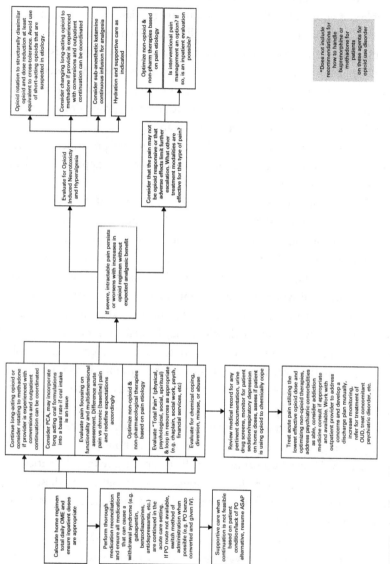

FIGURE 44.1 General Approach to Acute Pain Management in an Opioid Tolerant Patient

acute pain in an OTP is to calculate and compare total daily oral morphine equivalence (OME) utilization of the patient's home regimen versus their acute care orders and utilization. Continue the long-acting opioid when possible and ensure breakthrough doses are appropriate based on outpatient use and dosing prior to the consult. A full discussion on acute pain management in patients on opioid agonist therapy for opioid use disorder is outside the scope of this chapter and has been discussed elsewhere. Generally, it is best to continue the methadone and buprenorphine product (may break up total daily dose more frequently to optimize analgesic properties) and optimize all other strategies identified in this chapter.

Thorough medication reconciliation comparing the prescribed medication regimen with how it is taken outpatient should happen in tandem with evaluation of the opioid regimen. Once compiled, a comparison of these findings with the inpatient regimen in the context of the medical presentation of the patient should be assessed. The importance of an accurate and timely medication reconciliation cannot be overstated for a multitude of reasons. In the context of our pain and symptom assessment, we want to especially be on the lookout for use of medications or substances that can cause a withdrawal syndrome with abrupt cessation (e.g., benzodiazepines, gabapentin, antidepressants, cannabis, alcohol, etc.) and address any discrepancies quickly. Certain medications may be easily resumed inpatient if no contraindications are present (or the dose can be tapered when possible vs. abrupt cessation when medical management warrants discontinuation). Withdrawal from other agents, such as alcohol and cannabis, should be treated symptomatically.

When pain is opioid responsive and opioid requirements need to be elucidated during an acute pain crisis, utilizing intravenous patient-controlled analgesia (PCA) may be an appropriate first step. Ensure that the patient is continued on their home regimen of long-acting opioid or roll these morphine equivalents into a basal rate on the PCA if there are concerns about absorption or oral intake.

Converting AB's long-acting opioid regimen to methadone may be considered because it has the advantages of (1) being a potent opioid (may decrease pill burden); (2) is available in multiple preparations and can be administered via many routes of administration (oral, sublingual, via gastrostomy tube, rectal, IV, etc.) because its long half-life makes it a long-acting medication, not the dosage form; (3) it has three primary mechanisms of action for analgesia including opioid receptor agonism, NMDA antagonism, and serotonin norepinephrine reuptake inhibition (SNRI) activity; and (4) it is a preferred agent in patients with renal dysfunction. Organ dysfunction is an important consideration in pharmacotherapy selection. Due to the complex pharmacokinetics/pharmacodynamics and potency, methadone should only be prescribed by clinicians who are familiar with the nuances of dosing and monitoring. Furthermore, it is advisable prior to initiating methadone in an acute care setting to ensure that an outpatient prescriber can be identified who is willing to manage methadone for pain management.

Pain should be evaluated consistently, with a focus on functionality and multidimensional assessment specific to the patient's type of pain and other contributing factors, such as emotional distress, pain catastrophizing, and quality of life. It is important to differentiate between the patient's acute pain versus chronic, or baseline, pain. This provides a good opportunity to clarify and redefine expectations (e.g., it is not a reasonable expectation to improve pain below normal, baseline state) and focus on realistic goal-setting for the acute pain episode.

The optimization of non-opioid and nonpharmacologic therapies based on physical pain etiology is essential. Some examples for this thought process for AB are as follows:

- *Bone metastases*: Depending on imaging and scope, is she a candidate for balloon kyphoplasty/vertebroplasty for compression fracture (spine)? Is surgery an option if condition warrants (spine)? Is targeted palliative radiation an option? Would an interventional procedure such as a block followed by neurolysis or radiofrequency ablation be helpful? Are corticosteroids an option for acute bone pain (be mindful of effects on blood glucose because she seems to have uncontrolled diabetes at baseline, although this is not an exclusion for therapy. Work with primary team and nursing staff to optimize management and reduce risk of hypoglycemic episodes via a too strict correction protocol.) Is AB on (or has she been treated with previously) bone-modifying agents (bisphosphonates or RANK ligand inhibitors) to prevent further skeletal-related events and possibly assist with analgesia for bone pain? Keep in mind that she would not be a candidate for pamidronate based on renal dysfunction, and denosumab may be preferred over zoledronic acid for this same reason. Hypercalcemia may also be present with bone metastases and should be evaluated; osteoclast inhibitors would aid in treatment for this indication as well.

- *Pulmonary metastases*: Pain from lung mets may be somatic, visceral, neuropathic, or a combination thereof. A thorough assessment is imperative to determine an effective plan. Dyspnea, hemoptysis, and cough may also be associated with pulmonary mets and further contribute to pain, anxiety, and suffering as well as limit opioid dose escalation due to a higher risk of respiratory depression.

- *Pain from fungating breast wound*: A discussion of comprehensive wound care management and considerations is outside the scope of this chapter and can be found elsewhere. A few considerations for pain management that may be outside the "normal" acute care toolkit include topical opioids and ketamine with or without topical anesthetics, topical nonsteroidal anti-inflammatory drugs (NSAIDs), energy therapies such as Reiki and Qi gong, cognitive behavioral therapy, etc.

- *Neuropathic pain*: AB has several potential reasons that should be further investigated regarding neuropathic pain. She has known diabetic nephropathy so may also have some degree of diabetic peripheral neuropathy with or without any chemotherapy-induced peripheral neuropathy from previous chemotherapy (e.g., taxanes). Additionally, fungating wounds generally have a component of neuropathic pain due to nerve involvement throughout the area of the wound. Systemic treatment options should be evaluated in the context of organ dysfunction. Duloxetine may be the best option for AB as it is preferred in renal dysfunction (chronic kidney disease stage 3: no modification necessary; dose may be reduced by 50% if progresses to end-stage renal disease) and may help with her psychiatric comorbidities. Gabapentin may also be considered with appropriate dosage modification but would not have the benefit of treating AB's known concomitant symptoms. Depending on the extent of her spinal mets, she may have nerve pain related to nerve compression from a compression fracture, tumor impingement, etc. Treatment as listed earlier with kyphoplasty/vertebroplasty, surgical intervention, radiation, and interventional procedures may be of benefit.

Additionally, the four domains of "total pain" (physical, psychological, social, spiritual) should be evaluated to identify other interventions that may be useful to decrease patient suffering and assist with pain perception. Often these issues cannot be comprehensively addressed in the acute care setting. However, interventions can be initiated to provide some immediate benefit with a coordinated plan with outpatient follow-up and support to continue to address. A non-inclusive list of examples for AB may include

- AB has a known history of posttraumatic stress disorder (PTSD), anxiety, and depression so an evaluation of current and recent symptom severity and treatment is warranted. She also may be suffering from body image or intimacy issues from the sequelae of her cancer (e.g., fungating breast wound). Depending on the assessment, there may be potential to initiate an antidepressant and establish an outpatient support plan, such as psychotherapy, cognitive-behavioral therapy, physical self-regulation, etc. In the acute setting, would AB benefit from some targeted interventions from a social worker or counselor? Can her medication regimen (and outpatient follow-up) be further optimized by psychiatry? Can you lead her through a meditation or guided imagery exercise and encourage her and family to implement this a few times a day as part of the treatment plan?
- Is spirituality important in AB's life? Would she benefit from being seen acutely by a chaplain? If family distress is present, would her family benefit from a mutual visit as well?
- Are finances, insurance coverage status, etc. causing distress for AB and family? If so, a discussion with social work or financial counseling may be helpful.
- Is there distress about her shifting role in the family, her social circles, etc.? Is a counselor available to begin the process of working through these emotional struggles?

Evaluation for diversion, misuse, and abuse should be part of the comprehensive assessment. This should not delay treatment of the acute pain episode but may impact the discharge plan. Misuse is a therapeutic, intentional use of a drug in an inappropriate way (e.g., increasing an opioid dose to treat uncontrolled pain at home without being directed to do so by a member of the healthcare team). *Chemical coping*, or using opioids to treat a symptom other than what it is intended for (e.g., depression/anxiety) is also an example of misuse and is common in patients with complex disease states such as cancer. It may present an opportunity for input from psychiatry or addiction medicine consult services, if available, and the optimization of social work services to assist with patient support and care coordination. This evaluation needs to be approached in an unbiased manner using nonthreatening language. A thorough patient assessment can provide insight into what other symptoms need to be addressed. Education and clarification about the indication for opioids and what is being done to address the other symptom(s) can be helpful in this situation.

Utilizing certain NMDA antagonist therapies, such as subdissociative continuous infusion ketamine, to help decrease tolerance and hyperalgesia may be necessary to treat the acute pain crisis and reduce the underlying pathology. Methadone and dextromethorphan also antagonize the NMDA receptor to a lesser degree and have some positive evidence supporting efficacy in chronic pain and reversal of hyperalgesia. For AB, the selection of ketamine is optimal for several reasons:

1. It possesses a greater affinity for antagonizing the NMDA receptor, which is desirable for treatment of severe and intractable acute pain as well as combatting the effects of hyperalgesia and OIH.

2. It has shown swift benefit in decreasing symptoms of depression, and preliminary data are promising for its efficacy in the treatment of anxiety and PTSD. This is significant because chronic pain and depression are frequently encountered together. Moderate to severe pain that impairs function and/or is intractable is associated with greater depressive symptoms and worse outcomes, such as reduced quality of life, decreased work function, and increased healthcare utilization. Depression and PTSD in patients with pain is associated with worsened pain and impairment.

3. It can be used without dosage modification in advanced renal failure.

4. It has shown some utility as an adjunct analgesic in patients with obstructive sleep apnea (OSA). While we are uncertain of AB's status in regard to OSA, we know that she has some respiratory risk factors due to her pulmonary metastases.

Follow-up evaluation as to whether a patient's pain is improved, remains the same, or worsens with aggressive opioid escalation is an important next step. When patients are on chronic opioids and receive more opioids for acute pain, they are inherently at risk of developing opioid-induced neurotoxicity and/or OIH. If these conditions are present, increasing the current opioid dose in attempt to quell the acute pain will result in worsened pain and neurologic symptoms. Another reason that the pain may not be responding to escalating doses of opioids is that the pain is not opioid-responsive. While opioids used to be the cornerstone of pain management, we now know that certain types of pain are more responsive to non-opioid treatment modalities. It may be difficult to engage in a thorough pain assessment during a severe acute pain exacerbation, but location and a few descriptors in addition to the known medical history may be enough to give you a good hypothesis on the etiology to assist with therapy selection.

If an overall opioid dose reduction seems to improve pain, OIH is likely contributing to worsening pain, and we will want to take this into consideration when planning for the outpatient regimen transition. Sensitivity and response to a different opioid must also be considered. In addition to rotation of opioids and initiating a ketamine infusion (if appropriate), the optimization of non-opioid analgesic modalities should be implemented.

A final but critical step in acute pain management in an OTP is coordination of care. Ideally, decisions made in the acute care setting should be guided in part by outpatient follow-up. A few examples may include

1. Touching base with the provider who has agreed to prescribe methadone for pain outpatient and coordinating the discharge prescription based on time until follow-up appointment. If this provider is the same as the baseline prescriber, provide any updates about current medication regimen; changes to therapy and rationale; encouragement of controlled substance disposal (if pertinent); and any objective evidence of misuse, abuse, or

diversion (these should be communicated early to ensure that discharge is not delayed based on outpatient and inpatient provider collaborative plans and should include pertinent information for opioids and other drugs of abuse, such as alcohol, cocaine, etc.).

2. Ensure that any outpatient follow-up needs for total pain are established and communicated to AB prior to discharge.

3. If a compounded topical preparation is helpful for AB's wound pain, planning ahead to find an outpatient pharmacy that can fill the outpatient prescription, evaluating insurance coverage and out-of-pocket cost for the patient to ensure feasibility, and arranging for the patient to receive the prescription to avoid a gap in therapy are necessary. These conversations should be initiated several days prior to discharge.

KEY POINTS TO REMEMBER

- OTPs with acute pain have underlying factors, such as tolerance and hyperalgesia, that contribute to their pain experience.
- A thorough medication reconciliation, especially focused on pain and symptom medications, can help identify any initial discord between the home and acute care regimen.
- Pain should be evaluated by focusing on functionality and multidimensional assessment when possible. Acute and chronic pain should be differentiated, and setting realistic expectations and goals is paramount.
- Non-opioid and nonpharmacologic therapies should be optimized based on pain etiology and "total pain" (physical, psychological, social, spiritual) assessment.
- If severe, intractable pain persists or worsens with increases in the opioid regimen without proportional expected analgesic benefit, consider opioid-induced neurotoxicity, OIH, and that the pain isn't opioid-responsive.
- Develop your acute care plan with discharge in mind to ensure continued success in the outpatient setting.

Further Reading

Brant J. Holistic total pain management in palliative care: Cultural and global considerations. palliative medicine and hospice care. *Open Journal.* 2017;SE:S32–S8. doi:10.17140/PMHCOJ-SE-1-108.

De Andres J, Fabregat-Cid G, Asensio-Samper JM, Sanchis-Lopez N, Moliner-Velazquez S. Management of acute pain in patients on treatment with opioids. *Pain Manage.* 2015;5(3):167–173. Epub 2015, May 15. doi:10.2217/pmt.15.13. PubMed PMID: 25971640.

Lee M, Silverman SM, Hansen H, Patel VB, Manchikanti L. A comprehensive review of opioid-induced hyperalgesia. *Pain Physician.* 2011;14(2):145–161. Epub 2011, March 18. PubMed PMID: 21412369.

Loveday BA, Sindt J. Ketamine protocol for palliative care in cancer patients with refractory pain. *J Adv Pract Oncol.* 2015;6(6):555–561. Epub 2016, September 21. PubMed PMID: 27648345; PMCID: PMC5017546.

Macintyre PE, Roberts LJ, Huxtable CA. Management of opioid-tolerant patients with acute pain: Approaching the challenges. *Drugs.* 2020;80(1):9–21. Epub 2019, December 4. doi:10.1007/s40265-019-01236-4. PubMed PMID: 31792832.

Malzo M, Dawson KA. Opioid-induced neurotoxicity. *Am J Nurs.* 2013;113(10):51–56. Epub 2013, September 27. doi:10.1097/01.Naj.0000435351.53534.83. PubMed PMID: 24067833.

Schwenk ES, Viscusi ER, Buvanendran A, et al. Consensus guidelines on the use of intravenous ketamine infusions for acute pain management from the American Society of Regional Anesthesia and Pain Medicine, the American Academy of Pain Medicine, and the American Society of Anesthesiologists. *Reg Anesth Pain Med.* 2018;43(5):456–466. Epub 2018, June 6. doi:10.1097/aap.0000000000000806. PubMed PMID: 29870457; PMCID: PMC6023582.

Yoong J, Poon P. Principles of cancer pain management: An overview and focus on pharmacological and interventional strategies. *Aust J Gen Pract.* 2018;47(11):758–762. Epub 2019, June 18. doi:10.31128/ajgp-07-18-4629. PubMed PMID: 31207672.

45 Preexisting Implanted Pumps

Jane E. Loitman

Case Study

RC, a 54-year-old woman with metastatic ovarian cancer, omental caking, metastases to the liver, and constipation is admitted to your hospice with pain rated between 7 and 10/10. She has some nausea and mental clouding. During interdisciplinary team rounds, the patient's nurse reviews the patient's medication list with you, the hospice medical director, hoping for help in improving her pain control. You ask the nurse how much morphine the patient is taking. Morphine elixir was ordered yesterday; the patient took five 30 mg doses in the last 24 hours and her pain is down to 5/10. The records indicate that a "morphine pump" was placed 3 months ago at a rate of 2.6 mg/day. Her goal is to be comfortable but to be able to interact as much and as long as possible with her family.

What Do I Do Now?

To provide the most expeditious analgesia, it would help to understand the intrathecal (IT) pump, the dosage, and the relevance of the 30 mg breakthrough dose in relation to the current dosage.

An IT pump delivers medication into the IT space for those patients whom systemic therapy fails to provide improved analgesia or quality of life. This chapter reviews the considerations and practical concerns for using a preexisting, implanted IT pump to help providers to understand how to use these devices.

The World Health Organization analgesic step ladder, developed in 1986, was changed to include interventional, intraspinal, and neuromodulating therapies in 1994, to cover the approximately 10% of cancer patients who do not respond to systemic analgesics alone. Nonetheless, providers still work in the 1986 realm. In 2005, Reddy et al. found that approximately one-third of patients have poor outcomes, especially if they have neuropathic pain, incident pain, and mucocutaneous ulcers. The cost is prohibitive for payment with the hospice benefit though it is considered cost-effective after 3 months from placement. The greatest risk for adverse events and issues also occur in the immediate post-placement period. Pumps are frequently ignored when providers encounter patients with a device because they do not know what to do with them and simply continue to work with the original three-step ladder. Hospices will sometimes not accept patients with IT analgesia to avoid the need to work with the technology. Some data show that cancer patients receiving IT analgesia benefit and live longer versus those with parenteral analgesia (87% vs. 71%). There is less systemic toxicity from metabolites, less pill burden, and fewer side effects, and better analgesic control can be achieved within a 6-month period—important given hospice criteria. Refills and adjustments can easily be achieved bedside, and the relative cost is low.

This mode of delivery allows for lower doses of medication at the site of action. For instance, our case patient's morphine equivalent daily dose (MEDD) was decreased by 94% (from 18,600 mg/day to 876 mg/day), her pain scores decreased by 50%, and she became less somnolent, more interactive, and her functional status improved days after the pump was originally placed.

To work with this modality, one must understand how to adjust the dose, read the contents, and refill a pump with the assistance of a programmer.

Placing the programmer external to patient, over the implanted pump, can remotely interrogate the pump, which provides information about the medication, concentration, and rate as well as when a refill is needed.

MEDICATIONS

When considering the opioid analgesics in an IT pump, it is important to realize their equianalgesic comparisons and the limitations of these conversion methods (Box 45.1).

The US Food and Drug Administration (FDA) has only approved morphine, ziconotide, and baclofen for the use in an IT pump. However, for decades, hydromorphone, clonidine, bupivacaine, sufentanil, and fentanyl have also been used, alone and in combination. In fact, some cancer centers document that up to 40% of their patients receive IT drug combinations.

Some pumps have a patient-controlled analgesia (PCA) feature whereby extra doses at a specific rate or frequency are planned at a dose of 5–15% of the total daily dose. These can be administered over 15–45 minutes. A 2015 study showed that IT breakthrough doses reduced pain by 20% and was three times faster than with conventional medications.

A pump typically holds 40 mL, and the concentration impacts the frequency of refills. The FDA requires pumps to be refilled at least every 6 months, though refills in palliative care and hospice will likely be every 1–3 months. The Polyanalgesic Consensus Conference (PACC) reviews preclinical and clinical data to provide best practices to improve patient care and outcomes with IT therapy. To help with understanding drug concentration and range of rates, the PACC created recommendations for concentrations (Table 45.1).

BOX 45.1 **Intraspinal morphine conversion ratios**

300 mg oral morphine, equals
100 mg parenteral morphine, equals
10 mg epidural morphine, equals
1 mg intrathecal morphine

TABLE 45.1 **Polyanalgesic Consensus Conference (PACC) medication dosing and concentrations for intrathecal delivery**

Drug	Max concentration	Max dose/day	Initial dose/ day
Morphine	20 mg/mL	15 mg	0.1–0.5 mg
Hydromorphone	15 mg/mL	10 mg	0.01–0.15 mg
Fentanyl	10 mg/mL	1,000 µg	25–75 µg
Sufentanil	5 mg/mL	500 µg	10–20 µg
Bupivacaine	30 mg/mL	10 mg	1–4 mg
Clonidine	1,000 µg/mL	600 µg	20–100 µg
Ziconotide	100 µg/mL	19.2 µg	0.5–1.2 µg

If a patient's prognosis is less than a year, concentrations of morphine at 50 mg/mL or hydromorphone 100 mg/mL allow for titration with less concern for needing a refill.

Adjuvants are often added for neuropathic pain, and a patient may already have bupivacaine or clonidine present in their pump. These adjuvants can be very helpful with neuropathic pain. If using simply an opioid, and the patient continues to have inadequate relief, consider adding bupivacaine if the morphine dose is greater than 25 mg/ day or the hydromorphone dose is greater than 6 mg/day. You may start bupivacaine at 3 mg/day and increase as indicated and tolerated. If no relief is observed with bupivacaine, trial clonidine at 50 µg/day. If the clonidine reaches 850 µg/day, other adjuvants and analgesics can be trialed with the help of a team more accustomed to managing admixtures. However, one must work with commercial products and a compounding pharmacist, which can be expensive. Home infusion pharmacies may be different from institutional or retail pharmacies and may need to do what is considered *compounding medications* to achieve the desired concentration or to combine medications. Compounding requires compliance with mandates for a sterile environment and preservative-free medications. The PACC developed stepped recommendations for IT drug selection considerations (Table 45.2).

TABLE 45.2 Polyanalgesic Consensus Conference (PACC) recommended options for neuraxial treatment of cancer pain

Line 1	Morphine	Ziconotide	Fentanyl and hydromorphone ± bupivacaine
Line 2	Hydromorphone	Hydromorphone + bupivacaine or clonidine	Morphine + clonidine
Line 3	Clonidine	Ziconotide + fentanyl	Fentanyl + bupivacaine or clonidine
Line 4	Opioid + clonidine + bupivacaine	Bupivacaine + clonidine	
Line 5		Baclofen	

The medication directly infuses into the central nervous system (CNS), site of action, bypassing the first-pass effect and exposure in the gut (Figure 45.1). Similar to systemic opioid administration, IT opioid administration is measured in milligrams per day. The medication can take a full day to get from the pump in the abdomen to the brain.

For poorly controlled pain, the rate of flow can be increased, ultimately increasing the milligrams per day. If the medication is simply morphine, then the dose can be increased up to 15% of the daily dose. Generally, the standard of titration of no more than once a day as an outpatient or twice a day for inpatients is accepted. With an understanding of morphine use, most end-of-life FDA-approved analgesia can be managed while leaving the alternatives to the pain experts. If the patient already has a combination of medication, then increasing the rate will increase the daily dose of *all* medications, and one must pay particular attention to the total daily dose for each and be aware of toxicity. For instance, an IT infusion of morphine of 0.5 mg/mL and bupivacaine of 4.75 mg/mL may significantly improve the relief of refractory cancer pain although the adverse effects should be balanced and individualized. Side effects such as hypotension or neuro-muscular effects generally occur with doses of bupivacaine at 3 mg/day and clonidine greater than 20 µg/day.

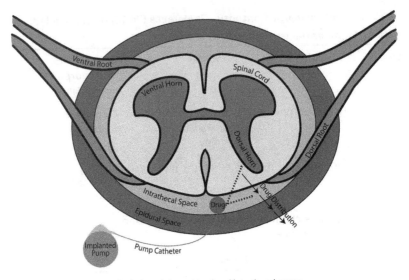

FIGURE 45.1 Transverse depiction of the epidural and intrathecal space.

REFILLS AND PROGRAMING

Changing the rate or refilling the pump is simple and can be done by nurses or physicians/independent practitioners. The clinician must go to the home or the bedside. For dose changes, only the programmer is needed. For refills, a kit, sterile gloves, and the syringe of medication(s) is needed. The manufacturer's kit contains the template, access needle, injecting needle, lidocaine, syringes to inject lidocaine and withdraw remaining medication, and sterile dressing.

The pump has both a computer and a reservoir that holds the medication (Figure 45.2). The pump's position can be easily palpable underneath the skin to understand the direction to place the template to locate the port for the reservoir. Once the area is cleaned in a sterile fashion, the template is placed over the pump and the middle of the port is accessed by the needle supplied in the kit. This needle is inserted into the opening in the template, through the skin and septum, and into the reservoir of the pump. Remove the anticipated amount of remaining liquid/medication from the reservoir with an empty syringe, switch syringes with the one containing the new medication, and inject the contents into the reservoir. The pump can now

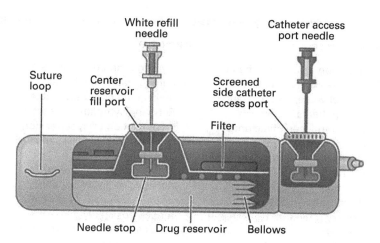

FIGURE 45.2 Side view of a pump that is internalized subcutaneously in the abdomen.

be reprogrammed with the new medication, concentration, volume, and rate. Programming is done with the programmer, and a new refill date will automatically be calculated based on the volume and rate. Planning for that date can help with preparation of the next medication, kit, and scheduling all around. It should be noted that the pump has an alarm that alerts the patient and caregivers that the pump needs to be refilled soon. There are always a couple milliliters of medication left in the pump should the refill occur after the alarm date, although the alarm can be disconcerting if not addressed expediently.

CONCERNS

Excluding technical or surgical problems, complications involving refills and pump management include those that can be anticipated and others with a relatively low probability of occurring (Table 45.3).

RETURN TO CASE

RC's morphine was titrated simply on three occasions prior to her death. She did not require more than two oral breakthrough doses per day or additional adjuvants, and only required one refill.

TABLE 45.3 **Adverse effects associated with intrathecal delivery of analgesics**

More common	Less common
• Granulomas at the catheter tip: 0.1–5% of patients after several years; less relevant in HPM patients.	• Overdose and/or withdrawal
	• Pump rotates 180 degrees, making the port unavailable
• Opioid-induced myoclonus, neurotoxicity, analgesia-metabolites- centrally mediated	• Rebound sympathetic reaction (hypotension or hypertension) from abrupt discontinuation of clonidine
• Delirium	• Refill outside of the pump resulting in overdose, although proprietary needle and septum reduce possibility
• Infection	
• Pruritus, constipation,	
• Urinary retention, weakness	
• Orthostatic hypotension (i.e., from bupivacaine)	• Medication preparation issues
• Nausea	• Programming issues

KEY POINTS TO REMEMBER

• The efficacy of IT analgesia has been demonstrated in malignant and non-malignant pain settings.
• Unlike nonmalignant pain, malignant and end-of-life pain can change quickly, and the adverse effects of systemic opioids interfere with comfort and quality of life.
• Since the cost benefit of placement requires forethought prior to the end of life, it behooves clinicians to take advantage of the technology if already in place.
• The more common adverse effects are similar to those with systemic opioids but occur to a lesser degree. The more severe risks are much less common.
• Training, planning, and having the entire team on board can make the use of a preexisting IT pump beneficial at the end of life.

Further Reading
Brogan SE, Winter NB, Okifuji A. Prospective observational study of patient-controlled intrathecal analgesia. *Region Anesth Pain Med.* 2015;40(4):369–375.

Bruel MD, Burton AW. Intrathecal therapy for cancer-related pain. *Pain Med.* 2016;17:2404–2421.

Coyne PJ, Smith T, Laird J, Hansen LA, Drake D. Effectively starting and titrating intrathecal analgesic therapy in patients with refractory cancer pain. *Clin J Oncol Nurs.* 2005;9(5):581–583.

Deer TR, Pope JE, Hayek SM, et al. The polyanalgesic consensus conference (PACC): Recommendations on intrathecal drug infusion systems best practices and guidelines. *Neuromodulation.* 2017;20(2):96–132.

Pittelkow TP, Bendel MA, Strand JJ, Moeschler SM. Curing opioid toxicity with intrathecal targeted drug delivery. *Hindawi, Case Reports in Medicine.* 2019;article ID 3428576.

Pope JE, Deer TR, Bruel BM, Falowski S. Clinical uses of intrathecal therapy and its placement in the pain care algorithm. *Pain Pract.* 2016;16(8)1092–1106.

Portenoy RK, Copenhaver DJ. Cancer pain management: Interventional therapies. *Pain.* 1995;63(1):65–76.

Reddy A, Hui D, Bruera E. A successful palliative care intervention for cancer pain refractory to intrathecal analgesia. *J Pain Symptom Manage.* 2012 July;44(1):124–130.

Smith TJ, Coyne PJ, Staats PS, Deer T, et al. An implantable drug delivery system (IDDS) for refractory cancer pain provides sustained pain control, less drug-related toxicity, and possibly better survival compared with comprehensive medical management (CMM). *Ann Oncol.* 2005 May;16(5):825–933. Epub 2005, April 7.

Smith TJ, Staats PS, Deer T, et al. Randomized clinical trial of an implantable drug delivery system compared with comprehensive medical management for refractory cancer pain: Impact on pain, drug-related toxicity, and survival. *J Clinical Oncol.* 2002;20(19):4040–4049.

Sylvester RK, Lindsay SM, Schauer C. The conversion challenge: From intrathecal to oral morphine. *Am J Hosp Palliat Care.* 2004;21(2):143–147.

46 Geriatric Pain Pharmacotherapy

Amelia L. Persico and Erica L. Wegrzyn

Case Study

An 83-year-old man with past medical history of chronic obstructive pulmonary disease (COPD), hypertension, urinary incontinence, and chronic pain secondary to severe osteoarthritis of the hip and knee and multilevel degenerative disc disease with spinal stenosis presents to the emergency department. He provides a written list of his current medications: extended-release (ER) oxycodone 30 mg twice a day, immediate-release (IR) oxycodone 5 mg three times a day as needed, pregabalin 150 mg twice a day, oxybutynin 10 mg twice a day, paroxetine 25 mg/day, diazepam 2 mg twice a day as needed, acetaminophen 650 mg four times a day as needed, diphenhydramine 50 mg every evening as needed for sleep, lisinopril 20 mg/day, diltiazem 120 mg twice a day, tiotropium Respimat 2.5 µg 2 puffs daily, budesonide/formoterol 160/4.5 µg 2 puffs twice a day, and albuterol MDI.

His chief complaint is a 72-hour history of altered mental status (AMS) with somnolence, nausea, constipation, and loss of appetite. He is afebrile, his complete blood count (CBC) is unremarkable, and his primary care provider has already ruled out urinary tract infection 2 days prior. On interview, you determine oxycodone IR was recently initiated due to increased pain.

What Do I Do Now?

This patient provides a prime example of the array of age-related pharmacokinetic changes that occur in the aging adult exacerbated by polypharmacy and anticholinergic medications. Our approach to this patient requires review of all potentially inappropriate medications (PIMs), assessment for drug-drug and drug-disease state interactions, and a focus on rational opioid therapy. We have identified three major potential medication-related causes for this patient's altered mental status: (1) high anticholinergic burden of current pharmacotherapy, (2) age-related physiological changes impacting pharmacokinetics, and (3) drug-drug interaction between diltiazem and oxycodone resulting in decreased phase I metabolism and increased active parent drug.

ANTICHOLINERGIC BURDEN

Anticholinergic medications are those that prevent acetylcholine from binding to muscarinic receptors, resulting in side effects such as constipation, dry eyes, dry mouth, confusion, and urinary retention. The Beers Criteria is generally considered the authority on anticholinergic and PIMs in the elderly. This patient's medication list includes five medications that are listed on the most up to date version of the Beers Criteria for their strong anticholinergic properties or central nervous system (CNS) depressant effects: diazepam, pregabalin, oxybutynin, paroxetine, and diphenhydramine. Concomitant use of multiple anticholinergic medications and CNS depressants could certainly be contributing to this patient's altered mental status (AMS) and constipation.

To reduce this patient's anticholinergic burden, an emphasis should be placed on sleep hygiene and cognitive-behavioral interventions in lieu of diphenhydramine. If pharmacotherapy is required, melatonin could be trialed. Transition to an alternative selective serotonin reuptake inhibitor (SSRI) could be of benefit as paroxetine is the most anticholinergic SSRI and is the only one that appears on the Beers list of drugs with strong anticholinergic properties. Although pharmacotherapy for urinary incontinence is inherently antimuscarinic, use of an extended-release (ER) oxybutynin product could mitigate some of the anticholinergic side effects.

Pregabalin is not considered to be highly anticholinergic; however, it is noted on the Beers criteria for its CNS depressant properties. Pregabalin is additionally notable in this particular patient due to the 2019 warning by the US Food and Drug Administration (FDA) regarding respiratory depression when gabapentinoids are prescribed concomitantly with opioids such as oxycodone. Caution is advised when using gabapentinoids and opioids concomitantly, along with the importance of weighing the risks versus benefits of rational polypharmacy while designing a targeted treatment regimen based on pain quality and presentation. Regardless, the additive effect of multiple anticholinergic medications along with pregabalin and oxycodone is likely to play a role in this patient's AMS.

Last, diazepam is not recommended in elderly patients due to its long duration of action, risk of cognitive impairment, and increased risk of opioid-induced respiratory depression when prescribed concomitantly with opioids. If benzodiazepines are required in an elderly patient, then those with a short half-life are preferred.

AGE-RELATED PHYSIOLOGICAL CHANGES IMPACTING PHARMACOKINETICS

Among the many impacts of the physiological changes inherent in aging are those in absorption, distribution, metabolism, and excretion of medications. Many of these changes are summarized in Table 46.1. These are a result of a gradual deterioration of the gastrointestinal (GI), hepatic, renal, cardiovascular, and respiratory systems. Slowing GI motility can decrease absorption of certain medications and increase risk of constipation. Distribution of medications is impacted by changes in total body weight, lean body mass, serum albumin, and total body fat. Medications that are highly protein bound or extremely lipophilic will be more impacted by these changes. Elderly patients with minimal adipose tissue and/or poor skin integrity can have unpredictable absorption of transdermal medications.

Reduction in hepatic mass and perfusion results in reduced first-pass metabolism and potential accumulation of active drug or toxic metabolites. This impact is multiplied in the setting of comorbid cirrhosis, chronic kidney disease, and chronic liver disease. A similar impact is seen when renal mass and function decline. One approach to avoid these metabolic concerns is to utilize medications which avoid first-pass metabolism and the cytochrome P450 system. Selection of medications utilizing phase II

TABLE 46.1 **Pharmacokinetic changes in the elderly**

Pharmacokinetic property	Physiologic changes with age	Clinical significance
Absorption	Increased total body fat	Often minimal
Distribution	Decreased lean body mass Decreased totally body water Slowing gastrointestinal motility Decreased albumin	• Increased volume of distribution and half -life of lipophilic drugs • Increased exposure to highly protein bound medications
Metabolism	Decreased hepatic mass Decreased hepatic blood flow Potential drug-drug interactions due to polypharmacy	• Increase in bioavailability of drugs subject to hepatic metabolism.
Excretion	Decreased blood flow to kidneys decreased renal mass and function	• Increased half-life and accumulation of active drug/active metabolites

metabolism can be advantageous, especially in those with hepatic or renal failure.

Changes in respiratory and cardiovascular health, such as hardening of elastic arteries and increased chest wall rigidity, increase the risk of respiratory depression in the aging population. Elderly patients are also at elevated risk of falls and are more susceptible to the well-known cognitive and sedative side effects of many pain medications.

Along with fall risk, it is important to consider corresponding bleeding risk and potential influencing factors. While this patient case does not mention increased bleeding risks, it is important to note that paroxetine's serotonin reuptake inhibition is associated with inhibition of platelet aggregation.

Traditional oral nonsteroidal anti-inflammatory drug (NSAID) use can also be particularly risky, despite superior evidence for use in osteoarthritis, owing to increased incidence of GI bleeds and inhibition of cyclo-oxygenase-1 (COX-1). Using a COX-2 selective NSAID can alleviate bleeding risk to some degree, however, increased thrombotic cardiovascular risks must be consider given the high comorbidities typical of this population.

RATIONAL OPIOID THERAPY IN THE ELDERLY PATIENT

When opioid therapy is indicated in an elderly patient, a careful assessment of the risks and benefits is required with attention paid to the pharmacokinetic and pharmacodynamic eccentricities of the aging adult as previously discussed. Patient-related factors to consider include hepatic and renal function, concomitant medications, type of pain (neuropathic vs. nociceptive), and respiratory stability, among others. Medication-related factors to consider include potency toward the mu opioid receptor, CNS activity, route of administration/formulations available, metabolic pathways, and presence of active metabolites. In all cases, the starting dose should be low and extremely gradual titration should be employed with a target of using the lowest effective dose.

Opioid medications that bypass phase I metabolism in the liver and are metabolized to inactive metabolites are subject to fewer drug-drug interactions and reduce the risk of accumulation of active/toxic metabolites. Thus, in elderly patients, hydromorphone, oxymorphone, levorphanol, tapentadol, or morphine can offer unique options for safer consideration relative to other opioids. However, clinicians should be aware that morphine is still subject to metabolism into morphine-6-glucuronide, which produces analgesia, and morphine-3-glucuronide which can produce neurotoxic side effects and can accumulate in patients with chronic kidney disease.

In this particular patient, his recently titrated oxycodone, which is subject to first-pass metabolism via both CYP2D6 and CYP3A4, could be contributing to constipation and AMS. Oxycodone is metabolized into two active metabolites, oxymorphone (via CYP2D6) and noroxycodone (via CYP3A4). Concomitant administration with a CYP3A4 inhibitor such as diltiazem can decrease metabolism of the parent drug resulting in accumulation of oxycodone. Potent CYP3A4 inhibitors include clarithromycin, itraconazole, phenobarbital, St. John's wort, phenytoin, and rifampin. This, coupled with decreased hepatic mass and perfusion, decreased GI motility related to old age, and concomitant anticholinergic medications could contribute to accumulation of oxycodone and result in AMS, somnolence, and constipation.

In addition to opportunities for de-prescribing and reducing anticholinergic burden, a transition to an opioid with reduced CNS activity, fewer drug-drug interactions, and lower rates of constipation could be beneficial. Given this patient's comorbid chronic obstructive pulmonary disease (COPD) and gabapentinoid use, he is also at increased risk of respiratory depression and could benefit from an opioid medication with reduced risk of opioid-induced respiratory depression.

The safest opioid option for this patient is buprenorphine, a partial agonist at the mu opioid receptor and antagonist at the kappa opioid receptor. Buprenorphine has lower intrinsic activity at the mu opioid receptor relative to other opioids, which improves its safety profile and reduces its impact on beta-arrestin; it demonstrates a plateau effect on carbon dioxide accumulation, thus reducing the risk of opioid-induced respiratory depression without compromising analgesia. Buprenorphine also has decreased CNS activity, with increased paraspinal activity and resulting in lower rates of somnolence and AMS. Finally, buprenorphine's unique activity provides decreased risk for opioid-induced constipation in this patient. Caution should be used in selecting the transdermal patch formulation for elderly patients with reduced subcutaneous adipose tissue due to potential alterations in absorption, and patients using buccal films should be counseled to wet the inside of their cheek with a sip of water prior to application of the film if they experience xerostomia. Of note, buprenorphine is also a CYP3A4 substrate, thus continued therapy with diltiazem could, theoretically, increase serum levels of buprenorphine. Given the enhanced safety profile allowed by buprenorphine's unique mechanisms as just outlined, this interaction can likely be well managed through monitoring alone with likely decreased clinical significance.

As always, an evidence-based, interdisciplinary, and multimodal approach to chronic pain management is recommended. Pain pharmacotherapy in the geriatric population is often confounded by multimorbidity, polypharmacy, and altered drug metabolism. However, an astute clinician can be counted on to consider the impact that the physiological changes of their aging patient can have on medication metabolism, assess for drug-drug and drug-disease state interactions, and minimize the anticholinergic burden of their patient's regimen.

KEY POINTS TO REMEMBER

- Aging impacts absorption, distribution, metabolism, and excretion of medications, which must be considered in therapy selection for elderly patients.
- Opioids that bypass phase I metabolism can provide an improved safety profile in elderly patients. These opioids are hydromorphone, oxymorphone, levorphanol, tapentadol, and morphine.
- Morphine is metabolized into morphine-6-glucuronide, which produces analgesia, and morphine-3-glucuronide, which can produce neurotoxic side effects and can accumulate in patients with decreased renal function.
- Anticholinergic medications causing constipation, dry eyes, dry mouth, confusion, and urinary retention can be particularly harmful in elderly patients. Many are considered potentially inappropriate medications on the Beers Criteria.
- The expertise of a clinical pharmacist can be extremely beneficial in pharmacotherapy selection for elderly patients, particularly those with polypharmacy, for a thorough assessment of drug-drug and drug disease state interactions.

Further Reading

American Geriatrics Society. American Geriatrics Society Panel on pharmacological management of persistent pain in older persons. *J Am Geriatr Soc.* 2009 August; 57(8):1331–1346.

American Geriatrics Society. American Geriatrics Society 2019 Updated AGS Beers Criteria for potentially inappropriate medication use in older adults. *J Am Geriatr Soc.* 2019;67:674–694.

Bettinger JJ, Wegrzyn EL, Fudin J. Pain management in the elderly: Focus on safe prescribing. *Practical Pain Management.* 2017;17(3):1. https://www.practicalpai nmanagement.com/treatments/pharmacological/opioids/pain-management-elde rly-focus-safe-prescribing. Accessed November 13th, 2021.

Klotz U. Pharmacokinetics and drug metabolism in the elderly. *Drug Metabol Rev.* 2009 February;41(2):67–76.

Marcum ZA, Duncan NA, Makris UE. Pharmacotherapies in geriatric chronic pain management. *Clin Geriatr Med.* 2016;32(4):705–724. doi:10.1016/j.cger.2016.06.007

Smith HS. Opioid metabolism. *Mayo Clin Proc.* 2009;84(7):613–624.

Index

For the benefit of digital users, indexed terms that span two pages (e.g., 52–53) may, on occasion, appear on only one of those pages.

Tables and figures are indicated by *t* and *f* following the page number.

Qi, 39, 61
Qi gong, 382
QTc interval prolongation
    methadone-induced, 152
    opioid-induced, 146–47

radiation therapy
radiopharmaceuticals
rational opioid therapy, 403–5
rectal administration of analgesics, 225–32
    absorption and bioavailability,
        228f, 228–29
    advantages and disadvantages, 226, 226t
    key points to remember, 232
rectal cancer, 269–76
rectal catheters, 231–32
rectum: venous drainage of, 228f, 228
referred pain, 54, 294–95
reflexes
    Chapman's, 54
    somato-visceral, 54
    viscero-somatic, 54
Reiki, 382
Relistor (methylnaltrexone), 169
remifentanil, 374
renal failure, 146
reverse sensitization, 100–1
riboflavin, 139
rifampin, 125t, 403–4
ritonavir, 125t

S-adenosyl methionine (SAMe), 55
Saunders, Cicely, 38
scar deactivation, 59–62
sedation, palliative, 243–50, 248t
selective serotonin-reuptake inhibitors
        (SSRIs), 81–82, 83
sennosides, 297–98
sensitization
    peripheral, 336
    reverse, 100–1
serotonin-norepinephrine reuptake
        inhibitors (SNRIs)

for breakthrough pain, 305–6
for neuropathic pain, 272
for pain in CKD, 359t
for pain in depression, 81–82, 83
serotonin syndrome, 114, 118
sexuality, 32
simvastatin, 125t
skeletal muscle relaxants, 115–16,
    305, 359t
skeletal-related events (SREs), 252
SMT (spinal manipulative therapy), 51–52
SNRIs. See serotonin-norepinephrine
    reuptake inhibitors
social domains, 28t, 32–33
sodium restriction, 346–47
sodium thiosulfate (STS), 320–21, 324–25
sodium valproate, 273t
somatic pain, 294–95, 302
somatoautonomic dysfunction, 52
somato-visceral reflexes, 54
spasticity, pain due to, 279, 280, 281
spinal manipulative therapy (SMT), 51–52
spinal nerves and innervations, 52, 53t
spirituality, 31–32, 383
squamous cell carcinoma, 173–81
SREs (skeletal-related events), 252
SSRIs (selective serotonin-reuptake
        inhibitors), 81–82, 83
St. John's wort, 403–4
stoicism, 29
stomal administration, 229–30
stress reduction, mindfulness-based, 18
STS (sodium thiosulfate), 320–21, 324–25
substance abuse, 147–48
Substance Abuse and Mental Health Services
        Administration (SAMHSA), 210
substance use disorders (SUDs), 210
sufentanil, 237t, 391, 392t
suicide, physician-assisted, 244
supplements, 131–38, 133t
support groups, 19
suppositories, 227, 232
surgical abdomen, 312

warfarin, 76–77
weakness, painless, 278
Western medicine, 33
willow bark, 133*t*, 138
windup phenomenon, 98
World Health Organization (WHO)
    contraindications to
      chiropractic manipulation
      therapy, 50
    pain ladder, 336–37, 390

wound healing: promotion of,
    322, 324–25
wounds, fungating: pain from, 382

X waiver, 210, 215

Yin and Yang, 39

ziconotide, 236, 237*t*, 391, 392*t*
zonisamide, 359*t*